ORDINARY MEDICINE

W9-BPO-122

Critical Global Health: Evidence, Efficacy, Ethnography
Edited by Vincanne Adams and João Biehl

AD Non Fiction
362.10973 K1626o

DISCARDED BY
MEAD PUBLIC LIBRARY

Kaufman, Sharon R. Ordinary medicine :
extraordinary treatments, longer lives, and where
to draw the line   9001109467

PRAISE FOR *ORDINARY MEDICINE*

"I devoured *Ordinary Medicine*. It gave me courage. It helped me delineate, sometimes for the first time, the interlocking forces and practices that have helped create an epidemic of unnecessary suffering at the end of life. Breathtaking in its scope, rigor, and intellectual range, this book will help readers take back control of their lives and deaths from the forces that have created an 'ordinary' end-of-life medicine that is far from ordinary."

—**KATY BUTLER**, author of *Knocking on Heaven's Door: The Path to a Better Way of Death*

"The recommendation by the ama to Medicare to begin paying physicians for discussions with patients about end-of-life care makes this new book by Sharon R. Kaufman particularly timely. She explains why the present health care system is biased toward excess treatment at the end of life and advocates a broad approach to health care reforms that goes beyond cost control to encompass social and ethical considerations."

—**VICTOR R. FUCHS**, author of *Who Shall Live? Health, Economics and Social Choice*

"Sharon R. Kaufman has made an important and disturbing discovery about the links between for-profit healthcare companies, so-called evidence-based medicine, doctors, and patients. *Ordinary Medicine* should be read, thought about, and acted upon by those who have the power to effect change."

—**VICTORIA SWEET**, author of *God's Hotel: A Doctor, a Hospital, and a Pilgrimage to the Heart of Medicine*

DISCARDED BY
MEAD PUBLIC LIBRARY

ORDINARY MEDICINE

Extraordinary Treatments, Longer Lives,
and Where to Draw the Line

SHARON R. KAUFMAN

DUKE UNIVERSITY PRESS *Durham & London* 2015

© 2015 Duke University Press
All rights reserved
Printed in the United States of America
on acid-free paper ∞
Typeset in Scala by Westchester Book Group

Library of Congress Cataloging-in-Publication Data
Kaufman, Sharon R.
Ordinary medicine : extraordinary treatments,
longer lives, and where to draw the line / Sharon
R. Kaufman
pages cm—(Critical global health)
Includes bibliographical references and index.
ISBN 978-0-8223-5902-9 (hardcover : alk. paper)
ISBN 978-0-8223-5888-6 (pbk. : alk. paper)
ISBN 978-0-8223-7550-0 (e-book)
1. Medical care—United States. 2. Medical
ethics—United States. 3. Medical care, Cost of—
United States. 4. Longevity—United States.
I. Title. II. Series: Critical global health.
RA395.A3K385 2015
362.10973—dc23
2014043465

Cover art: ERproductions Ltd. / Getty Images

9001109467

To the memory of
my father,
Bernard Kaufman Jr., MD,
1914–2008,
and to
Gay Becker,
colleague, friend,
1943–2007

CONTENTS

ACKNOWLEDGMENTS

This project would not have been possible without the permission, support, guidance and sincere engagement of many doctors, nurses, social workers, and other health care providers and patients and families. To protect the confidentiality of research sites and of individual health professionals, I thank them here anonymously. They know who they are. Doctors and all health professionals are under enormous time and administrative pressures today, and I thank all who helped with this project for so graciously taking the time to answer our questions and for allowing us to be present for intimate and confidential discussions. I thank them also for candid conversations, whether in formal interviews or on-the-fly dialogue, about their own treatment dilemmas, the changes they have seen in patients and medical practice, and the host of problems generated by a fragmented health care delivery system. My deep appreciation goes to the patients and families who welcomed us into clinic exams and into their homes for long interview conversations about the course of illness and treatment and the qualms about what to do.

The National Institute on Aging, an agency of the National Institutes of Health, supported this project in full. I thank the anthropologists, sociologists, psychologists, physicians, and nurses who evaluated my proposals and offered suggestions for strengthening the project. Sidney Stahl, my project officer at the NIA, provided welcome advice and important guidance over many years. This research was funded in two phases, by NIA Grant #RO1AG20962 and NIA Grant #RO1AG28426.

Three research associates, Lakshmi Fjord, Ann Russ, and Janet Shim, participated in different phases of this research. I thank them for their enthusiastic commitment, astute observations, probing interviews, and important insights. Their work expanded the scope and depth of this project.

For critical conversations along the way about the practice of medicine, the ethics of medical research, the problems new technologies generate for doctors and patients, the complexities of health care financing, and the vast reaches of the clinical research enterprise, I thank Joel Adelson, Scott Biggins, Alan Coleman, Sandra Del Grosso, Monica Freeman, Sharon Friend, Muriel Gillick, Roy Gordon, David Hayes, Al Jonsen, Barry Landfield, MaryAnn Landfield, Paul Mueller, John Roberts, Peter Stock, Michael Thaler, Alan Venook, and Richard Wagner. Their vast experience helped me understand what is at stake in medicine today, and their insights about the conduct of medical practice and how it has changed over the years, what has become standard and how, and the relationship of biomedical research to clinical practice contributed to my argument.

My colleagues and students in anthropology and sociology at the University of California–San Francisco, the University of California–Berkeley, and beyond offered lively conversation, encouragement, generous invitations, moral support, and good ideas at all phases of this project. There are far too many to thank individually. I have relished and benefited from our stimulating discussions about bioscience, medicine, technology, and anthropology and about the challenges of ethnographic research and writing. Thanks also to participants in the Life and Death Potluck for rewarding dialogue over many years. The creative work of my colleagues, students, and former students has enriched my own tremendously, and I feel blessed to be part of such an intellectually vibrant extended community.

My deep gratitude goes to Vincanne Adams, Lawrence Cohen, Doris Francis, Gelya Frank, Deborah Gordon, Barbara Koenig, Tom Laqueur, Margaret Lock, and Guy Micco for their friendship, insights, challenges, and conversations over many years about medicine and anthropology, research and writing, and what it means to be an anthropologist today. Additionally this project has benefited from the good colleagueship, exchange of ideas, and the inspiring work of João Biehl, Charles Briggs, Adele Clarke, Megan Crowley-Matoka, Sandra Gilbert, Cori Hayden, Martha Holstein, Lochlann Jain, Julie Livingston, Anne Lovell, Lynn Morgan, Adriana Petryna, Paul Rabinow, Tobias Rees, Lorna Rhodes, Lesley Sharp, Nancy Scheper-Hughes, Janelle Taylor, and Kathy Woodward.

I presented aspects of this project in many workshops, seminars, special lectures, and other academic venues over the course of nearly a decade. I thank the hosts, colleagues, and students at the following institutions for their invitations to present my work, for their gracious welcome, and for dialogue that helped move this project forward: UC Santa

Cruz, The Institute for Advanced Feminist Research; UC Berkeley, The Center for Health Research, The Townsend Center for the Humanities, and the Anthropology Department; University of Chicago, the Practice, Medicine and the Body Interdisciplinary Workshop of the departments of anthropology, human development, and social welfare; University of Washington, The Critical Medical Humanities Group; Cambridge University, the Royal Anthropological Institute conference Social Bodies; the Johannes Guttenberg University conference Reflections on Old Age and Ageing; the Newcastle University conference Ageing, Embodiment and Subjectivity; the British Sociological Association conference Body Work; University of Copenhagen, Center for Healthy Aging and the Anthropology Department; University of London, the Economic and Social Research Council; University of Leiden, the Leyden Academy on Vitality and Ageing; McGill University, Department of Social Studies of Medicine; University of North Carolina, Chapel Hill, the Center for Bioethics, Department of Social Medicine, and Department of Anthropology; and Stanford University, Medicine and Anthropology colloquium. I give special thanks to the organizers and participants in the 2011 Wenner-Gren Symposium, Potentiality and Humanness: Revisiting the Anthropological Object in Contemporary Biomedicine, for an especially rewarding conference. In 2009 I was honored to give the Benjamin Lieberman Memorial Lecture, sponsored by the University of California–San Francisco and the Mount Zion Center on Aging. The structure for this book began to take shape in that lecture.

Some of the material in this book first took shape in journal articles. I thank Lakshmi Fjord, Barbara Koenig, Wendy Max, Paul Mueller, Ann Russ, and Janet Shim for their support. Some of the ideas in chapters 1, 4, and 5 were initially developed in S. Kaufman, "Making Longevity in an Aging Society," *Perspectives in Biology and Medicine* 53 (2010): 407–24; S. Kaufman and L. Fjord, "Medicare, Ethics and Reflexive Longevity: Governing Time and Treatment in an Aging Society," *Medical Anthropology Quarterly* 25 (2011): 209–31; S. Kaufman and L. Fjord, "Making Longevity in an Aging Society: Linking Technology, Policy and Ethics," *Medische Antropologie* 23 (2011): 119–38; and S. Kaufman and W. Max, "Medicare's Embedded Ethics: The Challenge of Cost Control in an Aging Society," Health Affairs Blog, March 28, 2011, http://healthaffairs.org/blog /2011/03/28/medicares-embedded-ethics.

Portions of chapter 5 have been significantly revised and updated from A. Russ, J. Shim, and S. Kaufman, "'Is There Life on Dialysis?'

Time and Aging in a Clinically Sustained Existence," *Medical Anthropology* 24 (2005): 297–324. Other portions of that chapter are drawn and elaborated from S. Kaufman, P. S. Mueller, A. L. Ottenberg, and B. A. Koenig, "Ironic Technology: Old Age and the Implantable Cardioverter Defibrillator in U.S. Health Care," *Social Science and Medicine* 72 (2010): 6–14. An earlier version of chapter 6, in a different form, appeared as S. Kaufman, A. Russ, and J. Shim, "Aged Bodies and Kinship Matters: The Ethical Field of Kidney Transplant," *American Ethnologist* 33.1 (2006): 81–99. An earlier version of chapter 8, in a different form, appeared as S. Kaufman, "Fairness and the Tyranny of Potential in Kidney Transplantation," *Current Anthropology* 54, Suppl. 7 (2013): s56–66.

Patrick Fox and Wendy Max, codirectors of the Institute for Health and Aging, my home for many years at UCSF, have provided superb leadership in challenging times for public universities. I thank them for their steady support of my work and for important conversations about aging research and health care finance. Additional thanks goes to the talented staff at the Institute, especially Regina Gudelunas and Christie Chu, for their superb grants management and help with many things. They cheerfully and with great skill helped me navigate the always shifting bureaucracy of federal funding and university administration. Edwina Newsom fostered my work and life at IHA in ways large and small for many years. I am grateful to Lynn Watts for her perfect tape transcriptions and to Ann Oldervoll for her extensive Internet research and for compiling the bibliography. They were each a joy to work with.

I am lucky to have two wonderful academic homes at UCSF, the Department of Anthropology, History and Social Medicine in the School of Medicine and the Department of Social and Behavioral Sciences in the School of Nursing. I thank my colleagues and the staff in both places for their support of my work, for stimulating conversations about their own, and for their commitment to the importance of the social sciences on a health sciences campus.

Vincanne Adams, Tom Laqueur, Robert Martensen, and Stefan Timmermans carefully read an entire early draft of the manuscript and offered detailed comments. Their suggestions enabled me to clarify my argument and craft a better book. Jill Hannum's outstanding editorial skills helped me write more clearly and organize the book into its final form. The book is better for their good advice. I am delighted that Vincanne Adams and João Biehl wanted my book for the new book series, Critical Global Health: Evidence, Efficacy, Ethnography, at Duke University Press. Two anonymous reviewers provided superb suggestions for polishing the manuscript, and Ken Wissoker, editorial director, shepherded this book smoothly through the publication process. I am grateful to Susan Albury, Judith Hoover, and Willa Armstrong for the attention and care they brought to the publication process.

The untimely death of two of my closest colleagues occurred while I was conducting this research. Well before the field of medical anthropology was formally established, the physician and anthropologist Cecil Helman knew that anthropology had a great deal to contribute to medicine. His global understanding of the relationships among culture, health, illness, medicine, and healing have done a great deal to inform the discipline of medical anthropology and inspire students to embark on this career path. Gay Becker's work, interrupted by her death, on insurance and the social safety net in health care, illness and people's lives, and her career-long commitment to the importance of anthropology in promoting social justice inspired the analysis I present here. I dedicate this book, in part, to their memory.

Finally, I offer my heartfelt thanks to my family, Seth, Sarah, Avrami, Jacob, and Benjamin, for their constancy and good humor. They are the lights of my life.

The United States allows, even encourages,
the health care system to play many roles
other than improver of health.
—Daniel Callahan, *What Price Better Health?*

For any way of thought to become dominant, a conceptual
apparatus has to be advanced that appeals to our intuitions
and instincts, to our values and our desires, as well as to the
possibilities inherent in the social world we inhabit. If successful,
this conceptual apparatus becomes so embedded in common
sense as to be taken for granted and not open to question.
—David Harvey, *A Brief History of Neoliberalism*

INTRODUCTION
Diagnosing Twenty-First-Century Health Care

————

Medicine today comprises an unthinkably broad array of
knowledge and skills, professions, coalitions, and interest
groups, fears and promises, fantasies and soon-to-be-realities,
concrete and virtual institutions, folklores and sciences.
—Arthur Frank, *The Renewal of Generosity*

Medicine has changed radically over the past fifteen years. Some of those changes are obvious and dramatic and have provided welcome benefits. Who doesn't welcome the availability of cholesterol-lowering drugs, joint replacements and arthroscopic surgery, the anti-retrovirals that have made AIDS a chronic, manageable illness, and so much more?

Other equally obvious and dramatic changes, however, have become the subject of widespread lament: too much life-sustaining but death-prolonging technology is being used at the end of life; drug companies are paying physicians to promote their products; expensive tests, devices, and procedures are overused; drug costs, especially for cancer treatment, have skyrocketed, yet the new drugs don't necessarily offer better results than existing treatments. Most everyone who has had intimate dealings with the U.S. health care system of late can add to this list of obvious and well-publicized problems.

However, many equally dramatic and relatively recent changes within the U.S. health care delivery system are far less visible—indeed I contend that they are very well hidden. But although they function well below the radar of scrutiny, these changes have not just complicated medical practice and health care delivery but actually have altered their very nature. They have also altered how and what we *think* about health per se and about the options we have for controlling our life span and that of our loved ones. Therein lies the health care dilemma that patients, families, and providers by the millions face every day.

Today's Quandary: When, Where, and How to Draw the Line?

When faced with a life-threatening disease, most of us want the miracles of medicine to extend our lives into a vaguely perceived open-ended future. Yet we don't want to live too long, that is, into a medically prolonged period of suffering or suspension in some limbo, no longer who we were but not yet dead. The big problem, the intractable, increasingly apparent problem is that few know when that line between life-giving therapies and too much treatment is about to be crossed. The burden for knowing where that line sits, and then when and how to respond to it, rests first with doctors and the systems in which they work, yet neither the doctors nor the systems have been effective in recognizing it or foreseeing the consequences of crossing it. And so we find ourselves in a conundrum: the postwar baby boom generation grows older while confronting the old age of its parents; the oldest generation is living longer but not always better; and the widespread lament about *where* that line is located and what to do about it grows ever louder.

Thus the quandary for patients, families, and physicians is about how to live in the world of modern medicine and its life-giving tools, about getting the medicine we wish for but then having to live with the unsettling and far-ranging consequences.

This quandary, its origins, its drivers, and our troubled efforts to resolve it, are the focus of *Ordinary Medicine*. I focus on the ethical, cultural, and political forces driving health care delivery, forces that have made it difficult, if not impossible, to see the line between *enough* and *too much* or even to acknowledge that line's existence or its importance for patient care, medical practice, and the future of the health care system. Not only is this quandary often deeply unsettling for doctors, patients, and families, but it also lies at the crux of the impasse the United States has reached regarding health care reform. Only by *seeing* the way ordinary medicine works, the forces that shape the quandary as well as medicine's successes, can we hope to minimize that quandary and, in addition, work our way out of our untenable national situation.

Three Formative Developments

Three separate but interrelated societal developments that permeate the fabric of American society also control our health care quandary.

THE INCREASED ROLE AND INFLUENCE OF INDUSTRY

The first development is the rising power of the pharmaceutical and device industry, whose market-driven, market-expansion goals have a greater influence on the development and use of treatments than ever before. Industry largely determines which therapies will be investigated and which patient-consumer markets will be exploited. As a consequence its role in determining what doctors recommend and what patients ask for is also increasing. Biomedical research in the United States is a $100 billion enterprise that has approximately doubled in scope since 1999.

There has been a significant shift in the major source of research funding, from government to industry. In 1980, 32 percent of clinical research was funded by private pharmaceutical, medical device, and biotechnology companies. By the mid-1990s that figure had increased to over 50 percent; today it is 65 percent.

The clinical trials industry has mushroomed in recent decades. In 2000 the National Institutes of Health established a data bank of clinical trials information, ClinicalTrials.gov, listing some four thousand trials. By January 2014 its home page listed 159,000 ongoing clinical trials. Clinical trials have acquired strong influence beyond the laboratory. Since the turn of the millennium they have become a culturally prominent and powerful fixture in American life, further strengthening the role they play in ordinary medical practice. Patients *and their families,* increasingly adept at using the Internet to conduct research on diseases and treatments, have learned to view *participation* in clinical trials as disease treatment, as an individual right, and as the embodiment of hope.

THE PROLIFERATING NUMBER OF TREATMENT OPTIONS

The second development is the ever increasing number of treatment options to which doctors, patients, and their families *have access.* These readily available options (which are extremely difficult to say no to) contribute to the overuse of common therapies and diagnostic tools such as the MRI, colonoscopy, and cardiac defibrillator.

The increasing number of trials has generated ever more *evidence of therapeutic value.* Once this evidence is established for a new drug, device, or procedure it is allowed to go on the market. The evidence and the market presence explicitly influence not only what physicians recommend but also what patients learn to want. Unfortunately studies show that new treatment options do not necessarily offer patients better health or a longer life span.

New technologies for diagnosis and treatment, once they are approved for use by the Food and Drug Administration and reimbursed by Medicare and other insurers, are almost always accepted by physicians and patients. Once accepted, they become standard and their use often spreads beyond the population for which the technology was devised. For example, when the implantable cardiac defibrillator (ICD) was introduced in 1985 it was a "treatment of last resort" for very specific heart problems. By 2005 it had become a common surgical tool to stave off death, even for the oldest patients. Similarly the artificial heart pump (left ventricular assist device, LVAD) has shifted from being an experimental device intended for temporary use to being a standard long-term solution for end-stage heart disease.

AMERICANS' PERSPECTIVE ON AGING
AND THE TIMING OF DEATH

The third societal development orchestrating the health care dilemma is the profound impact our society's unrelenting prioritization of the use of new technologies has had on our perspective on aging and on death itself—especially with respect to the drugs, devices, and surgical procedures now available to treat what used to be end-stage diseases. In the United States today most deaths, regardless of a person's age, have come to be considered premature. Because medicine's tools can seemingly "add" time, the value of life has come to be measured, in large part, by its length. This has magnified our quandaries by reinforcing the desire for and rationality of intervening at ever older ages to extend life, regardless of the emotional and financial costs. The central role of high-tech life-prolonging treatments means life extension for many more older people, but it also means choosing among the available options, which often burdens patients and families with a heavy sense of responsibility for making the "right" choice. Will a treatment prolong the patient's life or simply prolong an unwanted kind of dying?

The apparent "good" of all new technologies and the burdens they create now meet an aging population. Over the past fifteen years the U.S. population in general, and therefore the patient population, has aged. In

2010, 13 percent of the population was over age sixty-five; 2 percent was over eighty-five. By 2050 those percentages will be 20 and 4 percent, respectively.

The surge of advanced treatments that keep lethal diseases at bay and our romance with new medical technologies go on relentlessly, with ever older persons on the receiving end and growing numbers of families caught in the tangle of emotional, financial, and organizational responsibilities of care. The particularly American ethos of "more is always better" underlies the high-tech and aggressive approaches to treatments. At the same time, fear, ambivalence, and complaints about *too much* proliferate.

The increase in the use of high-tech treatments for older patients is also reflected in ever increasing costs to the Medicare program and the nation. (Medicare is the federal program of health insurance available to persons sixty-five and older.) For example, the LVAD costs approximately $250,000—ten times more than the ICD. The number of patients over seventy-five who have been started on maintenance kidney dialysis has tripled in the past two decades, even though dialysis therapy does not necessarily improve quality of life or prolong life for elderly persons. Since 2001, when kidney transplantations from living donors first exceeded those from deceased donors, adult children have been donating their kidneys and parts of their livers to their parents and other older relatives with ever greater frequency.

————

Why bother to write a book about the quandary of crossing the line when so many millions of people in their later years have reaped the benefits of modern medicine? When so many have had their lives prolonged by cardiac procedures and cancer treatments? When so many live not only longer but better as a result of those treatments?

As a medical anthropologist, I have spent more than twenty years watching this quandary play out and asking why it occupies so much of American political debate and cuts such a wide swath through the public conversation about control over the time for dying. Mostly the quandary is experienced by older persons, their families, and their doctors. In 2002 I began to observe older patients in specialty clinics, where they were most often offered life-prolonging therapies. I listened to hundreds of patients, physicians, and family members deliberate about what to do and heard them express their hopes, fears, and reasoning. Thus I have had a ringside seat on the evolution of their dilemmas about crossing the line of "too much" and their desire to do everything possible to prolong life. Many patients ask their doctors what they themselves would do in similar situations, and doctors, notably, do not answer definitively.

I started tracing the themes that emerged in the clinic conversations about evidence and expectations, norms and standards, risks, hope and ambivalence, the urge to try everything and the demand to stop. The talk mostly settled on scientific evidence, standards of care, risk reduction, and necessary treatments, which led me to investigate how and why these have come to organize our "more is always better" approach to medicine. That quest, in turn, led me to think about the larger engines of the biomedical economy—the research and insurance industries (especially Medicare)—and their impact on what we do when life is at stake.

The Chain of Health Care Drivers: Four Invisible Controlling Factors

What emerged was my realization that there are unseen, determining forces, *a chain of health care drivers*, behind the dilemmas twenty-first-century American health care poses: Why do those of us caught up in the health care system often struggle so hard to decide what we want from potentially life-extending treatments? Why do we not know what to expect from them? Why do physicians prescribe specific treatments? Why do they sometimes go against their own professional values when making treatment decisions to prolong life? These quandaries are faced by millions every day—yet few if any of us can glean the lessons learned from the experiences of others. That is because the forces that determine the structure of the U.S. health care delivery system today are neither visible nor easily quantifiable, and what is hidden does not easily offer up the tools for understanding its nature. With those tools, doctors and patients might make different choices—choices that would promote significant system change.

Four primary drivers build on one another in a chain of events that governs medicine today. Those drivers and their effects on the practice of medicine and on the lives, health, and aging of all of us are the focus of *Ordinary Medicine*. Those drivers reveal the scope of our health care predicament and why we can't clearly see how to fix it. They show us what needs to be fixed and why. They are the key to restoring the primacy of the social good of medicine.

1. The initial driver is the biomedical research industry and its mushrooming clinical trials engine, which is churning out evidence of effective therapies at an unprecedented rate.
2. The committees that determine Medicare and private insurance payment policies evaluate that evidence to determine whether the therapy, device, or procedure in question should be reimbursable. If it is, physicians will prescribe it, insured patients will have access to it, and patients and families will want it.
3. Once a therapy is reimbursable by insurance, it almost instantly becomes a standard of care.
4. Finally, once therapies become standard, they also become ethically necessary and therefore difficult, if not impossible, for physicians, patients and families to refuse.

Health Care Drivers and the Ethical Field

The individuals seventy and older whom I sought out in high-tech treatment centers and the small, airless exam cubicles of community physicians' offices in several U.S. cities between 2002 and 2011 had life-threatening diseases.[1] Slowly over those years the determinative power of the chain of health care drivers became visible to me. And because I was observing human beings interacting in intimate and often desperate circumstances, what emerged was not just the structure of the chain but also its ethical underpinnings. It is a chain predicated on and imbued with ethical choices, political priorities, and economic commitments—in other words, it is based on and reflects cultural values. Not everyone's values, of course, but those that, through the political will of some, have become dominant in the health care arena.

These values dominate *all* of health care delivery today, not just health care for the elderly. Once one notices how strongly determinative these drivers are, however, it becomes perfectly clear that patients and families (and sometimes doctors) actually do not *decide* about treatments so much as they yield to procedures that the chain has made normal and ordinary. Everything I observed that affected patients and families on a human level—their options and rationales, emotions and ambivalence, their choices among the normal and normalized pathways of treatment and the ways that treatment goals impacted their experiences, sensibilities, and actions—proved to have these drivers and the values they represent as their common frame.

After spending many, many hours with physicians and older patients and their families, I also realized that the values and commitments that drive the entire health care enterprise—especially those of individualism, market-based approaches to health care services, and an instrumental or mechanistic view of medical "progress"—are so difficult to discern because they are exceptionally diffuse. Because they penetrate so much of American society and so heavily influence the patterns of biomedical research, medical treatment, and patient expectations, I think of them as forming an *ethical field*. This ethical field shapes health care policies, the development of biomedical technologies, and how evidence about treatment is produced and employed in clinical care. It is constituted also by what patients and families come to need and want. Ultimately the effects of the ethical field are seen in the physical caregiving tasks and emotional burdens placed on families. Its influence permeates every aspect of health care delivery and affects everyone: clinicians, patients, and families alike. Although it has grown increasingly dominant in recent decades, this ethical field has nonetheless already become, like the air we breathe, mostly unnoticed.[2]

Connecting the Quandary with "Ordinary Medicine"

The cacophony of voices and viewpoints I heard in the clinics—about whether to attempt to fix the body and with which tools, and about how to try to make patients "feel like themselves again"—led me to delve into the larger story, to learn why and how the problem of knowing when to stop treatment has been fraught with so much difficulty and has triggered such impassioned politics. I examined not only the components of the health care enterprise (evidence-based medicine, Medicare, etc.) but also the particularly American connections between individual rights and communal good and between politics and progress that characterize our contemporary society, drive the health care engine, and shape what happens to so many of us in later life.

I have coined the phrase *ordinary medicine* to serve as a shorthand reference that encompasses the wide range of features of the health care enterprise that must be looked at closely if we are ever to resolve the quandary about crossing the line. It reflects the hidden chain of connections among science, politics, industry, and insurance as well as the ethos that supports that chain. It emphasizes the fact that the driving features of our health care delivery system, and thus the practice of medicine and what we want from it, have become taken for granted and routine.

Ordinary medicine is vast and fragmented and offers no inherent facility, no clue or advice for physicians with which to evaluate when *more* is not better and for putting on the brakes. And so our wonderful ability to extend life with medical technique—into ever greater old age—is now inextricably intertwined with the emotional burdens and dilemmas families must shoulder because they are responsible for deciding where the line of "too much" is located and what to do about it.

Is this an untenable societal burden? I am convinced that our medical practices define the kind of society we have, by which I mean that they show starkly how the commercial enterprise of health care delivery has far surpassed the *social good* as a function and goal of medicine. The dominance of private industry, the emphasis on new technologies regardless of cost, and the lack of equity in the distribution of medical care have created a vocabulary that we use to describe ourselves as psychological and cultural beings. It is a vocabulary that conflates "being medically eligible for" and "needing" a liver transplant, an implantable heart pump, or defibrillator beyond the age of, say, eighty. This conflation is possible only because today's medicine provides those tools and because such procedures have imperceptibly become "normal" at ever older ages. Twenty years ago one could not "need" those therapies because they did not exist. Ten years ago few anticipated that older persons would become the growth market for such therapies.

Life-Extending Therapies for Older People: The New Normal

By 2002 I had already begun to look carefully at medical interventions that were clearly prolonging lives—and doing so for greater numbers of older people.[3] I chose to focus on therapies that were becoming more common for patients over the age of seventy because the intersection of life-extending treatments with an aging population had already become the double-edged sword of medicine. Treatments for and in an aging society, and Medicare payment for those treatments, were driving health care for everyone in the United States. The ability to extend (and the potential to extend) already older lives is at once miraculous, desired, and taken for granted and a significant source both of individual quandaries about what to do and of the national struggle about the goals and the good of medicine.

As I investigated the use of organ transplantation, cardiac devices and procedures, and aggressive cancer treatments for older persons (reflected in the many case examples throughout this book), it was clear that cultural notions of what was *routine* were continuing to change even as I watched. Increasing numbers of older people were receiving these and other potentially life-extending medical treatments, and many were in treatment for long periods of time. Many of them were able to live longer and better as a result. This is what we all want. Others, regardless of the extent of intervention, did not have their lives prolonged by treatments, or their life was prolonged but so were extreme disability and suffering. Still others faced guilt and ambivalence in moving forward with or stopping aggressive therapies and were unable to choose between those pathways. (Today it is not easily evident which of these three groups is the largest.)

In wanting to know how and why each of these responses, each of these outcomes had become so ordinary for an ever older cohort of patients, I began to understand that the answer to the problem of crossing the line for patients and families—and thus resolving the conundrum about the goals and good of medicine—lay somewhere within that very ordinariness. It is the ordinariness of today's medicine that needs to be examined—and altered—if we, as a nation, are ever to emerge from the impasse that is the fractured American health care system.

This ordinariness is in marked contrast with another development. For the approximately one-fifth of Americans who have Medicare insurance (those sixty-five and older), these life-extending treatments are generally available and relatively accessible. Their health care dilemmas center around which therapies to undertake and when to stop. Yet at least another fifth of our society (who are under sixty-five) has limited (often very limited) access to routine health care services. Their problems are different and are equally or arguably more pressing—for instance, whether to buy medications or groceries. Yet the problem about the confused goals of medical treatment is particularly apparent when we turn to the health care that older persons receive.

The Chain and Its Ethical Field: Shaping Medicine, Shaping Us

Medicine is part of society and can offer and deliver only what the science of the times and the political and economic priorities of the setting make available. Medical care in any location is influenced by what patients expect and by how access to it is determined and organized. In addition to being shaped *by* particular social and historical circumstances, the contours of medical practice and the organization of health care delivery themselves shape societal goals and norms and individual expectations about what is fixable and should be fixed, and among whom.

Ordinary medicine—the chain of health care drivers and the ethical field that supports it—matters because it is a profoundly influential shaping tool in our society. It not only determines which therapies are available but also affects how and why we say yes (or sometimes no) to specific therapies. The chain and the ethical field are the mechanisms by which treatment standards become social standards. They are the governing agents of doctor and patient behavior. They chart our senses of obligation and responsibility to the ill among us, guide our expressions of love and duty, and are the source of our quandaries about where and when to draw the line. Ordinary medicine shapes our most personal experiences of growing older and, ultimately, undermines medicine's ability to function as a social good.

We have come to the point where every day in hospitals and clinics, at bedsides and kitchen tables, before and after receiving therapies, the hope of potentially life-prolonging treatment comes up against the possibility of a prolonged, unwanted kind of living and dying. An eighty-six-year-old man succinctly summarized the dilemma to me at one clinic I visited. Two years earlier, following a third heart attack, he had received an automatic implantable cardiac defibrillator:

> After I passed out and was taken to the hospital, the cardiologist said I should get an ICD. He said he wouldn't be doing his job right if he didn't say that I needed an ICD. He told me the two stents I had previously were blocked. So I agreed and he put it in. Now it seems the ICD has prolonged my life a little bit. But the longer it prolongs my life, the more other things are happening to me, that it can't correct. And you know, all the medicines, all the treatments, have side effects, and some of them are pretty bad. So which do you want? The question is, do you want to have the other things that are going wrong and the side effects, or do you want to end it all? And when? I haven't given up on medicine, but the body wears out and there's nothing you can do about that.

The Disconnected Worlds of Health Policy and Medical Practice

This patient was caught up in a situation I found all too common during the years I spent conducting the research that led to this book: it often seems that the policy and clinical worlds exist on different planets. While the chain of health care drivers dictated that he "needed" an ICD, the clinical picture—"all the other things that are going wrong and the side effects"—is much more complicated, nuanced. While listening to patients, families, and physicians interact in clinics over the years, I also attended health policy lectures at my university and read numerous policy reports about Medicare reform and the state of health care delivery. It became clear that policy analyses dwell in the world of charts, statistics, and projections. They report trends in services, illnesses, payments, and costs, and they concentrate on quantification—numbers of patients, diseases, medical errors, hospitalizations, nursing home and clinic visits, costs of treatment, trends in government and private insurance spending, and so on. They create models, algorithms, and programs for better health care delivery and cost-effectiveness and focus on the organization of service delivery, cost sharing, coverage, and eligibility standards. If we can only reduce or streamline or add something to or eliminate something from the system, the reports tend to emphasize, then our costs will go down or at least not rise as quickly, services will be more efficient, and perhaps patients will be served better.

In the clinic, on the other hand, doctors and nurses are doing what they think is best for *this* patient right *now*. Their decisions depend on clinical and scientific evidence, technical skills, the diagnostic and treatment tools available to them and to the patient, their overall level of experience, and what they know about the patient's condition and life. Their goals are to treat disease, reduce risks, and prolong the life in front of them, or at least to make that life more comfortable.

Occasionally the worlds of policy and the clinic meet in a way that is visible to many, and the results are broadly regarded as positive. Recent examples include the use of checklists to reduce infections in hospitals, the consolidation of services and financial arrangements in "medical homes" and physician groups in order to reduce costs and the fragmentation of care, attempts to standardize treatments that have been proven effective, and the broadening of the spectrum of treatments that are included in some hospice coverage.

However, with regard to the expanding array of lifesaving therapies for older persons, it seems that the policy experts do not know what goes on in the clinic with respect to the difficult choices to be made, standard treatments, the press to treat, or the demands of physician and family responsibility. Because policymakers do not attend to those things, they cannot take into account the deeply rooted connections this book examines: connections between, for example, individual responsibility and technological innovation, between medical necessity and Medicare reimbursement, between doctors' recommendations and the clinical trials industry.

Clinicians, on the other hand, have not been and cannot be concerned primarily (or at all) with cost savings (though many are turning some of their attention to costs now). They cannot alter deeply rooted practice patterns on their own; in fact many physicians and nurses have told me that there are alterations they cannot make but "society" should make. Such changes might, for example, address whether to admit very old persons who are nearing the end of their life to hospital intensive care units for aggressive therapies; whether to start kidney dialysis for frail, demented, and/or very sick elderly persons; whether to implement age restrictions for organ transplantation; whether to suggest repeated rounds of chemotherapy for those at advanced ages.

The clinical world's interconnected yet often unseen entrenchment in powerful economic, political, and social forces determines the practice of medicine and the lives of patients, and it is one reason why health care reform has been so elusive in the United States. Its disconnection from the policymaking world has bothered me for a long time. By showing how the links in the chain connect to escalating expectations about health and life in old age, I hope to open a passageway for communication between the two worlds.

The Intersection of Ordinary Medicine and Our Aging Society: Progress or Postprogress?

Employing the most sophisticated medical treatments for octogenarians, nonagenarians, and older has come to seem normal, ordinary, and necessary. Almost unthinkable thirty years ago, these developments are now taken for granted at the same time that increasing numbers of patients and families pay a price in suffering and in the disquiet that accompanies the feeling, the knowledge of having crossed the line.

As a result our society has arrived at a point where choosing not to undergo heart surgery, chemotherapy, or organ transplantation, for example, or deciding against a feeding tube, implantable cardiac device, or kidney dialysis when one is eighty or beyond often seems somehow suspect—to patients, families, and doctors alike. Physicians' thinking, health care financing (which is driven by our system of Medicare reimbursement), and the culture and structure of medical treatment all point toward saying yes when the newest therapies and diagnostic tools are offered. Saying no to potentially lifesaving therapies seems like refusing to take the path of progress that medicine has trod for the past two centuries and must be explained and justified to oneself and others because it does not seem rational or ethical. As things stand now, for those who have Medicare insurance, it is simply *easier* to start receiving therapies than to say no to them, thus pushing doctors, patients, and families toward ever more intervention.

These developments have led me to characterize U.S. health care, ordinary medicine, as exemplifying what I call "postprogress." If progress refers to the long-held Enlightenment idea and ideal that rationality and its tools can unequivocally improve life and reduce suffering, then postprogress characterizes today's medicine and the quagmire it often creates, especially regarding the prioritizing and effects of ever more technology use in our aging society. Postprogress acknowledges that the value of life prolongation has come up against the dilemma of extending the life span past a point that people want. Postprogress suggests that technical ability and more and more interventions, while they extend wanted life for many, also bring with them existential quandaries about one's own relationship to medicine, to suffering, to *more* life, and to the apparent control that can be exercised over the timing of death. Medicine's abilities and interventions are accompanied as well by societal concerns about the present and future financial solvency of the health care delivery system. Postprogress is our uneasy, pervasive, contemporary condition.

————

My first task in this book is to trace the sources and effects of the chain and its ethical field so that its diffuse locations in American institutions, technological developments, clinical practice, and consumer health care desires can be better understood. My second task is to analyze the ways the socioethical changes taking place in medical care and the systems that support it are affecting the quality of our individual experience. On the way I explore some of the difficult issues facing health care delivery today (especially certain new technologies and procedures and their open-ended use) and a few of the ways age does and does not matter. I also touch on elements of clinical, policy, and bioethics discussions that get minimized or erased in the face of the lure of life-extending treatments.

Thus *Ordinary Medicine* is an account of the four parts of the determinative chain of health care drivers and the ethics and politics that surround it. I describe how medicine for the elderly shapes health care for everyone. I trace the effects of the chain on the sensibilities of the patients, families, and doctors I met on their journeys through the health care system. Nearly every reader of this book will recognize elements of their own journey through our health care system.

Chapter 1, "Ordinary Medicine in Our Aging Society: The Dilemma of Longevity," describes the chain of connections among science, industry, and insurance that defines our predicament and shapes how treatments emerge, become available to patients, and then are deemed to be wanted and necessary. The chapter also introduces the field of ethical choices that is inherent in the operation of this chain. Such ethical choices determine the goals of clinical research, which therapies are considered appropriate, and how doctors and patients respond. For example, Medicare reimbursement policies do not provide cost constraints or age limits for certain treatments, and there is an imperative for doctors to offer treatments to patients that they would not choose for themselves. Importantly, because broad-based ethical choices both underlie and are embedded within the chain, their role as drivers of U.S. health care is hidden and remains largely unexamined.

Focusing on the point where medical technology and our aging population intersect, this chapter describes how the chain of health care drivers strengthens the bureaucracy of medicine, heightens the importance of risk awareness in medicine and society, and reinforces the rationality of extending life at ever older ages with more and more interventions. Taken together these developments create the predicament introduced in this chapter and central to the book: patients, families, and physicians all find themselves caught up in a system in which *more* and *yes* are so entrenched that saying no to it involves negotiation, pleading, and grappling with deep emotional consequences.

Chapter 2, "The Medical-Industrial Complex I: Evidence-Based Medicine, the Biomedical Economy, and the Ascendance of Clinical Trials," examines two components of the vast engine of biomedical research from which therapies emerge: the phenomenon of evidence-based medicine, that is, the proactive and transparent application of the best (and newest) published scientific research findings about medical treatments, and the business of clinical trials. These two components are the apparatuses of truth-making in medicine. They define what counts as "good" medicine. Through them research findings from experimental studies are converted into best evidence for treatment. That conversion is the first of the four transformations that constitute contemporary medicine. It affects all the others and thus affects what happens to patients and families.

Chapter 3, "The Medical-Industrial Complex II: Access, Industry, and the Clinical Trials Phenomenon," shows how evidence from clinical trials emerges, how those findings determine insurance reimbursement patterns and then treatment standards, and how those in turn organize the work of physicians. This chapter ends with a look at the specter that hangs over these engines of innovation and evidence: the fact that the pharmaceutical and biotech industries and the for-profit market for technologies all have a growing impact on shaping research agendas, and thus on shaping treatments.

Chapter 4, " 'Reimbursement Is Critical for Everything': Medicare and the Ethics of Managing Life," turns to the Medicare insurance system, whose reimbursement policies and decisions convert best evidence into available treatments—the second transformation in the chain of health care drivers. Beyond their role as the gatekeepers to treatment for those sixty-five and older, Medicare reimbursement decisions organize the next two transformations in the chain as well. Once a therapy is eligible for reimbursement, it almost instantly undergoes the third transformation and becomes standard for everyone; then, in the fourth transformative move, it becomes necessary. That is, reimbursement legitimates which interventions *should* be employed to treat which conditions. Medicare dictates the way treatment practices unfold for millions of persons in the United States. Its policies are instrumental to the ways seniors experience old age and dying and everyone else experiences what to need, want, and expect from medicine.

Chapter 5, "Standard and Necessary Treatments: The Changing Means and Ends of Technology," shows how the press for new technologies in U.S. health care complicates the goals of medical practice in our aging society. In examining three types of treatment—the implantable cardiac defibrillator, kidney dialysis, and liver transplantation—I show how technological innovations and interventions become standard and necessary. I show also how they influence our thinking about which conditions are the logical, rational targets for particular therapies, which patients need them, and what we come to want from them. Questions about how to measure successful treatment and what constitutes therapeutic benefit loom large here, and each patient's story illustrates the quandary of determining how one should live in relation to the tools of medicine as one grows old.

Chapter 6, "Family Matters: Kidneys and New Forms of Care," demonstrates how patients and families become caught up in the world of kidney transplantation, especially living donor transplantation. Living kidney donation, in particular from an adult child to a parent, has become a normal cultural practice and a routine social fact that, for many, guides how love and obligation are expressed. As scientific evidence emerged that transplants from living donors have comparatively high success rates and that transplantation can be and is successful in older persons, that evidence provided the basis for expressing love and obligation through living donation.

The world of transplantation is just one arena in which today's medicine shapes love, obligation, and other sensibilities about how to live. Chapter 7, "Influencing the Character of the Future: Prognosis, Risk, and Time Left," examines four decision-making moments regarding treatment options. I show how prognosis and risk assessment organize doctors' practices and patients' and families' experiences with respect to remaining time, the control of time, and the relationship of medical interventions to "time left." By offering prognoses, medicine instructs us to imagine different future scenarios, and then it insists that we choose among them.

Chapter 8, "For Whose Benefit? Our Shared Quandary," returns to the example of kidney transplantation because it so dramatically illustrates how fairness, realized in equitable access for all, has been reinvented in our aging society through medical procedures. The growing demand for kidneys among older patients has created a fairness and access problem because older persons are receiving an increasingly greater proportion of the total number of available deceased donor kidneys, which contributes to greater scarcity for younger patients in need. The ordinariness of organ transplantation at older ages links issues of scarcity and the right to health with notions of the public good and a broadened conception of public health.

In my conclusion, "Toward a New Social Contract?," I emphasize how our predicament is emblematic of other trends in American society. How we shape the values and directions of the health care delivery enterprise will determine—and reveal—the kind of society we create in the coming years. Because the trends that have brought us to this point are entrenched and ongoing—especially the dominance of private industry in health care services, the priority given to technology use regardless of cost, and the lack of equity in the distribution of medical care—they continue to derail the practice of medicine, indeed the entire health care delivery enterprise, as a social good.

My investigation of how our cultural values, including political and economic forces, shape the chain of health care drivers has two primary goals. One is to show how much those drivers determine about medical care and thus about contemporary life. The other, by extension, is to try to shed needed light on how the very logic, the unexamined ordinariness of ordinary medicine, impedes the kind of health care reform Americans say they want—reform that would bring preventive care, chronic care, and basic acute care services to more people while, at the same time, reducing costs.

The work of medicine, the burden of responsibility that patients and families shoulder about crossing the line (to potentially more life or death), and the existential and societal question about how to live in relation to medicine's tools all urgently demand that we give deep consideration to our heath care enterprise's reigning logic, its organizational drivers, and the values that support it. By unveiling the hidden workings of our predicament, I hope *Ordinary Medicine* will facilitate steps toward establishing a renewed sense of trust in U.S. medicine and an understanding of what has led to our current impasse. My interactions in the clinics I visited over many years made it clear that our untenable health care enterprise affects us all very deeply and that the case for fixing it is strong. What also became clear is that in order to fix it, we must understand clearly why the system—as it affects our aging society—is so badly broken. The answers are to be found here.

PART I

THE QUANDARY AND UNEXAMINED ORDINARINESS OF

TWENTY-FIRST-CENTURY MEDICINE

1

ORDINARY MEDICINE IN OUR AGING SOCIETY
The Dilemma of Longevity

In the furthering of a genuinely modern culture, it is the aging who actually
have pride of place; they are where the action is, for they are something
historically new as a large population sector.
—Gerald J. Gruman, "Cultural Origins of Present-Day 'Age-ism':
The Modernization of the Life Cycle"

Americans' involvement with medicine and its techniques has deepened
dramatically as a result of the monumental changes over the past decade
and a half in the practice of medicine and in the entire U.S. health care
industry. Nowhere is this revealed more starkly than at the place where
life-extending medicine and ever greater age intersect.

Although few appear to have foreseen our current predicament, it was
inevitable that medicine would collide with age.[1] Today, while our health
care dilemmas are evident for patients at every age, they are more sharply
defined for those in later life. Much of medicine is oriented around aging:
treating its symptoms, confronting its challenges, and preparing for it
with a wide array of preventive and future-oriented interventions. Disease prevention and symptom control for those in midlife and beyond
are taken for granted by health care professionals and active health care
consumers alike; they have become essential components of good health
care.

The ongoing cycle of watching, waiting, testing, and treating that
characterizes good medical care for all and that affects so many older
persons is accompanied by more health-related tasks and duties than
ever before. There are more specialists involved in one's care; more clinic
visits, tests, and test follow-ups; more insurance paperwork; and, at every

juncture, *more decision making*. There are more medications, more surgeries, more dilemmas about what to do. How did we get here? What is driving the ongoing changes that fuel our dilemmas?

Ordinary Medicine: Mrs. Walters's Predicament

The taken-for-granted, mostly unexamined contemporary situation in which we find ourselves attempting to do the very best we can as doctors and patients is what I call *ordinary medicine*. This chapter introduces the chain of ordinary medicine's drivers, the ethical commitments and political decisions that undergird it, and the links among the drivers, the decisions, and the reality of our aging society. The chain of health care drivers is what determines what the clinic delivers, what patients expect, and why the quandary about the line has become so pervasive.

That quandary is well illustrated by the example of Mrs. Walters, whose difficult, and increasingly common, situation exemplifies many elements of the intersection of old age and life-extending treatments.

I first met Martha Walters, age eighty-eight, in 2008 during her third hospitalization in as many months for severe heart failure, a growing problem in the United States. During the previous hospitalization (at a different hospital from the one in which I met her), physicians had implanted a pacemaker and automatic cardiac (or cardioverter) defibrillator—now considered an ordinary, routine treatment—telling her that without that device, she would die. The ICD monitors heart rate and rhythm and recognizes the onset of life-threatening cardiac arrhythmias. When it detects an abnormal rhythm, it delivers timed electrical discharges or shocks to the heart muscle, thereby disrupting and ending the life-threatening situation.[2]

A month after that episode I arrived at the hospital to find Mrs. Walters sitting up in bed. She was both friendly and cheerful while staff came and went from her room. Her ICD had just been deactivated. This was done because, following a long discussion with the cardiology team, the palliative care team, and her daughters, Mrs. Walters had learned that the purpose of the ICD was to shock a lethal cardiac rhythm into a normal one. This would prolong her life but not ease the many other symptoms she was having. After much discussion, Mrs. Walters and her family felt comfortable about not pursuing what all considered to be "heroic" life-prolonging interventions, and they arranged for hospice care. Together the doctor, patient, and family drew what they considered to be a clear line: no obvious heroics. Yet they remained oblivious to the fact that her cardiac pacemaker too would sustain Mrs. Walters's life, though it did not prevent life-threatening problems.[3]

I encountered Mrs. Walters again eighteen months later in a cardiology clinic exam room. She was about to turn ninety and was obviously despondent. Four months earlier she had been "discharged" from hospice because, I was told by her daughters, she was "too healthy." But since that discharge she had been hospitalized three times for life-threatening cardiac episodes and other problems. Her most recent hospitalization had been four weeks before this clinic visit. One of her daughters informed me, "If my sister and the doctors hadn't been at her bedside [in the hospital] and taken care of her heart condition, we would have lost her." Now that they were removed from the structure of end-of-life hospice care, with its clarity about allowing death to arrive, the family was pursuing life-extending treatments. Their earlier sense of where they would draw the line had vanished, and they were following the ordinary pathways of medicine, which, unless someone intervenes, does not acknowledge a line indicating "too much."

Mrs. Walters had barely been out of bed since her most recent hospitalization and had deteriorated rapidly. Her daughters, distressed that she was losing the desire to live, wanted to shore her up emotionally and physically. Sitting on the exam table, Mrs. Walters cried, "I don't want to do anything. I just want to go to sleep and get it over with. I don't think I'm going to get better." When the physician arrived, he adjusted her medications and confirmed that she was to continue to have her pacemaker checked every three months.

Mrs. Walters found herself between the rock of her own (and her family's) ambivalence about whether to pursue lifesaving treatments or palliative care and the hard place of being shuttled by the system between end-of-life hospice and rescue medicine. Though the deactivation of her ICD ensured that she would not be "shocked" back to life (and ongoing heart disease) if she had a lethal cardiac event, her pacemaker and repeated hospitalizations kept her alive. Her situation exemplifies *ordinary medicine* at work.

Ordinary Medicine's Underlying Drivers

Throughout this book I make reference to the chain of drivers that creates ordinary medicine's structure and delivery. The chapters that follow address each link in detail. The chain appears to be rationally, logically based, but, as we'll see, it operates on a foundation of ethical judgments and political decisions. These inform the practice of medicine today and speak to patients, families, and doctors through the logic and reason—the rationality—of science, evidence-based medicine, and standards of care. It is highly ironic that while we mostly ignore—or cannot see—the underlying ethics and politics, like Mrs. Walters and her family we struggle mightily with the problem they engender: *where, when, and how to draw the line.*

The chain of connections, the backbone of the biomedical enterprise in which American health care is delivered, follows a fixed order of progression, and each part of the chain influences the next part. It begins with scientific innovation, which then links to testing on patients in studies, to the accumulation and evaluation of research evidence, and finally to insurance reimbursement and the setting of standards and protocols. At each link a *transformation* occurs that makes it possible for the move to the next link to happen seamlessly and, most tellingly, unnoticed.

The first element in the series is the massive enterprise of biomedical research that underlies today's evidence-based medicine. The first transformation takes place there when, based on research findings, scientific evidence is created that shows whether a treatment is beneficial. While all kinds of research take place, the most highly valued form of evidence is produced from clinical trials. Once evidence of treatment benefit has been created, the second transformative move occurs. This time it happens within the matrix of Medicare payment policies, which converts experimental evidence into available, paid-for therapies. In the third transformation, the vast majority of reimbursable treatments instantly become standards of care. The next transformation, which largely goes unrecognized, is the ethical inflection that is given to those standard-of-care practices and turns them into *necessary* interventions that are difficult, if not impossible, to refuse. In other words, the standards become standard.

This entire chain of transformations governs all of medicine today, and it gives rise to the social and individual predicaments we face. There is also a fifth transformation, which occurs within and among us, the patients and families, because ordinary medicine's chain has altered and continues to shape our relationship to the body, the future, and our deepest commitments to family. The treatment scenarios presented throughout this book illustrate this fifth transformation as patients, families, and physicians contemplate crossing the line. Their deliberations are set up by the drivers that define the health care enterprise, and those drivers ensure that, as in Mrs. Walters's case, any ambivalence about how much treatment is too much is coupled with a system-wide culture and bureaucracy that always move the patient toward life-extending treatments.

Ordinary Medicine's Ethical Field

Significantly, and as I will continue to emphasize and illustrate, *ethical* commitments and judgments are what underlie the seeming rationality of the health care drivers and the connections among them. All features of the continuum, from basic science through to health care delivery, are built on prior cultural and political decisions, prior political and economic motivations. This is what I refer to as the "ethical field" that surrounds any idea for a treatment as it progresses from the beginning to the end of that continuum.

Traditionally ethics in the realm of health care, known as bioethics, has been understood as referring to the content of difficult clinical *choices*, such as whether to withhold or withdraw treatment. Bioethics-based solutions have, for example, stressed improved communication between doctors and patients in order to clarify treatment goals. The ethical field I examine here is far more diffuse. The ethical field is foundational to the drivers of health care delivery that make new drugs, devices, and procedures compelling, determine patients' needs, and define necessary treatment. So my purposes here are best served by referring not to ethics but to what I conceptualize as the ethical *field* that forms the bedrock of the biomedical economy and the marketplace and infuses all of ordinary medicine.

Becoming "Ordinary"

For every ambivalent Mrs. Walters, there is another patient who aggressively pursues treatment in the hope of staying alive, and there are others (though far fewer) who firmly reject treatment. And for every ambivalent family, there are those who urge the patient to ask for (or even demand) any and all life-prolonging measures. This spectrum of options is the result of a particular confluence of diverse elements that stem from and work with the chain of drivers. These elements include the central role that high-tech treatments have come to play at older ages, the growth in industry-funded research and the clinical trials business, the emphasis on commercial interests and new technologies, the vernacular of "preventive maintenance" and "risk awareness" that characterizes so much of middle-class life, and the patient expectations and family responsibility that are tied to treatments. Together these have given rise to the perfect storm that is the predicament of ordinary medicine.

In one sense I intend the term *ordinary medicine* ironically, for there is nothing usual or customary or inevitable about this transformative constellation of developments or about the fact that ethical judgments underlie all the links connecting the parts of the health care enterprise. Nonetheless the ways medicine is practiced, the hidden drivers behind that practice, and the sensibilities that result are all truly ordinary now. Ordinary because of the widespread assumption that the discoveries of biomedical science most always produce useful therapies and that we should have a right to all those therapies, regardless of cost or age. Ordinary because high-tech interventions are employed so routinely for older patients, both with and without scientific evidence of their effectiveness. Ordinary in that the successes of medicine influence us to think that the body is infinitely fixable and life is infinitely extendable. Ordinary because we have come to expect that organ transplants, cardiac devices, aggressive chemotherapy, and complex surgeries will cure us of disease, relieve us of debilitating symptoms, and thwart death, regardless of age or severity of condition. After all, those interventions have become routine for those in later life and are entirely unremarkable as medical facts. Ordinary because all of this has become standard, normal, rational, and ethically appropriate. My term *ordinary medicine* is thus only partly ironic.

Developments in Treatment, Technology, and Research:
How Standards Become Standard in an Aging Society

An example of the making of ordinary medicine can be seen in the way life-extending medical treatments first emerged and were then taken up in new, expanded ways. Many such treatments played a central role in the lives of the patients and families I met in clinics and interviewed, and thus they feature prominently in this book. For example, since the beginning of the twenty-first century, ICDs such as Mrs. Walters's have become a commonly used tool that is now considered necessary in order to stave off death. The left ventricular assist device (LVAD), an artificial heart pump, has shifted from being an experimental device used temporarily for patients dying of heart failure to being considered the logical, longer-term or permanent solution for growing numbers of people with end-stage heart disease.[4] More older people than ever before are routinely receiving maintenance kidney dialysis for end-stage renal disease and aggressive interventions for cancers of all sorts. Living kidney donation exceeded deceased donor donation for the first time in 2001; liver transplantation for primary liver cancer has become standard-of-care treatment; and increasing numbers of older people are receiving these transplants.

The very fact that the U.S. population is aging contributes to (and also results from) the changing patterns of medicine. In 1970 fewer than 10 percent of Americans were over sixty-five (9.9 percent); fewer than 1 percent were over eighty-five; and only 20.4 million people were enrolled in Medicare. In 2010, 13 percent of the population was over sixty-five and about 2 percent over eighty-five. According to projections for 2050, those percentages will increase to 20.2 and 4.3, respectively.[5]

In 2010, 47.2 million people were enrolled in Medicare,[6] which pays for 80 percent of acute medical treatments for those sixty-five and over. The aging of the population affects Medicare payment policies, the reimbursement policies of private insurance companies, consumer expectations and demands, and clinical trends. There is no question that Medicare reimbursement policy is the gateway to life-prolonging treatments for eligible U.S. citizens and legal residents. It enables access to treatments that many would not otherwise have. Medicare policy is dynamic: it responds to emerging research findings about new, potentially life-prolonging interventions and pays for those new treatments experts consider to be safe and effective.

Well into the twentieth century it was common for people to die in their fifties and sixties, and compared with today, fewer people lived into their eighties and beyond and fewer expected that they would do so. The pressing medical goal for a great part of that century addressed the prevention of death among children and those in young adulthood and midlife, including those who were dying as a result of diabetes, heart attacks, renal disease, or cancers. Only relatively recently, during the later twentieth century, did preventive measures, early detection, and curative treatments for those and a host of other conditions become so stunningly effective. The major result has been that diseases that previously were fatal because there were no effective interventions for them have been transformed into treatable conditions that can be managed for years or even decades, thus enabling and accompanying the aging of the population.

These developments in treatment and technology occurred in an environment of health care delivery that also underwent significant shifts in the first decade of the new millennium, each shift taking place at a particular link on the chain. Private industry funding of biomedical research, which in the 1990s surpassed funding from the National Institutes of Health, began to dominate the research funding stream. There was an explosion in the number of clinical trials that were conducted, accompanied by a heightened cultural sense of their value. As a result of such trials, a steadily increasing number of drugs, devices, and procedures were deemed safe enough and beneficial enough to be put on the market, and the Medicare program paid for many of them. The prices of some potentially lifesaving drugs skyrocketed. New websites enabled patients to become savvy health care consumers, yet at the same time the web and advertising campaigns gave misleading information. The decade's undeniable trajectory was toward more patients and families wanting more treatments than ever before, regardless of the cost.[7]

The increasing use of life-extending therapies in later life is motivated by and linked to both the infrastructure of the biomedical research enterprise and the growing influence of private industry. Medicare reimbursement policies, while enabling older citizens to gain access to treatments (and to hospice care), also generate the widespread disquiet that accompanies those treatments.

Fueling that disquiet and connecting the structures of science, industry, payment, and treatment are the powerful and elusive forces of the ethical field, which drives what makes a therapy be considered appropriate and necessary, what can and should be paid for and why, and which goals research and therapy should strive for. Thus there is no pure rationality or objectivity to the logic of the chain of health care drivers, the logic of ordinary medicine.[8]

The Chain-Based Logic of Staving Off Sudden Death: The ICD

That today's taken-for-granted medicine is able to cure disease and routinely turn fatal conditions into chronic conditions is uncontestable. What is far less clear is that ordinary medicine's ethical field and its logic also make the treatments that can achieve these ends *necessary*, thus fostering new choices, dilemmas, and demands. This is how our existing system of institutions connecting science to standard treatments and to payment for them operates. In a very general sense, patients and their families know this. They presume and hope that their doctors will "keep up with the research," weigh the evidence, and then decide what is right for them.

What is not well understood is the fact that the *chain itself* has become the overarching framework—the conceptual *and empirical* apparatus—for what is deemed right and appropriate in the creation of treatments and the delivery of medical care. Research evidence that is inextricably tied to insurance eligibility, standard making, and necessity *shapes* how we act in relation to treatment options, how we think about the norms of later life, and what we come to want from medicine.

The ethical concerns that such a shaping mechanism raises are clear: Where does responsibility lie? What are the relative roles of families, doctors, and the insurance industry in providing treatment? Yet what is not obvious is the determinative ethical-political field—our particularly American ethos that places individualism among the highest values and measures progress largely by new technologies and market forces—on which the shaping framework is based. This is the field that has given moral weight to the "more is better" ethos in medicine and has helped to make staving off a quick death (the kind many if not most of us claim to want in late life) ordinary, despite the attendant monetary and psychological costs. The increasingly common use of the ICD offers a telling example. There is no question of the unequivocal "good" of this device for preventing young people from dying. Yet today more than 110,000 patients in the United States receive ICDs each year.[9] Most persons with ICDs are older and sicker with underlying cardiac disease, and the electrical shocks from ICDs do not necessarily extend an older person's life or improve its quality.[10] Indeed, as happened to Mrs. Walters, the ICD transforms the possible and immediate risk of death into the near certainty of progressive, more advanced heart failure.[11]

The ICD is being implanted more frequently because research evidence has paved the way for it to become standard care, because Medicare pays for it, and because treatment for the risk of dying, even in late life for those with end-stage heart disease, has become so important in medicine. Once the idea of extending even the oldest, sickest lives with this or another such device has been conceived and the tool made widely available, the idea and the tool become an ordinary part of the medico-socioethical landscape. *Yet the effects of this logic most affect the oldest patients.* Consider Sam Tolleson, who, like some other patients with ICDs, lived a long time enduring the pain of the device's shocks and the knowledge that his debility was being prolonged.[12]

Mr. Tolleson: Saying "Stop"

At eighty-eight Sam Tolleson had been living with cardiac disease for twenty-five years by the time I met him and his frail, mostly bed-bound wife in their apartment at a retirement residence. Tall and thin, with piercing blue eyes and a head of thick white hair, he used oxygen and walked slowly, bent over his walker. He graciously welcomed me to sit down and chat and then moved toward his own favorite chair, grumbling that the tube connecting the oxygen tank to his nasal cannula was always getting twisted and it was driving him crazy. His first heart attack and cardiac bypass surgery occurred when he was in his mid-sixties. When he was eighty he suffered another heart attack, and when he awoke in the hospital, he was told that physicians had implanted a cardiac pacemaker device that included a defibrillator function. The physicians were following standard practice, doing what was appropriate both to stabilize his heart rate (the pacemaker) and prevent sudden death from a future heart attack (the defibrillator, or ICD). Mr. Tolleson noted that it wasn't until sometime after getting the defibrillator that he learned what it would do.

About two years before we met, when he was eighty-six and had progressing cardiac disease, the implanted defibrillator began to shock his potentially lethal cardiac rhythms back to normal. Over a period of several months, Mr. Tolleson was shocked fifteen times. "There is no question," he said, "that those shocks extended my life. It's very likely that one of those episodes, without the defibrillator, would have been my last." The first ten shocks, he reported, were "spread out, over weeks." But when he received five shocks in one day, he decided that he had had enough. "They were more and more painful. The very thought that I was going to have another one, I couldn't take it."

So he made an appointment to have the defibrillator part of the device turned off. This choice is highly unusual. It simply does not occur to most patients or their families that the device, once placed under the skin, can easily be deactivated and that patients can make that choice. Most physicians never discuss that possibility with patients.[13] Mr. Tolleson noted, "Both the doctor and the technician [from the device company] were reluctant to turn it off. But I convinced them. They didn't really try to talk me out of it. But the conversation was long enough so that they could know for certain that that was what I wanted to do."

When I asked if he felt relieved after having deactivated the device two years earlier, he said yes, but added, "I'm apprehensive too. Since I turned it off, I've probably had a dozen cardiac episodes—rapid heartbeats. . . . The pacemaker part of the device is still on. And the recording device corroborates that I have had these episodes. When they first started, I went to the emergency room, panic-stricken. But it's become old hat. I quit reporting them to my doctor or my kids. I do tell my wife. . . . Yesterday afternoon I had an episode, a big one, in the middle of my afternoon card game."

He went on to say that at about the time he deactivated the defibrillator, his doctors "wanted to put me on [kidney] dialysis. And I wouldn't do it. And that distressed the family too. The family was very upset with me. I have three children, and they all cried. I had to talk with them about it, and I felt terrible after I talked with them." He continued, "Perhaps I should just have done what they wanted me to. But life is getting harder all the time."

Mr. Tolleson died two days after our conversation.

When he received the dual-function device in 2000, Mr. Tolleson was considered an "appropriate candidate" for implanting the defibrillator-pacemaker combination, according to evidence from medical studies. At that time the medical and reimbursement criterion for defibrillator implantation was an experienced incident of cardiac arrest or documented arrhythmia. Mr. Tolleson was certainly eligible for the device. Scientific evidence, routine reimbursement, standard of care, specialist expertise, industry's goal to sell devices, and medicine's mandate to extend life are all strong forces, and taken together they led to the understanding that Mr. Tolleson should have the device. Yet for him its placement had longer-term existential effects. He was caught, for a time, in the quandary of ordinary medicine: whether to continue the treatment or to stop.

Eventually Mr. Tolleson found himself needing to defend his decision to turn off the defibrillator, both to his family and to medical staff. He realized he had crossed the line he did not wish to have crossed: extended life but with pain and suffering. For those in later life, such dilemmas are becoming increasingly common.

Yet I interviewed scores of individuals over seventy-five who were glad to have an ICD that "shocked" them back to life once, twice or more often than that, who did not mind the pain that accompanied extended life. Some of them did not have the device implanted when their doctors suggested they should and waited, sometimes for years, to do so, yet all were pleased and relieved finally to have one. A small miracle of modern medicine, the ICD will be a recurring subject in later chapters as well, for it serves a crucial role as an exemplar of the kinds of quandaries life-extending treatments open up, the implications of postprogress medicine.

Risk Awareness and the Obligation to Longevity

Two things have increased along with the median age of the U.S. population: the desire for medicine's interventions well into advanced age and doctors' ability to treat diseases in later life, to intervene in some way to make life more comfortable and to stave off death. Surgical procedures are safer, and many are less invasive than in years past. Medications to treat many conditions are more effective. Better diagnostic tests enable early detection and thus earlier treatment of diseases that could become life-threatening. Today patients faced with serious illness in later life most often want to be treated and opt for the newer treatments. They are opting for greater longevity.

This is fueled by the fact that most people today know something about chemotherapy, radiation, and surgery for cancer and have friends and relatives who have undergone those therapies and whose lives (may) have been extended because of them. Almost everyone knows someone with a pacemaker or a more complex cardiac device or someone who has had cardiac bypass surgery, recovered well, and as a result lived years, perhaps decades longer. More older individuals and their families read about all kinds of therapies in the media and conduct their own Internet searches, and they have come to understand that standard medical care now means continuing to treat disease well into old age. The promises of laboratory science, with their seeming potential for cure or remission, are part of the fabric of American life. Breakthroughs in stem cell research and application are always felt to be just around the corner, as are the cures that many assume will follow when the genetics of different cancers are more thoroughly understood.

The almost-here quality of medical discoveries and the hope invested in drugs and devices that offer a potential magic bullet are fueled by the politics and economics of the research enterprise itself and by the media. Both of these entities link new and experimental treatments to long-held and tenacious ideas of open-ended scientific progress.[14] Robert Butler, the founding director of the National Institute on Aging, quipped, when he was eighty years old, that "80 is the new 60,"[15] reflecting our changed cultural understanding of life course expectations and echoing similar remarks now in circulation ("50 is the new 40," "40 is the new 30," etc.). Given this prevailing perspective, those who are in their later years see no reason not to partake of the available bounty and promise, especially now that death-defying, symptom-controlling interventions have become so commonplace among them.

There is no doubt that increasing risk awareness (and the uncertainty that both underlies and results from it) is driving a great deal of health care delivery today. Like the increasing hope invested in clinical science, increasing risk awareness also leads to a demand for more information and interventions. Yet more information and increased surveillance of the body in order to control risk do not lead to less risk. On the contrary, the more one learns and knows, the more risks one is aware of. The demand for more intervention requires that we balance competing desires: we want to know how to live longer yet not live past the point when pain and suffering overwhelm our well-being or our ability to find meaning in life.

Within this context, exercising one's obligation and commitment to health and longer life becomes a complex, challenging enterprise at any age, but especially so at advanced ages. Health promotion has become a meaningful social practice, a central aspect of contemporary thinking, particularly for a vast middle class.[16] Over the past thirty years or so, risk management has come to play an ever larger role in medicine and in health care consumers' thinking about medical intervention. Ulrich Beck, Anthony Giddens,[17] and other social theorists have described the ways in which *risk* as a way of knowing and risk assessment as a technique for living constitute the structural conditions of life in our postindustrial society. Political values now in the ascendancy in the United States reinforce the emphasis on individual rather than government responsibility for risk reduction. Medical practice, being part of the sociopolitical landscape, responds to that development.

It is through individual risk assessment that both health and health care are now largely understood as risk reduction,[18] but it was not always so. Over the past three decades risk has shifted from an epidemiological notion of disease rates to being a condition of uncertainty located within a person. It has been transformed from a statistical entity to a near-tangible problem and has become a clinical concept used by doctors to treat patients. As such, it is at once a medical idea, a state of lived experience, and a symptom of future disease.[19]

According to that logic, once a risk has been assessed, something must be done to reduce it. And because health risks have increasingly been conceptualized as individuals' problems, the solutions to them are therefore considered to reside in individual strategies for behavior change or clinical intervention. The upstream causes of disease, from pollution to poverty, and the kinds of political action required to address them are de-emphasized in medicine and in neoliberal society, both of which stress instead individual responsibility for disease prevention and health promotion. So, as individuals, we are expected to *decide* on prevention and health maintenance strategies for ourselves and our family members and act on our decisions. Failure to do so is, without question, understood by many to be a moral transgression.[20]

For example, screening (for high cholesterol, diabetes, heart disease, cancer of the breast, prostate, colon, etc.) is considered important because it enables us to calculate our individual risk numerically, and the resulting risk scores become the basis for whether treatment is needed.[21] The debates over whether and when to screen, how often, and with which techniques have spilled over from medical conferences and journals onto the front pages of newspapers because screening technologies, imperfect as they are, have become so central to medical risk reduction and so central to our societal desire to enhance longevity.

The plethora of clinical tests that are now available—for assessing cardiac, cancer, and genetic risks—illustrates this trend in health promotion and risk reduction. Clinical medicine has come to rely more and more on the numbers, scores, and scans that are generated by diagnostic tests and on procedures that enable ever more finely tuned interpretations of disease states and bodily conditions. It is in terms of these results and scores that doctors, patients, and the public learn to understand what constitutes health and illness and learn to weigh the risks and benefits of future treatment options. More broadly we come to think about the body and how we can extend our lives in terms of our numbers. Blood pressure and cholesterol measurement, prostate-specific antigen test numbers, kidney creatinine levels,[22] cardiac ejection fractions, mammogram and CT findings, stages of cancer, white blood counts, liver function scores, and so on are all *representations* of the extent of disease and degrees of health and risk that have come to matter to us deeply. We organize what we want from medicine, say yes or no to treatments, undertake the care of others, and consider the future in terms of such representations, which did not exist in such profusion until relatively recently. They focus our attention on the self as a biological being and on our individual responsibility for improving our own health with the tools of medicine.

In her book *Statistical Panic* the cultural theorist Kathleen Woodward provides a cogent analysis of the ways our "society of statistics" provokes panic by focusing our attention on the experience of always being at risk, mostly by knowing "our scores"—a shorthand phrase almost everyone recognizes by now. She and others note that we are all at risk all the time, "that to be normal is to be in a state of risk." Clinicians in some fields work to "treat" risk itself.[23] The practice, for example, of performing double mastectomies prior to a diagnosis of breast cancer and based solely on genetic analysis and family history is perhaps the most well known and extreme response to risk awareness.[24] Growing numbers of individuals with family histories of cancer or genetic disease now desire presymptomatic, subclinical identification of risks in order, they hope, to preempt the manifestation of disease.[25]

In our risk-aware world, medicine's tools and physicians' discussions with patients make risks real by locating them (using statistics, scores, and scans) in our bodies—and thus in our lives. At the same time, those tools are to be used to minimize risks if patients and the public take them seriously and decide to use them. There is more risk to be aware of because technologies enable us to see and understand it as never before and to do so ever earlier in the course of disease. For example, people are now diagnosed with prediabetes, prehypertension, and borderline high cholesterol.[26] The more risk we know about, the more things we can (and therefore must) do to avoid and ameliorate it. This is one of the ironies of medicine today.

The tools and the talk emphasize that risk is everywhere, acting on the body and the disease, threatening our expectations about longevity, and a great deal of today's medicine aims to guide patients to minimize, thwart, or avoid risks. Much of the burden of doing so settles on those in later life who face life-threatening and end-stage diseases.

II: ORDINARY MEDICINE: SHAPING THE DOCTOR-PATIENT RELATIONSHIP

We have neither an easily agreed-upon metric for clinical
excellence nor a metric for misery.
—Charles Rosenberg, *Our Present Complaint*

As anyone knows who has entered a hospital, sat in a clinic, had a drug prescription filled, waited for diagnostic tests and results, or dealt with insurance paperwork, the delivery of medical care today encompasses a great deal more than the doctor-patient relationship. That relationship itself, while still claimed by most to be the essential and most important feature of medical care, has been fraying for many years. It has been reconfigured by layers of administration and oversight, by the use of technology, and by government, industry, and activist citizen input and negotiation regarding what constitutes evidence, risk, best treatment, and the right to treatment.

Beginning in the 1960s players from outside the medical profession entered the health arena and transformed the delivery of medical care into a business, a fragmented, "bureaucratically-crafted" infrastructure,[27] a technology-driven enterprise and an insurance nightmare. The challenges to trust in the doctor-patient relationship were accompanied and facilitated by the increasing impact of "strangers at the bedside"[28]— the lawyers, bioethicists, activists, government regulatory bodies, and new, formal means of oversight—all of which became structurally integrated into medical care during a dramatic period of change between the mid-1960s and mid-1970s. In that earlier era the new, nonmedical players arrived on the scene after some alarming conditions of medical research on human subjects were exposed,[29] ethical conundrums brought about by a scarcity of lifesaving resources emerged, and a new technology, the mechanical ventilator (or breathing machine), raised the question of who should authorize the timing of death. The historian David Rothman documents three ways in which the scope and content of medical care were reorganized during those years: by the replacement of relatively autonomous physician authority with a new commitment to collective and public decision making; by a new reliance on formal practices surrounding decision making, especially the medical chart, which became a legal document as well as a means of communication among health specialists; and by the creation of new documents of ethical principles and policies, all shaped by outsiders—bioethicists, legislators, government commissions, judges—to frame the doctor-patient relationship.[30]

Medicare arrived as well during those years, funding medical education, including specialty training, and reimbursing physicians for the care they provide—most significantly, for the procedures they perform. Since that era bureaucratic forces and their impacts on what physicians are able to do have become stronger. For example, regulations about hospital length of stay, the pricing and availability of drugs, insurance coverage rules, reductions in Medicare reimbursement for physicians, information technologies and computer-generated algorithms for treatment, shifting treatment standards, and the burgeoning clinical trials industry, to name a few features of contemporary health care bureaucracy, have shaped how doctors and nurses practice medicine. Those bureaucratic forces are influenced more than ever by financial interests, and they affect how patients understand what to want.

Evolving Expectations and Dilemmas

The "bureaucratically crafted infrastructure" and reconfigured doctor-patient relationship that are part of ordinary medicine *shape our sensibilities*. They frame how we think about what to do and what to want as well as our longings and emotional claims on one another and our ambivalent feelings about the value of some treatments at advanced ages. This was certainly true of the patients I met during my research, including Mr. Tolleson, even though he eventually chose to buck the system.

While all of medicine in the United States is based on the connections and transformations I describe, for those with both access to Medicare insurance and the ability and wherewithal to get to a clinic, ordinary medicine organizes patient expectations and ambivalence about longevity and the often twinned promise and problem of *more future*. Without both the means and the desire (often stimulated by a family member) to get to a doctor's office or medical center for diagnosis and treatment, patients could not begin the journey to complex, life-prolonging treatments. Both are necessary in order to receive the health care I describe. The patients and families I observed and spoke with had all taken that first step and then faced the question of how and whether to live in relation to medicine's tools, capabilities, and potential.

Before, during, and after diagnostic tests and the ensuing procedures, many patients pondered what sort of future would unfold for them if they proceeded with this or that therapeutic option, if they chose aggressive treatments, if they decided against any medical treatment at all. Many were forced to confront the (often overwhelming) complexity of procedures and an array of choices at the same time that they had to consider the seriousness of their disease. Some agreed to go forward with treatments not out of personal desire but because their children or spouses wanted them to continue living. Many debated within themselves and with family members *how much more time* they wanted to live and whether the *extra* time that medicine *might* provide was worth it in relation to the strain and suffering, guilt and obligation caused by disease and by further therapies. The cases of Mrs. Walters and Mr. Tolleson offer but two examples.

Families, for their part, mostly wanted their ill relative to pursue treatment, though they sometimes wondered if treatment would shorten rather than lengthen life and create more rather than less suffering. I met hundreds of family members—worried spouses, sometimes also frail and with medical problems of their own, and adult children who had taken the day or week off from work or had flown into town to accompany a parent to the doctor. Sometimes as many as six or seven relatives were in attendance at the clinic. Sometimes, faced with the array of therapy options, a son or daughter would cry out to a nurse or physician, "Help me! What should we decide?" Regardless of long discussions with health professionals, many felt that they were jumping blindly into treatments they feared but that their relative should nonetheless have. Sometimes they were *never* sure if they had done the right thing for their loved one.

Families worked hard to care for their sick relative, to keep him or her alive before and after treatments. In the complex world of health care today, this entails helping the patient schedule and receive procedures in different medical centers and doctors' offices, a process that can continue for years. It involves organizing and keeping track of insurance paperwork; managing wounds, surgical incisions, medications, diets, and exercise programs; and, crucially, ensuring that everything is done correctly so the patient will not die. In order to do all of this, family members rearrange their work schedules, quit their jobs, and enlist relatives and neighbors to assist with child care and any number of household chores.

In the end most patients and families with access to an array of medical services want to keep their options open, and so they agree to treatments that will enable them to do so. They all have high expectations of medicine's capabilities. Yet I found that, mostly, they do not know what to want in terms of specific drugs or procedures, do not decide on or choose specific therapies. What they do want is to keep hope alive, and thus they mostly go down the pathways suggested by health professionals that they feel will add life, will leave no stone unturned—gestures that are meant to show love and concern for one another.

In contrast to patients and families, who hold onto their expectations of medicine's capabilities and struggle in the moment to understand what the doctor is telling them, physicians act strategically. They think about what needs to happen now and what will happen next. They want to give the best care possible, in terms of both life extension and comfort, for the patient in front of them. So they are guided by the evidence contained in consensus reports and clinical trials findings and by the truths that the patient's body provides through the scores revealed in scans, chemistry panels, and other diagnostic tests. They want the "facts" (which are changing constantly) to direct treatment choices. At the same time, they are mindful of the need to let patients decide what to do. The dance they do in clinic conversations—discussing what they consider to be necessary therapies and why, yet urging patients to speak their mind about what they want—makes up a great deal of clinical work today. Mostly unvoiced, however, and especially relevant when the patient is old, are the kinds of problems that arise after the decision is made to move forward with treatments because those treatments open the door to additional treatments and to other problems.

Weighing the "Choice" between Death and the Demands of Longevity

Among the predicaments that today's ordinary medicine puts us in is entanglement with a new obligation to longevity. We think about mortality and longevity today *in relation to* medicine, its treatments and its potential to shape a longer life. It has become difficult if not impossible to think about them in any *other* way because our personal decisions about longevity and mortality result from the political, economic, and structural dimensions of a vast and impersonal health care enterprise.

Because medicine so powerfully shapes the late life of millions, and because we are talking about *life*, it has become commonplace for those on the receiving end of interventions and their family members to gauge the worth of life *in relation to* medical treatment and to consider *how much more life* would be worth undertaking how much more treatment. These are widespread preoccupations for millions of patients and families as they experience that balancing act, that weighing of the worth of more life against the worth of more treatment, that judgment about crossing the line. It is a balancing act that, if not unique to the contemporary era, has certainly intensified of late, and it signifies a relatively new kind of medicoethical relationship that now infuses private, personal deliberations about what to do.

The disconnect between the worlds of health policy and the clinic comes into clear view here: the world of health policy does not take the balancing act or its effects into consideration. The policy world leaves almost entirely unexplored the connection of that weighing to the transformations that underpin our health care delivery system and to our national dilemmas about health care equity, cost cutting, and the goals of medicine. Those who work in the clinical world often are not aware that the options they provide to patients can incite profound preoccupation about obligation, love, and the worth of more life. Clinicians often do not see that the choices they offer to patients—choices they are obligated to offer in our era of patient-centered care, individual autonomy, and shared decision making—represent an off-loading of ethical responsibility onto those patients and their families, that is, off-loading onto those with the least ability to understand prognosis, the purpose of specific treatments, and the implications of crossing the line.

Mrs. Dang: Guided to Accept a New Liver

Consider, for example, the dilemmas sometimes triggered by liver transplantation, one of the most complex and costly procedures performed today and, for those with certain conditions, a treatment considered appropriate and necessary well into advanced age. And why not? Older people are more likely than younger people to develop liver conditions that transplantation can cure or treat. Older people are the ones who *need* that intervention; it can extend their lives. The normalcy of that kind of response is just one illustration of how the rapidly shifting norms of medicine have changed us. What was extraordinary two decades ago is unsurprising and logical today.

The story of Mrs. Van Dang, her family, and her liver transplant provides an example of how ordinary medicine operates and how patients and families come to think of recent developments in medicine as so normal. Her story, as it unfolded, was one of many that enabled me to see the chain of health care drivers, the forces that guided her to yes. Mrs. Dang and her family also struggled with that inescapable element of ordinary medicine: the quandary of the line.

Mrs. Dang's story offers a glimpse into how the authority of Medicare policy, which is based on scientific studies of clinical evidence, becomes embedded in physician, patient, and family feelings of responsibility for using the most sophisticated techniques of medicine to extend life and how families imagine and practice responsibility.

Two of Mrs. Dang's three daughters brought her, at seventy-two, to a liver clinic in a major medical center because her chronic liver disease was becoming more advanced and her local doctor suspected cancer as well. In three clinic visits over an eight-month period I saw the patient and family move from ambivalence about undergoing such a major intervention to acceptance of it in order for Mrs. Dang to live.

At the first clinic visit the surgeon said Mrs. Dang would be in "good enough" shape to withstand the stress of transplant surgery, and he guided the family to think about the future. He urged them to make a decision about moving forward, saying, "I think she would have a tough year and then she could live nine to fifteen years with no problems." Another physician, a liver specialist, told the family, "She has enough problems with the cirrhosis that she should be put on the national waiting list for a donor liver. It's a good idea to do that now." The physicians were guided by experience, clinical evidence, and prognosis. Mrs. Dang was concentrating hard on the doctors' words, and she did not want a transplant.

As I walked with the family out of the clinic, one of Mrs. Dang's daughters said, "I need to ask my mother if she wants to live ten more years." This kind of statement, common today, is thinkable only because clinical evidence has paved the way for Medicare to cover liver transplants, which can cure lethal disease and extend life for years. Medicare began reimbursement for transplantation in the case of liver cancer in 2001. Mrs. Dang was fortunate to be diagnosed and treated after that year. The survival statistics are compelling. It would not be rational *not* to have a transplant. The surgeon's words encouraging the patient and family to consider five, ten, fifteen more years of life without liver disease inspired the daughter's proposed question to her mother, which was couched as if one could know the date of one's death and then add ten years to it. The surgeon's words positioned the family to consider an open-ended future for Mrs. Dang, as if she and her daughters could prognosticate about both her death *and* her extended life as specifically and confidently as did the physicians.

At their second clinic visit six months later, the liver specialist presented the family with the numbers: 10 percent of patients die in the first year; 90 percent survive at least three years. And he said, "I think she would benefit from a liver transplant." Both the numbers and his words reflect the clinical evidence. The family walked out of the clinic in a state of extreme ambivalence.

Two months later, after Mrs. Dang had turned seventy-three, I sat with the family in the clinic waiting room as the daughters confessed that they were burdened by the thought of a transplant, worried that transplant surgery would shorten rather than lengthen their mother's life. They were ambivalent because age mattered to them. Was a new liver worth the risk at her age?

The concerns of Mrs. Dang's family are well founded. I learned from liver specialists that about 30 percent of those who do survive a liver transplant experience a range of complications, some of them quite serious. The normalcy of liver transplantation is what is presented, and that normalcy becomes a normative expectation. While physicians may mention to patients the variability of actual outcomes, that topic generally is not emphasized in clinic conversations, and so it is mostly absent from patient and family calculations about what to do.

One of Mrs. Dang's daughters posed a now frequently debated question, one that reflects the often unvoiced problem of who, ultimately, is responsible for the outcomes of procedures that may but may not actually extend life: "If you have cancer and decide not to treat it, is that suicide? I don't think so, but I wonder. If I think my mother shouldn't be listed for transplant, is that murder?" Such reflections, in which families feel the moral weight of guilt and complicity, as if they could be "killing" or "saving" a loved one, are common.[31] Yet they are largely overlooked in the cultural conversation about health care delivery and reform. Families come to feel that the onus is entirely on them. The weight of that perceived burden of killing or saving is a downstream effect of the value placed on technological innovation and its legitimacy, as conferred first by Medicare reimbursement policy and then by what becomes standard practice.

By now three physicians had advised Mrs. Dang to have the transplant, and the daughters were inclined to follow that advice. Mrs. Dang wasn't sure what she would do, but she was no longer completely opposed to a transplant. A few minutes later in the exam room, the doctor said, "I feel strongly that a transplant is the best chance to save her life." And Mrs. Dang replied with confidence, "I've made up my mind. It's okay. I'll do it to live." The physicians' calculations about the risk of death without a transplant and chances for survival with a transplant became the reason for her to go forward and the reason for her family to support her decision.

Thus Mrs. Dang headed toward a liver transplant because standard clinical pathways, the logics of treatment and its reimbursement, and professional and familial obligation all led her toward that outcome. The physicians were guided by clinical evidence, Medicare guidelines, and their mandate to save life. The family's conversion to viewing transplantation as a solution to the patient's cancer occurred through several means. The physicians' repeated talk about the future, especially the words "I think she would benefit from a transplant," made the patient and family more comfortable with the idea that a transplant was appropriate. Over time they became socialized to the normalcy of the procedure. It became the logical and right thing to do, the appropriate path to take. *Logical* because her disease would progress and become the cause of her death, perhaps quite soon, and a transplant could cure the disease, preventing death. A great deal of clinical evidence shows that to be the case. *Right* because saving life is the highest priority, because the family wanted to make *that* choice, and because for patients in the United States with Medicare or other insurance it can be done as a matter of course. And, finally, *appropriate* because the links among the political, economic, and clinical structures that shape the pathway to transplant are, mostly, not seen by participants in the system.

Mrs. Dang recovered easily from her transplant surgery, aided by significant amounts of care from her family. She felt well and, following several months of recovery, was able to live independently and resume the activities she enjoyed. Her positive outcome highlights the complicated ethical terrain of ordinary medicine. Successes such as hers—and there are many—reinforce the sense of appropriateness of this procedure. The price we pay is the deepening quandary of where and when to stop.

The Ethical Field Revisited: The Health Care Enterprise
and Society's Values

The case of Mrs. Dang provides an example of how the ethical field shapes what happens in the clinic. Thinking about ethics as a field, as part of a broad sociostructural terrain, has not been adequately scrutinized by health consumers, providers, or those in health care policy for its capacity to shape treatment priorities in our aging country. But such a field nonetheless infuses the chain that determines "evidence" of benefit and Medicare insurance reimbursement criteria and thus organizes clinical practice, patient need, and necessary treatment. Again it is the seeming rationality of each piece of this enterprise that masks our ability to see that the connections within the system are ethically driven in the first place.

One reason for this is that the language of evidence, standards, and necessary treatment—the language of rationality—does not raise what have traditionally been understood as ethical or values-based concerns. Thus ethics continues to be thought of as a topic that is *outside of rather than determinative of* the realms of scientific outcomes data, Medicare payment criteria, and treatment necessity.[32]

As a result of this displacement, debates about health care reform, especially on the topic of potentially life-prolonging therapies for older persons, have settled in the political arena and focus almost entirely on cost cutting. Reform is stymied, some suggest,[33] because cost cutting has been equated with rationing and "death panels." In the public conversation ethics itself has come to rest almost entirely within the realm of costs; therefore discussion on the topic is limited to the quagmire of cost cutting and rationing.

My own argument goes much further. While it is true that in the U.S. political debate ethics has come to be associated with costs, that is by no means the root of our reform dilemmas. Rather because the ethical field shapes how choices are made all the way along the line, including within the chain of health care drivers, any efforts to effect change or reform must consider and grapple with the *prior* commitments and priorities that are reflected in the connections and transformations within the chain. The rising cost of therapies that so occupies reformers occurs only at the end of the chain and is merely one effect of the drivers and transformations, each of them forged by ethical choices, that I describe.

The case of Mrs. Dang illustrates some of the ethical field's parameters. The case of Mr. Carter offers another example, this one of a patient's expectations of lifesaving treatment, as well as the angst that families experience regarding how to express care when faced with life-threatening disease and the risks of intervention. In neither case does concern about cost feature in the tangle of health care structures, imperatives, diagnostic procedures, and dilemmas in which the families find themselves.[34]

Mr. Carter: How Treatments Shape Expectations

Taken together, Mr. Adam Carter's liver disease, the chain of logic about medical eligibility and treatment, his family's involvement, and his own emerging expectations provide a further example of the workings of ordinary medicine. While he waited for a deceased donor liver to become available, Mr. Carter was compelled to undergo various treatments in order to prevent his liver cancer from spreading. If the cancer did spread beyond the liver, it would make him ineligible for a transplant according to Medicare reimbursement rules. Such treatments, and the fact that they will be paid for and are accessible, shape the expectations and claims of older patients, their families, and most of us who will undoubtedly be patients in time. His treatment scenario and outcome reflect the confluence of state-of-the-art medicine, Medicare reimbursement policy, the choices we are given, and the kind of anxieties that follow.

When I met the Carters in 2009, seventy-two-year-old Adam Carter was very ill with advanced liver disease. He had been diagnosed with hepatitis C seventeen years earlier, and over several years had suffered through forty-two of a recommended forty-eight weeks of interferon therapy.[35] Lying on a couch in his living room, he told me, "Every week you continue, you become more invested in it. You desperately want to cure it. So though I was getting sicker and sicker, I was more deeply committed each week." He stopped when the side effects made him too ill to continue. The hepatitis C virus did not disappear.

In 2003, when he was having more symptoms of liver disease, he was sent to a major medical center, where the doctors placed him on the national liver transplant list. "I knew that hepatitis C could turn into liver failure," he recalled. "At the time my wife and I thought, what a great thing to have transplant as a possibility in your back pocket. Isn't this wonderful, if it should be necessary. It seemed so remote . . . and I thought I was of the age where I may never need a transplant." But liver cancer developed. He had been diagnosed with two tumors, and now they were growing larger.

One cannot receive an organ transplant immediately following diagnosis. One must wait, either on the national waiting list for an organ from a deceased donor or for someone to volunteer to be a living donor. Meanwhile, as a temporary measure while he waited, Mr. Carter's tumors would be targeted and treated to keep them small enough so they would not spread beyond the liver. If that happened, he would no longer be medically eligible, according to Medicare insurance reimbursement rules, for a transplant because, with cancer in other parts of his body, a liver transplant would not cure his disease.

I heard the word *eligible* often while I was conducting the research for this book. Medicare reimbursement guidelines, developed by the committees that set Medicare payment policy, govern who among older citizens in the United States is eligible for financial reimbursement for medical procedures, including liver transplants. Eligibility is key to how physicians plan treatments and how patients consider them.

"So," Mr. Carter told me, "I had the electrical current treatment and chemo three times, every couple of months, because the tumors kept growing. It was the only way I could get a transplant."[36]

His wife told me, "By 2008 he was getting more and more debilitated. Then they asked if Adam could find a living donor, because that would be quicker than waiting on the list. And we would get into these awful arguments because, first, he wouldn't send the living donor information packets to our relatives. I wrote to Adam's sister, and it's the only time she never replied. And then our daughter said she would be a living donor. And I thought, Oh my god, I cannot stand the thought of that. I was so torn, so upset. We had such horrible arguments. Because Adam would say, 'I want a liver.' And I said, 'I don't want both of you having that kind of surgery, that risk.' It was hell."

"It was pretty clear that I wasn't going to take anything from a relative," Mr. Carter chimed in. "What a decision—going to a relative and saying, 'They're gonna take half your liver, and it's just as serious an operation for you as it is for me. . . .' How can you? It's the most difficult thing."

"But you wanted one so desperately," Mrs. Carter countered, "you would have taken it from her. . . . And then of course our daughter took forever to get her blood tested, and that was a very stressful time. I nearly lost my mind, and thank god she wasn't the right blood type."

After the debilitating and ultimately unsuccessful hepatitis c therapy, years on the national transplant waiting list, and the ablation and chemotherapy treatment that kept him medically eligible for a transplant, Mr. Carter felt that he deserved an organ. It was the only way he would survive. The ethics of the system and the operational logic that enabled him to move from one therapy to the next while he waited for a transplant supported his view. (An alternative ethics might propose that after all that time and use of significant resources, Mr. Carter would have exhausted his claim on the system. Or, as some patients do, he could have made a personal decision that he had had enough treatment and would not have a transplant.) He worried he would not be considered strong enough, at seventy-two and with severe disease, to withstand the operation. But two weeks after our conversation his name came to the top of the list and he received a liver from a deceased donor. In the ensuing months his recovery was swift and everything he had hoped for. He resumed many of his old routines. To his physicians, his pathway through the course of treatments was ordinary, unremarkable, simply the way medicine works. They were, of course, pleased with his recovery.

Mr. Carter's positive outcome exemplifies medical progress; a decade before, a liver transplant was not the standard of care for his condition. Given our society's political and technological commitments over many years, why would we deny two hundred years of medical progress and limit these and other life-prolonging treatments? Yet the direction that progress has taken in the U.S. health care system has opened up complex ethical territory about how to be a good family member, how to think about one's own *normal* life span and what to do to achieve it, how to distribute scarce, expensive resources in an aging society, and whether limits on progress can be instituted at all. All of this is now ordinary.

Personal Sensibilities Confront the Postprogress Predicament

We are in an era of patient-centered medicine in which patient and family alike are expected to be paramount in the decision-making process. Within our current system reimbursement of a treatment by Medicare insurance gives rise to the understanding that that treatment is appropriate, ordinary, and the right thing to do. However, the fact that others have been treated successfully, along with the prospect of a successful treatment for oneself, also contribute to a distinct form of modern anxiety, which the situations and sensibilities of the Dang and Carter families reveal.

Over time Mr. Carter came to embrace a perspective that might be characterized as follows: After all the treatments I've been through and all the suffering those treatments caused, I deserve a transplant. And also, because taking part of someone else's liver is sound medical therapy, I can, if necessary, seek a part of your liver in order to live. And you will feel obligated to think about donating it to me. I will have to consider whether I want you to do so.

The idea that one deserves treatment—because it is available, because it saves life, and because the successes of medical techniques along with reimbursement for them encourage patients to do whatever is necessary to extend life—comes up against the responsibilities and obligations of others and to others. This idea does not exist in a vacuum, outside of relationships. In Mr. Carter's case, the physicians' responsibilities were to guide him through the thicket of interventions that would prevent the spread of liver cancer while he waited for an organ and to guide his family to consider who could volunteer to be a living donor in case his condition deteriorated before a deceased donor organ became available to him. The Carter family was placed in an uncomfortable position: they had to consider whether or not to solicit a volunteer living donor and then decide which family members to approach. They questioned whether asking for such a volunteer was the right thing to do in the first place. They had to weigh the value of Mr. Carter's health and (potential) extended life against the health, and possibly the life, of another, perhaps younger family member. The Carters were both caught in the web of emotions, options, and obligations that accompanies this and other life-extending procedures. That web is now an insidious part of standard medicine and is unavoidable for families; certainly it was fraught with turmoil for the Carters.

Mrs. Dang's daughters expressed a different sensibility. They pondered the ramifications of supporting or opposing transplant surgery for their mother. If they supported the idea, they worried that she might die in surgery or suffer a great deal afterward or that they would be greatly burdened by her postsurgery needs. If they did not support the treatment, they confronted the issue of whether they would be contributing to her death, would be complicit in causing the end of her life.

Despite the varying sensibilities and anxieties that their examples reveal, both Mrs. Dang and Mr. Carter illustrate the successes of medicine, the kind of medicine that fulfills the ideal of progress. Yet, as everyone is well aware, treatments that can cure so miraculously coexist with others that manage disease and prevent dying but also extend the duration of advanced disease. Mrs. Walters's story provides one such example. Cancer and heart disease are the two leading causes of death in the United States and are the major conditions affecting older people, and both these conditions have been transformed in recent decades by therapies that stave off death. Maintenance dialysis for end-stage kidney disease also falls into that category. Such medical techniques and their promise, along with our own expectations, have by now taught us two things: that we do not have to die from those conditions, at least not yet, and that there is no set point at which we must, or should, stop pursuing treatments. And so *deciding how long to continue treatments that cannot cure disease has become a major societal preoccupation.*

Because the quandary of when or whether to stop has become so pervasive, and because the American health care enterprise is now so broken, the issue for me has been to examine how in an aging society life-extending therapies have gotten caught up in the perfect storm of ordinary medicine, how and why they bring increasing numbers of patients and families, indeed our entire society, to face the quandary of the line.

I am not seeking to make a case for or against the *use* of these or any other therapies by patients of any particular age. I am not interested in questioning the good of any of medicine's successes or of any patient and family decisions. Rather my interest in the examples I present is in mapping how ordinary medicine unfolds for different players and in describing how standards become standard. How do physicians think through patients' options, explain their risks to them, create the parameters for the living person in front of them of the standard treatments and the scientific evidence? How does the fact that older patients often consider *time left* in relation to time already lived affect their approach to undergoing complicated procedures with long recovery periods? What range of dilemmas does ordinary medicine instigate for family members? These are among the everyday, on-the-ground manifestations of ordinary medicine my examples map, and only by understanding them can we better confront the consequences of our postprogress predicament.

It bears repeating that our medical practices define the kind of society we have and, by extension, that because those practices have changed over the years so has the society. The chain of institutional and bureaucratic forces that determines the ways medical goals are established, treatment patterns emerge, and our existential decision-making quandaries are formulated has another, even more far-reaching effect: it shapes our desires and anxieties about medicine in general and about living longer in particular. I would go so far as to say that it has altered, and continues to shape, three vital components of what it is to be human: the relationship between the body and the self, how we understand time and the character of the future, and our most intimate family commitments. Thus it profoundly influences how we relate to those we love. It has shaped as well not just medicine's relationship to old age but also the very experience of growing old in the United States.

The chapters that follow describe in greater detail the cultural sources of our entanglement with longevity making, the work of and connections among our health care institutions and their effects on doctors, patients, families, and American life today. The cases I present exemplify the degree to which that powerful set of activities remains unrecognized for its role in governing how we understand options in the clinic, what to wish for, and how to think about our striving for longevity. Progress or postprogress?

PART II

THE CHAIN OF HEALTH CARE DRIVERS

2

THE MEDICAL-INDUSTRIAL COMPLEX I

Evidence-Based Medicine, the Biomedical Economy,
and the Ascendance of Clinical Trials

———

The vast engine of biomedical research is where the chain of forces that shapes health care delivery and patient experience begins. In the 1990s a confluence of two phenomena, both of which had existed for decades, strengthened the biomedical research world's impact on the health care delivery enterprise. First, the notion of evidence-based medicine (EBM), the proactive and transparent application of the best published scientific research findings about medical treatments, became a stronger influence than in previous years in determining standards and values in health care interventions. Second, the clinical trials industry grew exponentially. The infrastructure and organization of these two phenomena, these huge apparatuses of truth making in medicine, have come to prioritize the thinking of many doctors and patients about what constitutes appropriate treatment and responsible medicine. This confluence of evidence-based medicine and clinical trials, combined with their cultural capital in the health care delivery enterprise, is a major force buttressing ordinary medicine and driving the quandary of when, where, and how to draw the line.

New drugs, devices, and procedures must be tested on people in research studies before they are approved for widespread use. The outcomes of those studies are transformed into scientific evidence documenting good or improved therapeutics. The conversion of research *findings* into *best evidence* for treatment is the first activity, the first link that connects scientific innovation to physicians' work in the clinic and to patients' and families' expectations about treatment. That initial transformation of findings into evidence affects all the other transformations that follow.

Evidence-based medicine is grounded firmly in the "new medical-industrial complex" that was first described in 1980 by Arnold Relman, then editor of the *New England Journal of Medicine*. Inspired by President Eisenhower's earlier coinage of the term *military-industrial complex*, Relman used his similar phrase to articulate the ways science, medicine, profits, and politics were becoming entangled together and were beginning to have a growing impact on health care policy. Relman defined that new complex as "a large and growing network of private corporations engaged in the business of supplying health-care services to patients for a profit."[1]

Relman described the most notable players in the profit-driven private health care sector at the time: proprietary hospitals and nursing homes, diagnostic laboratories, home care and emergency room services, and proprietary hemodialysis centers. Together those entities produced about $40 billion for the industry in 1979. Relman's concern was that this already large and growing complex would create overuse of procedures and technologies at the expense of care; fragmentation in the delivery of care and services; the use of procedures that are unnecessary, inefficient, or simply not the best; and conflicts of interest for physicians. He also felt it would exert undue influence on national health policy. At the time Relman was not troubled by the "old" medical-industrial complex, the pharmaceutical and medical equipment companies (he never mentioned medical device companies), noting that they had been around a long time, were socially useful, and "in a capitalistic society there are no practical alternatives to the private manufacture of drugs and medical equipment." He was primarily concerned with the problem of how to fund the need for modern health care technology while simultaneously protecting equity, access, and the quality of medical work and patient care. The worries he articulated were about the corporatization of heath care, the rise of the medical marketplace at the expense of physicians' autonomous judgment, and ultimately the demise of medicine as a social good.[2]

Relman was prescient of course. While he was not alone in his predictions, no group of citizens or indeed government policy has emerged in the intervening thirty-plus years with the moral force or broad authority to stem the tide of the growing commercial business of health care. No laws, social movements, or developments in medicine itself or in the American political landscape have had the power—yet—to curb the increasing encroachment of the private sector into research, technology development, therapeutics, and insurance reimbursement. The proliferation of technologies and health care services, along with the drive for profits within that complex, have escalated substantially since Relman first expressed his concern. Today EBM and the clinical trials industry are firmly intertwined with the medical-industrial complex. And the cultural authority that evidence-based medicine enjoys keeps it deeply connected to that increasingly corporatized and commercialized complex and to the political and economic commitments on which it rests. As we will see, insurers, physicians, educators, researchers, medical specialty groups, patients, and those who would reform health care delivery all want evidence-based medicine; that is, they all want a scientifically organized basis for medical practice—for medical progress. Who could be against that?

Evidence-based medicine and the clinical trials industry are what set the groundwork for how doctors and patients understand appropriate treatments and how patients and families consider what to do.

From Research Findings to Evidence for Best Treatment: The First Transformation

The contemporary health care enterprise has its foundational scientific and therapeutic sources both in basic biological research, conducted in laboratories, and in clinical research studies to test products or procedures on people. Clinical trials, experiments that use sick patients or healthy volunteers, are today considered the benchmark of medical research. The outcomes of those studies—for example, determining whether a drug or device works and is safe, the extent to which it works, on which kinds of patients with which conditions it works best, and how serious are the side effects—are used to determine the evidence on which new treatments are based. Those outcomes are used also to determine whether existing treatments can be expanded safely to include new patient populations, populations that were never tested in research studies. That is how the findings of clinical research are transformed into evidence for best treatment.

Today that evidence accumulates more rapidly than ever before, in large part because the well-financed pharmaceutical, device, and biotech industries contribute so substantially to its creation. Because existing drugs, devices, and procedures are always being compared with newer products and techniques, what constitutes the best evidence for a treatment is a topic that is always in development. In recent years the rapid proliferation of research study results has led to more new treatments than ever before and to the expanding use of existing treatments among populations not tested in research, especially older persons.

How does this play out in medicine today? The history of the automatic implantable cardiac defibrillator, the small electronic device that Mrs. Walters and Mr. Tolleson received, provides a good example of the conversion of research findings to evidence for treatment and how that evidence is then taken up by physicians in practice.

When it was initially approved by the U.S. Food and Drug Administration in 1985, Medicare provided limited coverage for the ICD, framing it conceptually at that time as "a treatment of last resort" for patients who had documented episodes of life-threatening arrhythmias or cardiac arrest.[3] But in 2003 the floodgates burst open. A series of clinical trials conducted between 2002 and 2005 and sponsored variously by the National Institutes of Health (NIH) and the device industry showed that the device provided survival benefits for increasingly lower risk populations, that is, for a much broader range of persons who had had heart attacks and showed certain measures of declining heart function.[4] Those trials and their results expanded the number of patients who would be considered medically appropriate for the device in terms of their cardiac function and symptoms, who would likely benefit from it according to the clinical trials outcomes data, and thus who would be eligible for Medicare reimbursement for the device and its placement.

The implantable cardiac defibrillator is simply one example of the perfect storm that is ordinary medicine. In this case the rationale for expanded ICD use was determined by many elements: the industry's organization of research protocols to show survival benefit for more kinds of patients, the cultural value of those trials' results in producing a truth about medical progress, the public's desire for more treatments, physicians' mandate to save life, and the politics of limitless payment for those with Medicare insurance.

The use of the ICD reveals how the evidence produced by clinical trial findings affects physicians' work by creating the treatment standard for practice; by expanding what is thought to be "treatable," in this case, by reconceptualizing risk as a condition that deserves treatment; and by minimizing or ignoring the salience of advanced age when considering the use of the device. The 2002–5 ICD trials enrolled mostly persons in their sixties, with only small percentages of enrollees beyond the age of seventy (although some trials were open to individuals up to eighty).

Overall the results of those trials did not show an explicit ICD benefit for older persons. Nevertheless during that short timeframe the ICD came to be considered more broadly within the medical community as a means of primary prevention of sudden cardiac death, even though some physicians expressed reservations about such expanded use, claiming that specific clinical trial results did not provide adequate evidence for the expansion.[5] Nonetheless over the span of that trials period the ICD came to be seen as appropriate for use among a broader cohort of patients, and quickly thereafter it came to be considered ordinary, if not standard, for a substantially larger population of older and lower risk patients.

Some of the practitioners we interviewed were among those who had reservations about expanded ICD use, and they reflected on the pressures created by the confluence of emerging evidence and an aging population. A cardiac specialist who implants devices said, "It just seems that we're all going to die, and many eighty-five-year-olds are not healthy. I mean, they are going to have the arrhythmia risk. I feel like it's a technology I'm being asked to utilize that prevents the type of death that might occur naturally in someone from the age of eighty-five and beyond. It may not be ideal to prevent that. That is, arrhythmia death is actually maybe one of the nicer exit strategies for all of us, after a certain age."

From New Evidence to "One More Tool": Physicians' Changing Perspectives

Such pressures on them aside, however, physicians also explained that the changing evidence, as it emerged from the 2002–5 clinical trials, altered their thinking about appropriate use of the device.[6] One physician who implants ICDs remarked:

> Now we've come all the way to the point where we realize, scientifically, that you can put an ICD in someone who's never had a cardiac event at all, without doing any other testing, but just bring them in from the office and put it in. Because at some point they may face this arrhythmia risk, and, scientifically, they'll be better if they have this than someone who doesn't have it. We've all grown to accept that. So I think I've changed in terms of my thinking about what's treatable or when it should be treated.
>
> I really see a difference compared to when I was in training. And the reason it's so clear to me is I remember, in training, being confronted

with the notion of putting a defibrillator in an eighty-year-old patient and thinking that that was just the most extreme circumstance. How could we justify preventing sudden death in an eighty-year-old person? And now it's commonplace because the evidence has accumulated. Now my threshold—I have more of the incredulous reaction to someone who may be over ninety. I feel it changing, and I feel me changing as well.

Yet he and others noted that the broadened, more relaxed criteria for device implantation placed increasing emphasis on the *existence of the risk of sudden death as a scientific reason for employing the device*. Not only did research show that the device would provide survival benefit for people who already had suffered a life-threatening cardiac event or who showed various measures of declining heart function, but clinical trials also were subsequently organized to show that the risk of death alone was reason to implant the device. Clinical trial evidence had reconceptualized risk per se as a condition that can and should be treated. By 2004 this development proved morally disquieting for some, as new findings emerged that recalibrated what constituted standard treatment for using the device. One physician reflected at that time:

The science already shows that every person who has had a cardiac arrest would potentially be considered a candidate for an implantable defibrillator. So I'm asked to see anyone that's had a cardiac arrest and try and decide whether they should have the defibrillator. The other clinical criteria would be someone who has a demonstrably weakened heart muscle—and we use actual numerical ejection fraction criteria [the amount of blood pumped out of the heart with each heart beat]—who has had some degree of nonsustained arrhythmia. Now the most aggressive approach, which is currently happening as we speak, is that patients are simply recognized as having a moderately weakened heart muscle, and they may have never had an arrhythmia before. They may be just statistically enough at a risk for sudden death. They've never had a heart attack or any event at all. And now we're being asked to accept those patients for implantable defibrillator placement, just because they've reached a numerical cut-off, with an ejection fraction of 35 percent. You simply can go straight to an implantable defibrillator. So whatever my ethical, moral dilemmas were, they may be increasing now because I'm being asked to consider simply anyone and everyone who has a weakened heart muscle for this technology.

Adding to the broadened criteria for device placement is the fact that those with weakened heart muscles are generally older people. This physician continued:

Age is not a widely discussed criterion that some doctors, patients, and families use to exclude themselves from consideration before I ever see them. But once I'm asked to see them, it's usually because the internist or the general cardiologist has made a determination that, whatever the age, they still want this arrhythmia to be aggressively managed with a defibrillator. It becomes very controversial sometimes, and maybe that's one of the sources of my personal unrest. Sometimes I disagree. But it's very tricky to sit down with an eighty-eight-year-old patient or their loving family—and by now they've heard about this technology—and to say, "You know, he does meet the clinical criteria, but, really, at his age, it may not be the right thing in this case. If he were to have a dangerous arrhythmia—that's the way people pass quietly in their sleep. That may be a natural moment at the end of the person's life." Sudden death is actually a pretty good way to go. So it may not be something that we want to jar your loved one awake with.

That's a very hard discussion to have because they may think you're not on their side, or that you're not offering expensive technology, or you're rationing. So if you're going to get into that, you'd better be ready, and you'd better be able to walk the line in a very delicate way and say, "Now, of course, I'm very happy to offer this to you, but let's think carefully about whether it would feel right under these circumstances."

It's just sort of a vague judgment that this person's eighty-eight, and they seem mentally alert, but you just get a sense, boy, they've been through so much. . . . I've found my way into an area of medicine that I, on the one hand, believe in, but on the other hand, it doesn't leave me feeling great about what I'm doing in terms of utilization of technology. I'm glad the technology is there, but it seems I'm asked to use it at times when I'm not perfectly comfortable. Wouldn't the surgeon say the same thing about some of the people they're asked to do bypass on? I think so. Wouldn't the coronary specialist say the same thing? I think that's the nature of this project, to say there's a discomfort zone, and for me, it seems to invade my time with some frequency.

Another physician, less troubled by the trend toward implanting devices in older, sicker patients, expressed a different viewpoint:

Some doctors just recognize they can't really predict the future, so why sweat it? Why try? Just do what you know to do. The patient *qualifies* [according to evidence-based and reimbursement criteria], so go with what you know, and get it over with. And there'll be a cancer doctor to worry about that metastatic cancer. But don't try to get in on that because you're going to just stumble. Because push comes to shove, if the family pushes you and the patient pushes you, you can't predict whether it's going to be six months, twelve months, eighteen months. One of the biggest problems that we get into as physicians is that we say, "Your loved one has six months to go, less than six months to live." And who wants to be part of that miscalculation? So I think a lot of my colleagues just say, "I'm not even going to sweat that. If they qualify, if they meet the criteria, let's go."

There is no doubt that evidence supporting the device's expanded use—to emphasize the reduction in the risk of death rather than treatment of specific, life-threatening symptoms—provokes quandaries. One physician noted that ICD use has become one more tool in the "extravaganza of cardiology" and the "technology parade" that have become so normalized for persons in later life:

One of the scenarios that troubles me the most is that the patient that comes into the hospital, they arrive with a heart attack, they're rushed to the heart room, the blockage is identified, and they have an appropriate intervention with a stent. They have other blockages that are not causing their acute problem but will be a problem later. They then have a discussion about the need or the role for bypass. They go to bypass surgery. They then have some extra beats noted on the heart monitor because they're monitored; they do have a weakened heart muscle. They're felt to be at risk for future dangerous arrhythmias. And then I get called, and I'm just part of this two-week extravaganza of cardiology where we basically pull out all the stops. And the person leaves, having had three separate types of intervention, ending with a device that is very expensive but of proven scientific benefit and value. But sometimes we do all of this for someone who's very old. I become party to a technology parade where I'm the last part of it, which basically eliminates any potential of margin savings benefit to the hospital. I obliterate that as part of a desire to simply take care of patients. The reason that we do it is because you couldn't have gone through all of this and not also cover that base. If you're going to offer this sort of aggressive open-heart surgery procedure, then you surely would offer them something as easy—even though it's expensive—as an implantable defibrillator.

But that's where the ethical dilemma starts. I'm not sure that's what the patient wants. But we're very powerful in our ability to convince them that that's what they should have, *according to what the studies show*. And I believe in these studies. We definitely convince eighty-somethings to go through all of this. And you let them go, then, from the hospital, never really knowing, except by some study or inference, whether you've really made them live any longer, whether they're just miserable at home, whether it was worth it.

How did we get to this point? What conditions paved the way for this kind of medical treatment to be conceived, emerge, and flower? It was not inevitable.

The Genesis of Today's Relationship between Research and Therapeutics

Scientific research has always been a driving force of medicine, and the quest for the scientific basis of medical treatments has motivated researchers, clinicians, and medical reformers for centuries. But a new configuration of state-sponsored investment in biomedical science was forged with the creation of the National Institutes of Health in 1946. Postwar prosperity enabled both such investment and the public's "vision of progress without conflict" that motivated and supported it.[7] The U.S. Congress and the public became convinced that if great sums of money were devoted to biomedical research, diseases of all kinds could be cured, and beginning in the 1950s they united overwhelmingly in support of massive government funding for basic biomedical research. This united front exemplified a new cultural awareness supporting the use of government funds to promote the health of the nation. It ushered in an era of public optimism about the partnership of government and science in the service of medical progress.

Paul Beeson, a physician who rose to national prominence as an academic clinician, teacher, and researcher after World War II, described to me forty years later the postwar mood of the nation. The United States was characterized, he noted, by the conviction that the "good" embodied in the sciences would change all aspects of life for the better and by the confidence that large sums of money were the answer:

> It was abundantly demonstrated during the war that if you put enough money into a big problem you could solve it: radar, jet propulsion, penicillin. Government researchers developed a good treatment for malaria, because our troops were going into malaria areas. In war ads in the magazines, General Motors would say they were making tanks now, but just wait 'til after the war and see what our new automobiles are going to be like. The whole country was anxious to channel money out of wartime expenditures and into good living. There were a lot of influential people in Congress who saw that things could be done to improve the nation's health if enough federal funds were put into it. The NIH, a branch of the public health service, began to give out large grants to the universities of the country. All of a sudden we had this big explosion of academic medicine—in surgery, medicine, whatever—with full-time departments growing.
>
> When I was at Yale [1952–1965] a big burst of new money came in, and we could expand so rapidly. We could build labs and we applied for huge grants. People were saying, "Don't you want some more money?" It was that kind of time.[8]

More than twenty years of unprecedented growth in government-sponsored medical research followed. Between 1955 and 1960 support from Congress increased the NIH budget from $81 million to $400 million.[9] By 1965 the NIH was by far the single most important source of research funds for university and medical school investigators,[10] and it continued to dominate the funding of biomedical research into the 1980s.

There has been broad consensus since the end of World War II that biomedical research is essential to improving individual and population health around the globe, and the NIH remains the largest federal funder of such research, accounting for $29 billion dollars in research support in 2007.[11] In many universities at which basic biological research is carried out, the NIH is still the single largest source of research funds. The growth in the biomedical sciences and in drug development after World War II was facilitated by direct political pressure on Congress by lobbying groups determined to find a cure for cancer. Finding a cure was a major political goal throughout the 1950s and 1960s, and industry-government partnerships, such as those that enabled military developments in wartime, were considered to be the best way to ensure rapid progress.[12]

As research funding and opportunities expanded, many researchers saw the need to establish standards specific to laboratory and clinical research methods. By the end of the 1950s some clinician-investigators already considered the randomized controlled trial (RCT) to be the gold standard for scientific experimentation.[13] In an RCT participating patients or healthy volunteers are assigned randomly to one of two groups. One group will get the experimental treatment; the other will get either a placebo or the standard treatment. Researchers then compare the outcomes and determine, based on their findings, whether the experimental treatment is better than the standard (or no) treatment and how much better in terms of cure, remission rates, and the time to death.[14]

Testing a new therapy against a placebo, the standard treatment, or no therapy at all means withholding the experimental treatment from one group—in effect, rationing that treatment in the service of greater medical knowledge and (potentially) better treatments in the future. The value of such withholding can be accepted only when physicians acknowledge the gaps in their knowledge about diseases and therapies. During the 1950s one advocate for the method of randomized trials summarized this perspective: "It is the physician's duty to do his best for his patients, and if he believes that there is some evidence in favor of a certain treatment, he will feel bound to use it. If, however, he is acquainted with the requirements for valid proof, he will often see that what looked like evidence is not evidence at all, and he will feel free to experiment."[15]

The RCT soon achieved wider recognition among medical researchers, especially those in academic medical settings, as an objective, quantitative technique for measuring the safety and effectiveness of the new drugs that were rapidly becoming available. Those who pushed for standardization in research methods were motivated to produce "scientific," that is, statistically valid therapeutic knowledge as a means to control the criteria by which doctors made treatment decisions for their patients. The rise of the RCT and the importance of statistical methods thus shifted authority regarding treatments away from individual doctors onto a research method. From its inception the RCT was criticized by some researchers and clinicians who were not convinced that statistical analysis was the key to better research design or patient treatments, but it nonetheless began to be perceived as *the* standard for determining the most *truthful* scientific research outcomes and, by extension, the most (and least) effective therapies in terms of patient care.[16]

New treatments continued to emerge, and the value of the RCT increased during the period of postwar government expansion in medical research. The issue of the standardization of treatments became increasingly important. Academic-based physician-researchers were the first to realize that physicians' individualized traditions for determining and trying out new therapies needed to give way to standardized approaches in order to best serve patients and to educate doctors, and they advocated strongly for the use of organized, randomized clinical trials to evaluate new interventions. As academic medicine departments in universities grew, so too did the clinical trial enterprises based there. The importance of quantification and especially of statistical validation in research was further facilitated by the NIH, which began to demand objectivity and quantification of experiments and their results.[17]

Guidelines for evaluating the safety and effectiveness of treatments emerging from experiments on human subjects did not become a matter of governmental and public concern until the sudden increase in 1962 of severe birth defects from taking the drug thalidomide. Already in widespread use during the 1950s among pregnant women in Europe to treat morning sickness and risk of premature delivery, the drug was being evaluated by the Food and Drug Administration at the time of the increase, although it was also being administered to American women enrolled in drug industry studies.[18] Once they learned of the link between thalidomide and infants born with missing limbs, U.S. officials delayed FDA approval, averting a more widespread disaster. That incident led to stricter requirements for drug manufacturers to prove both the safety and therapeutic efficacy of their products.[19] The FDA developed tighter regulations for approval of drugs, and the thalidomide scare institutionalized the randomized controlled trial as the scientific gold standard for drug safety and approval. By the late 1960s the RCT had become mandatory for FDA approval of drugs in the United States, and it became the preferred research tool for evidence-based evaluations of all therapeutics.

By the late 1970s it had become standard in most of the other Western industrialized countries as well.[20]

During the 1960s some academic physicians were already arguing that much of medical practice lacked "the scientific qualities of valid evidence, logical analyses, and demonstrable proofs."[21] They reasoned that without standardized terminology and procedures, medical practice would never be able to correctly follow the rules of scientific method. For example, "every aspect of clinical management can be designed, executed, and appraised with intellectual procedures identical to those used in any experimental situation. . . . At the bedside, exactly the same principles of scientific method [can be seen to apply as] are used for any other experiment."[22]

By the late 1960s and into the 1970s academic-based physicians were subtly reconceiving the practice of medicine from the inside. Medicare, which arrived on the scene in 1965, contributed to the expansion of academic medicine (as Beeson noted), thereby strengthening the shifts undertaken by academic practitioners. Medicine was no longer understood as the practical application of a science located elsewhere; rather it was becoming a scientific activity in and of itself, grounded in epidemiological and statistical reasoning.[23] That shift was (and still is) accompanied by physician and consumer complaints that a standardized "cookbook" approach (as many critics have called it) to treatment de-emphasizes or ignores the actual patient and his or her problems and that evidence-based therapies derived from experiments on relatively small and homogeneous populations simply are not appropriate to the conditions of each and every patient.

It was in the late 1980s when I interviewed Beeson and six other influential physicians who had been at the height of their careers in the 1960s and 1970s. I asked each of them about the changes they had seen in medicine during the twentieth century, and their responses at the time provide insight into the evolution of ordinary medicine. Each of them noted, among other things, that an occupation long guided by the ideals of duty, empathy, care, and charity had become guided more explicitly by scientific and technological developments and the implementation of reimbursement. Here is how J. Dunbar Shields, a community-based internist, depicted Medicare: "It has taken care of some people who probably were not getting good medical care. But it has had some disadvantages too. There's no more charity work done. Doctors now collect anywhere from 96 to 99 percent of their bills. Of course they complain that they are not paid enough by Medicare. And indeed they probably are not. But Medicare has taken out of medicine the pleasure that doctors had in doing work for nothing. And it has made everybody more money-minded."[24]

While these physicians welcomed the ability to effectively treat more diseases, and to do so with less invasive techniques, they worried about the demise of the individualized care and sense of duty that they felt were essential to the doctor-patient relationship. They spoke about how technology had complicated if not usurped the ability of the doctor to know the patient and the family and to communicate with both.

Perhaps the iconic practice of their era was the house call, which doctors in practice prior to the 1960s noted was a superb mechanism for getting to know the patient in the context of the family. But house calls lost their value with the increasing reliance on objective diagnostic criteria located in doctors' offices, clinics, and hospitals and on effective drug treatments. Care was replaced by cure and treatment; duty was replaced by cost-effectiveness. Reflecting on these issues, Shields noted, "My son Joe makes absolutely no house calls and never has. I talked to him about it, and he said, 'Dad, I just can't do that. Suppose I leave my office and make a house call across town. In modern medicine, we have to have our tools. I can't do any of the things I want to do to this individual out of the office. In order to do the most for my patients, I just can't afford to do house calls.' And he's absolutely right. That is right for all doctors now."[25] Beeson noted how technology changed hospital care during the 1970s:

> In intensive care—which is really the most exciting part of modern medicine, everyone is thrilled about putting catheters in and measuring pressures here and there and measuring blood gasses all the time—the talk is of "the numbers": "What are the numbers on Mrs. Jones this morning?" And you list her oxygen, CO_2, sodium and potassium and you talk about what you are going to do to correct those. If you go and stand in an intensive care unit, you will see a team of four or five people, and they look across the patient and talk to one another about the numbers. But the patient is listening, and it is so important to put a reassuring hand on the patient's arm and look him in the eye and say something. Instead of that, they talk about the numbers and then go on to the next patient. This is one of the sad things about the technological aspects becoming so dominant in patient care.[26]

"The most exciting part of modern medicine," Beeson's words reveal, had become the technical things one could do to get numerical diagnostic results. By that time standardized measurement tools had become highly valued in their own right, not merely as aids with which to understand disease and the health of a patient but as a primary focus of medical treatment and care. In addition these physicians and others noted the increasing speed with which medicine replaces one set of truths with another and the fact that the questions and answers of medical research were becoming focused ever more narrowly. They predicted that the resulting transience of medical knowledge—the impermanence of medical information generated by the very pace of the biomedical science revolution—would fundamentally alter the practice of medicine. They were right.

When these doctors were in training in the 1920s and 1930s, the body of relevant knowledge was contained in textbooks; little new knowledge that altered day-to-day practice was being produced. The culture of medicine was characterized by its continuity and highly limited powers. Beeson told me, "I have just been looking at the 1931 textbook of medicine that I studied and practically memorized, and it is quite clear from underlining and margin notes that I thought this was about 'it,' and that I would be using that dogma for the rest of my life."[27]

In marked contrast the anthropologist Melvin Konner, a medical student in 1981–84, describes how, in just those four years, the increasing pace of scientific and technological innovation supplanted previous ways of understanding disease, treatment, and the body:

Liver transplants, previously a rarity, have become relatively practical and commonplace. The immunosuppressant cyclosporine has dramatically altered the success rates of all kinds of transplants. Traditional antacid therapy for ulcers has been laid aside in favor of systemic drugs like cimetidine, which within two years of its approval became the most frequently prescribed drug of any kind in the United States. Calcium-channel blockers, a completely new class of drugs, were approved and became a mainstay of cardiology. Noninvasive widening of clogged arteries in the heart began to rival bypass surgery as a treatment method for one of our most common serious illnesses. AIDS, a new and fatal disease, was identified, shown to be taking on dangerous epidemic proportions, and likened to a virus not just of a species but of a whole biological category previously not considered to be among the causes of human illness. Lithium, an extraordinary simple elemental substance, overtook antischizophrenic drugs as the treatment of choice for intermittent forms of psychosis. Alzheimer's disease was recognized as the leading cause of senile and presenile dementia and a major health problem of our time. The basic science of recombinant DNA became an essential part of every physician's knowledge, promising as it does a vast variety of new and powerful drugs, as well as the imminent prospect of that science-fiction therapy, "gene surgery." Magnetic resonance imaging—known also as nuclear magnetic resonance, or N.M.R.—became the gold standard of radiology, promising to replace CAT scanning (itself a quite new modality) in several important areas of diagnosis. And in vitro fertilization made the transition from a science-fiction laboratory technique to a proven and accepted method of treatment for infertility, making hundreds of "test-tube babies" a reality. These are only a few highlights of the new knowledge discovered or made practical while my graduating class was attending medical school. In most cases they were not, and could not be, taught to the students who graduated the year before we entered.[28]

The problem, then, became not only how to teach the "skills needed to evaluate and master the always-emerging new knowledge" but also how to standardize the evaluation and administration of the new, so rapidly emerging treatments.[29]

Beeson, Shields, and the other physicians I interviewed in the 1980s were concerned primarily with how the effects of specialization, more technology, and the new reimbursement structures would affect the doctor-patient relationship, and their remarks were prescient regarding the change in that relationship. They did not, however, predict the extent to which the developments in research, practice, and the business of health care—especially the authority given to the elements that make up the EBM matrix—have organized medical treatment. Those developments have become the default setting for health care delivery in the United States.

The Ascendance of Evidence-Based Medicine

The origin of contemporary evidence-based medicine is a 1985 medical text that showcased clinical epidemiology as a preferable, more science-based approach to the practice of medicine.[30] Thus it began as an innovation in medical education, designed to transform medical practice by standardizing the interpretation of clinical data and by replacing idiosyncratic clinical preferences for treatment with the findings of scientific research. The authors of that text, medical educators themselves, devised systematic guidelines (also called protocols and algorithms) as teaching tools, and they formulated the concept of evidence-based medicine in order to encapsulate a more comprehensive, science-based approach to clinical work.[31]

In a subsequent article, published in 1992, those authors wrote, "Medical practice is changing and the change, which involves using the medical literature more effectively in guiding medical practice, is profound enough that it can appropriately be called a paradigm shift."[32] That article goes on to describe the methodological tools and advances specific to EBM: use of randomized controlled trials to assess drug efficacy, meta-analysis, articles on how to do literature searches, textbooks on clinical epidemiology, and vehicles such as professional journals to disseminate evidence. A key feature of this new paradigm, the authors emphasize, is the reduced value given to individual physician authority in comparison to previous eras of medical education.

By the 1990s the problem of standardizing treatments was becoming a dominant preoccupation for medical educators and doctors in major research centers because, as Konner's account makes overwhelmingly clear, new drugs, devices, and technological developments in medicine and surgery were arriving on the scene with greater frequency than ever before. The sociologists Stefan Timmermans and Marc Berg have presented the situation numerically: "In the 1990s, an estimated 2 million medical articles were published yearly in more than 20,000 biomedical journals, more than 250,000 controlled trials of health care therapies had been conducted, and more than $50 billion was being spent annually on medical research."[33]

Which treatments were best? Were new therapeutics better than those that already existed? How much better? With more interventions of all kinds available, how could the profession of medicine address the issue of variations in medical practice and achieve consensus about best therapies?

Evidence-based medicine is now an umbrella term defined as the "conscientious, explicit, and judicious use of current best evidence in the care of individual patients."[34] Today most evidence-based medicine comes from patient-centered clinical research.[35] The goal of EBM—as a range of techniques and practices unified "by the pursuit of a new approach to medical knowledge and authority"[36]—is to show which scientific methods and experiments present the most truthful, reliable findings about safe and effective treatments. The many beneficial procedures and therapies of the past two decades—many of which enable greater longevity—serve to reinforce the view that useful treatments emerge from evidence generated in systematic research studies, especially from the randomized controlled clinical trial.

By the year 2000, according to the American Association of Medical Colleges, 88 percent of U.S. medical schools had embraced EBM as a central tenet of their curriculum in a "quiet, educational revolution."[37] Rather than being taught to follow the practices of experienced clinicians, medical students were taught to seek and review published evidence.

Evidence-based medicine quickly had a societal effect much broader than originally envisioned because it filled a growing need. The standardization of treatment approaches was becoming a major concern in the financing and organizing of health care delivery systems, and for several reasons: health care costs were rising; there was growing demand for accountability in public and private business; governments and private insurance schemes in industrialized countries needed to justify the basis on which they reimbursed treatments. In the face of these developments, government officials, policymakers, practitioners, and health care consumers all wanted assurances that mechanisms for evidence of treatment safety and effectiveness existed and were put in place. Those concerns remain today, and the phenomenon of evidence-based medicine has come to play an increasingly central role in shaping biomedical research agendas and guiding health policy. In addition EBM has become increasingly important over the past two decades in determining insurance reimbursement and thus the treatments patients actually receive. Today EBM serves as a tool for accountability, efficiency, effectiveness, and cost control in health care delivery systems in the United States and elsewhere.[38] And, importantly, it serves as a standard-setting device for what is now referred to as "best medical practices" in clinical treatment (that is, the standardized approaches to evidence-based, guideline-organized care delivery).

Evidence and Generalizability: The Randomized Controlled Trial and the Limits of Evidence-Based Medicine

All of the outcome studies, practice guidelines, and teaching tools within the vast EBM matrix have a single goal: to provide a stronger scientific foundation for clinical practice, for the delivery of medical care to patients. Yet evidence-based medicine omits from its scientifically based (and especially numerically based) matrix the social, messy, nonscientific features of health care delivery that influence what doctors do and what happens to patients. Erased from the public face of EBM is the fact that evidence is sometimes ignored when physicians and patients make treatment choices, that physicians sometimes go against their own better judgment and acquiesce to patients' demands, that treatment guidelines and policies do not always follow scientifically generated evidence. Also erased are the ethos of individual rights and personal choice and the market pressures with which EBM is intertwined.

The authority afforded the RCT, the hallmark method of EBM in the culture of medicine today, is built, perhaps surprisingly, on a practice in which only a very small percentage of patients actually participate in clinical trials. Fewer than 3 percent of cancer patients participate in cancer clinical trials for new therapies, for example.[39] And clinical trial results are based on a careful selection of patients with specific characteristics of health and disease.

Although the authority vested in the trials influences much of medical practice, the generalizability of trial findings to large patient populations is questionable. Ordinary medicine mutes or ignores the question of generalizability, and this fact engenders one of its profound effects in our aging society. Whether treatments that benefit some trial participants will also benefit a larger and more diverse group of patients, especially the elderly—those with multiple health problems who would not have been eligible to participate in trials—is a dilemma doctors often confront, as we saw in the case of the ICD.[40] Added to that dilemma is the great variation in the health, physiology, and functioning of those in later life and thus the associated uncertainty regarding treatment outcomes among older patients.

Furthermore few treatment guidelines recommended by official medical organizations for specific treatments emerge from what is considered level 1 evidence, that is, evidence from randomized controlled clinical trials. (For cancer, for example, RCT-based guidelines number approximately one in fifteen.) The reason is that those trials are expensive to conduct, take many years to complete, and often are never completed. Sometimes their results are contested or proven wrong in subsequent trials. Finally, there will never be enough evidence from clinical trials to answer all the questions about what to do that emerge for patients and doctors in the clinical setting. Thus most treatment and clinical practice guidelines are the result of expert consensus committees, whose members meet to evaluate all kinds of scientific studies in addition to randomized clinical trials. In fact the most widespread application of EBM is in establishing clinical practice guidelines, which the Institute of Medicine defines as "systematically developed statements to assist practitioner and patient decisions about appropriate health care for specific clinical circumstances."[41]

The limits to the evidence in EBM are exposed in the decision-making process of expert guideline committees, not because those committees ignore or minimize the science in their deliberations but rather because their decisions must also consider the effects of economic pressures and research agendas on their guideline recommendations. For a start, evaluation of scientific studies includes discussion about which treatments are likely to be covered by insurance. One of the highest priorities of expert consensus panels is to assure that treatments they recommend will be reimbursed by government and private insurers; otherwise doctors will not prescribe them and patients will not receive them. So their evaluations must take into account what insurers will ultimately accept as eligible for reimbursement. The insurers themselves cannot be expected to wade through the volume of clinical studies produced in all medical fields in order to independently evaluate benefits and thus make their decisions about reimbursement.[42]

Additionally the complex relationship (to be discussed shortly) between private industry and government-sponsored research regarding what kinds of clinical trials to conduct and the goals of those trials is ultimately reflected in the kinds of evidence that are produced (that is, benefit of a new treatment or evidence of benefit of an existing treatment for a broader population of patients) and then in the treatments that become available and are recommended. Simply put, in research, industry is motivated by profit to look for indications of broader applicability for a drug or device. Academic researchers funded by the NIH, on the other hand, want to follow their own agendas, which only sometimes overlap with industry priorities. As one oncologist stated, "Pharma wants to create drugs with big markets; academics want to figure out who benefits and who doesn't by studying biomarkers." Experts who create treatment guidelines can evaluate only the scientific evidence in front of them, and more and more often that evidence comes from research studies that are designed, funded, and organized by industry sponsors.

Patient and family expectations also play a role in devising expert panel guidelines. One member of a consensus committee told me succinctly, "Guideline committee members know what patients want. They know what patients expect, and they go along with that. Their decisions are based on science but informed by what patients expect, and they do expect to receive treatments."

All these factors weave through the framework of evidence-based medicine and illustrate that even when scientific evidence and generalizability are limited or absent, the therapies purportedly evaluated by EBM *become standard*. The framework of the RCT is considered the authoritative basis for transforming research findings into patient treatments, despite those often messy components.

———

The randomized controlled trial now undergirds and directs health care delivery more explicitly than ever before. Practicing physicians are mindful of this at the same time that they are aware of the limitations of new study results. In our interviews they articulated the ways that evidence is in play in practice—how it lives and works in the clinic—as they spoke about EBM's effects on their own sense of hope, on treatment protocols, and therefore on what they do. For instance, an internist who specializes in geriatrics noted, "As each new intervention comes along, we try it because it helps us think that we're intervening. But many of these clinical trials haven't been around long enough. When a new intervention comes on, it has been shown to work in the cases studied. But in the long run, several years, a five-, ten-year study, and in epidemiological studies, it may not make any difference at all. And look at the hormone replacement studies. Sobering." A cardiologist reflected, "In our hospital and in many, the treatment algorithm is primarily angioplasty. So from the point of view of a whole hospital culture, it's a very invasive cardiology approach. All the emergency room doctors and all the cardiology house staff and faculty are of the mind-set here that there's an aggressive approach to patients with heart attacks. There's a written practice guideline saying anybody with a suspected heart attack goes to the cath lab [for angiograms and then for subsequent angioplasty and other procedures]. That's the treatment plan."

The RCT and the evidence-based medicine phenomenon are designed to guide clinical judgment about the use of treatments, not to dictate to or replace it.[43] Yet in framing clinical possibilities, both the RCT and EBM sometimes set up dilemmas for doctors. One cardiologist echoed sentiments I heard from others as well: "There is an illusion that you're going to make the patient better with intervention, and it can be a real illusion. People that are ill with multisystem illness, elderly, demented, where one of the options is death—which would be a welcome option—so no, I don't always proceed. And I think those are some of the most difficult decisions, not only for me, but for many of my colleagues."

Clinicians work within many parameters to make guidelines that they feel are appropriate to their patients' conditions. Their approach to these guidelines is practical: they follow recommendations and standards that they consider useful, or potentially so, for each individual case. Most patients assume this, and no patient would want otherwise, though when it plays out in the clinic, patients may not realize that this is what is happening.

In the clinic standard protocols guide how clinicians talk with their older patients about treatment goals in relation to the prospect of greater longevity. In the examples below of conversations in cancer clinics, the oncologists—like clinicians in other specialties—first interpret the complexities of research evidence for each patient's condition. They then guide the patient to undergo what they think is the best of the treatment strategies that have standards established in guidelines. All physicians today have more tools at their disposal than ever before to do something at all disease stages and more evidence to draw from regarding which treatments to pursue, but this is particularly true of oncologists. Cancer can be diagnosed in very early stages now, and different kinds of therapy (chemotherapy, surgery, radiation) and different lines of chemotherapy can be tried over months and years. In a cancer clinic patients can face a staggering array of information and options.

One oncologist told a woman who had been treated previously for invasive bladder cancer, "You're a healthy eighty-four. . . . The good news is, from the CT scan of a few months ago, you do not have cancer spread elsewhere. Looks like we need a new CT scan. . . . There are two ways to approach this. We need to do a pathology review, to confirm that it's only on the surface. I recommend washing the inside of the bladder out with a medicine, BCG [intervesicle therapy]. Studies show if you wash inside the bladder with this drug, the surface cancer can go away for six weeks. Then if all goes well, you can do it again. It's hard work, but if you don't do the wash . . . [his voice trails off]. In the long term, in about half the patients, we will have to go on and remove the bladder. I'm going to recommend we do the wash."[44]

In another clinic an oncologist had the following exchange with an eighty-year-old man with prostate cancer. The doctor began by saying:

> You don't have that many other medical conditions. There is nothing I can see to keep you from living until ninety or even a hundred. . . . Plus your Gleason grade is high.[45] We need to decide between surgery and radiation. You already met with a urology oncologist, and now you will need to meet with a radiation oncologist. If you do surgery and we find that cancer has spread outside the edge, we would then do radiation. You started hormone therapy this week. The hormones should knock down your PSA.[46] Surgery should cut your PSA completely. Radiation takes longer to get the PSA down. If you do surgery, you can do radiation after, but you can't really do surgery after radiation because of the scarring that results from radiation. Since you have a relatively aggressive cancer there may be a need for radiation after surgery. So your options are surgery, then radiation. . . . I wouldn't recommend external beam radiation only, but external beam and brachytherapy.[47] You'd have external beam radiation for five weeks, then the seeds. You'd be on the hormones two years. The main point of the hormone therapy is to improve the effectiveness of the radiation. . . . On the hormone therapy you have to be careful to do cardio exercises and weight lifting because the hormones affect the bones. Another problem with radiation is that it causes scar tissue in the bladder, which heightens the risk of bladder cancer ten years out.

When the patient responded, "But I'm eighty! Ten years out!," the oncologist reassured him, "If I didn't think you'd be around in ten years, I wouldn't suggest you do a treatment." The patient then asked what would happen if he did nothing and was told, "You wouldn't know for some time, maybe five to ten years, before it's a clinical problem. If you have symptoms then, we can't cure it. Now we can cure it. Unfortunately, metastasized prostate cancer is not a good way to go."

That oncologist's focus on projecting and helping to ensure his patient's future is a logical response to recent tables of mortality statistics that provide average life expectancy numbers not only at birth but at any given age. (A person may have an average life expectancy at birth of eighty years. However, upon reaching the age of eighty that person's average life expectancy is nearly ninety.)

That oncologist's prognostic stance is also reflected in this exchange at a follow-up exam for a ninety-six-year-old woman three weeks following her surgery for metastasized cancer of the uterus. After the patient reassured him that she'd "had no aftereffects, no pain whatsoever," the oncologist emphasized prevention of disease recurrence: "We did get all of what was in the bowel. But when you're at stage 3, surgery is not the cure-all. There's a 50 percent chance or greater that the cancer will come back. We don't know how long that will take. Maybe months, maybe years. So the discussion we need to have is, what's the next step? Chemo, radiation, or watch and see? Right now, we're looking at doing what is as minimal as possible. If you were young and healthy, we would suggest chemo or radiation. But are these worth the potential harm to you from side effects? That's a decision we'll make together. With chemo there's a longer survival period and a longer time before the cancer comes back. But it's a quality-of-life decision. What limits the chemo is the side effects. It's case by case. And that's part of what you decide." Asked by the patient's daughter whether he always recommends chemotherapy, the doctor responded, "We always offer it. My bias is that chemotherapy would be harder than it would be worth. I don't know what we're going to gain. I'm leaning toward radiation. . . . You'll need to be examined every three months."

Like their colleagues in other specialties, these oncologists are performing a balancing act on their patients' behalf. On the one hand, clinical trials and the resulting best practices greatly influence what physicians do and how they think about treatments. The guidelines shape and also constrain physicians,' and therefore patients,' choices. On the other hand, guidelines are a means by which practitioners pursue their own goals for patient treatments; they are not an end in themselves. Guidelines developed in academic medical centers perhaps carry more practical weight there. Most patient care, however, is in the hands of community physicians, among whom there is enormous variation in practice. The sheer array of possible options led one oncologist to remark, "The problem is that when you get five oncologists discussing a case, you get six opinions about what to do."

In addition many studies document that clinicians in many areas of practice simply ignore evidence-based guidelines in their recommendations to patients.[48] Reasons for this include, among others, that the physician is unaware of the guidelines or disagrees with them; the guidelines' applicability to actual patient care is or appears to be limited; and, quite simply, some patients have a preference for treatments that to them indicate hope, regardless of evidence.[49]

Other studies show regional variations in the use of diagnosis and in treatments of all sorts—from cardiac stent and ICD use to renal dialysis for end-stage renal disease to hospice referrals. These studies indicate that the variations depend on the concentration of specialists and subspecialists in a given town or area, on physicians' style of practice and economic incentives, and on the local availability of expensive services. Researchers at the Dartmouth Atlas of Health Care, which tracks regional variations in the way health care is delivered in the United States, have found that "people are more likely to be 'diagnosed' with a disease when their physician or hospital treats them more intensively." Their work looks closely at such questions as these: "Why do some primary care physicians order more than twice as many CT scans as their colleagues in the same practice? Why are the rates of coronary stents three times higher in Elyria, Ohio, compared with nearby Cleveland, home of the famous Cleveland Clinic?" They find that regional variation is determined largely by physicians' utilization of services (that is, the amount of treatments doctors give to patients), not by differences in regional insurance reimbursement rates, socioeconomic status of patients, overall patient health, or other factors.[50] Regional variation in physician treatment practices illustrates the limits of evidence-based medicine in actually shaping national standards uniformly.

Nevertheless evidence-based standards and guidelines, developed from constantly emerging clinical trial evidence and other outcome studies, continue to coordinate and shape the work of health professionals. As the physicians said regarding the ICD, those standards transform ideas about what can be treated and in whom, at the same time that they may generate tension between standard care and ideas about ethically appropriate care. Furthermore, as we will see later, standards and guidelines influence popular opinion about what should be treated and with which technologies.

Research evidence is also one source of a sometimes profound anxiety that patients and families feel when considering how to proceed. Debates are increasingly common, both within and beyond the health professions, regarding what is actually "best" as we grow older. The debates are charged and are important because taken together, and in the context of an aging society, the treatment protocols, practice guidelines, consensus reports, therapies, and so on that fall under the EBM umbrella constitute an enormous truth-making regime that determines medical practice and thus what happens to patients. The various parts of the EBM matrix have themselves become a science,[51] shaping a great deal about the goals of medicine and guiding health care consumers' relationship to medical intervention. Yet there is no absolute agreement about the algorithms that constitute EBM, and even if there were universal agreement, the EBM matrix cannot eliminate the quandaries it has contributed to and fostered—including and especially the quandary about crossing the line of too much treatment.

THE MEDICAL-INDUSTRIAL COMPLEX II

Access, Industry, and the Clinical Trials Phenomenon

————

Struggles over what constitutes therapeutic benefit and who—or, in the case of evidence-based medicine, what—has the authority to determine it are hardly new, but today those struggles are accompanied by the political problem of access. The issue of access has proven problematic on many fronts: researchers' need for access to funds to carry out their studies, industry's need for access to FDA approval in order to market medicines and devices and make profits, the influence of Medicare reimbursement policies, and consumers' need for access to available therapies.

Industry's Growing Influence on the Biomedical Research Enterprise

There is no doubt that the privatization of services by the medical-industrial complex that Arnold Relman described more than three decades ago has shaped the landscape of contemporary health care delivery and contributed to the development of the problems he foresaw—primarily how to both fund the need for the modern technologies and protect equity, patients' access to therapies, and the quality of care. Those problems have had far-reaching effects. Since the 1980s and 1990s the burgeoning medical marketplace has anchored and dominated the chain of connections and transformations that is the backbone of U.S. health care delivery. That marketplace often stresses efficiency and profit above optimal treatment and actual care, as many are aware.[1] For example, it organizes the common fifteen-minute time slots in which doctors and patients attempt to carry on their conversations and exams; it creates the computerized algorithms into which patients' problems and treatments must fit; and, as Relman foresaw, the marketplace thwarts the social good of medicine.

Biomedical research in the United States has doubled since 1999, to the point that today it accounts for about 4.5 percent of total health expenditures.[2] In recent decades a significant shift in the major source of research funding has also occurred, from government to private industry—pharmaceutical, medical device, and biotechnology companies—whose share jumped from 32 percent in 1980 to over 50 percent by the mid-1990s to approximately 65 percent today.[3]

This shift in the major source of support is complicated by the fact that the boundaries between public and private funding of biomedical research are hard to draw clearly and perhaps always have been. Basic biological research may begin with funding from the NIH; then molecules discovered at universities through that support are taken up for therapeutic development by the pharmaceutical industry or biotechnology firms. Yet pharmaceutical companies sometimes also fund basic research, and academic institutions also participate in the marketing of new therapeutics.[4] Some research represents collaboration between the NIH, collaborative university and hospital groups, and industry sponsors. However hard it may be to draw a line between private and public funding of biomedical research, industry contributions to academic research rose by 875 percent between 1980 and 2000.[5] The fact that industry is contributing more and more heavily to the total pot of funding has repercussions for the kinds of research undertaken and thus for patient treatment patterns.

Ultimately the shift in the funding source affects the kinds of questions we ask about our obligations to our own longevity and to those we love. Profit-driven, backed by huge resources, and pressured by stockholders' demands, pharmaceutical companies and more recently device companies have become more involved in all stages of the biomedical research enterprise and more aggressive in their involvement. Choosing the research topic and designing the study so that their product will appear beneficial in comparison to standard treatments, to deciding which kinds of patients will make the best study subjects, moving clinical trials from universities and major medical centers to private contract research organizations, ghostwriting and publishing articles that show the favorable but not the negative findings, using physicians as marketing tools, lobbying the FDA for approval and mounting massive public advertising campaigns—all of these activities have escalated since the turn of the millennium.[6]

Total federal funding for biomedical research increased by $200 million (0.7 percent) between 2003 and 2007. In contrast, support from pharmaceutical, biotechnology, and device companies increased from $40 billion in 2003 to $58.6 billion in 2007, an increase of 25 percent. The industry that funded the most research in 2008 was the pharmaceutical industry. Yet between 2003 and 2008 that industry grew by only 15 percent, while biotechnology companies grew 41 percent and medical device firms showed the largest rate of growth at 59 percent.[7] In the decade beginning in 1994 total industry funding for biomedical research increased by 102 percent. The growth rate for device companies was 264 percent, exceeding both the pharmaceutical (89 percent growth rate) and biotechnology (98 percent) sectors. Analysts of these trends wrote in 2011, "Driven by demand, total medical spending on devices has increased at a rate that is several times that for health services and twice that for drugs."[8] In that decade pharmaceutical companies increasingly emphasized clinical trials research rather than new drug discovery, designing studies that attempt to show that their existing products work for an expanded market of new groups of patients rather than spend the huge sums new product development requires. All of this impacts what happens to patients and to patients' expectations of medicine.

In addition to the fact that there is no question that industry money is enabling research and driving research agendas, industry sponsors also pay university departments much more to conduct a study than does the NIH. One university cancer researcher provided an example in 2011 of how this works. He reported to me that a National Cancer Institute study to test a drug would pay his academic department $2,000 per patient enrolled in the study; a pharmaceutical company funding the same study would pay $15,000 per enrolled patient. Because it costs $4,000 to $4,500 per patient for an academic center to conduct a clinical trial, he noted, the department or group conducting the research loses money if the trial is sponsored by the NIH, putting clinical trial researchers not funded (at least in part) by industry at a distinct disadvantage.

Many have noted that industry sponsorship of medical research opens questions about what constitutes reliable data and evidence in the first place. Some scholars note that the impacts of industry-sponsored research can be divided into two categories. First, there are problems related to the "*subtle* impact of industry interests on the design of a study, its conduct, and the interpretation of data."[9] Second, there are the more serious problems of the manipulation of research data, selective publication of findings, and ghostwriting. More thoroughly than ever before, in recent years industry involvement in research has blurred the line between the practice of science and the marketing of products. This undercuts the very basis of evidence-based medicine. Two analysts of this phenomenon go so far as to state, "In fact, insistence on the need for EBM—with its over-emphasis on one particular methodology of establishing evidence, i.e. the randomized controlled trial—gives financial interests unprecedented power to shape medical practice."[10] Others emphasize that the entire scientific enterprise has become subject to being used as part of industry marketing campaigns.[11]

Not all biomedical research dollars are spent on randomized clinical trials, of course, and EBM encompasses more than clinical trials within its scientific matrix. But because of the explosion in the number of clinical trials being conducted, the centrality of the clinical trials enterprise to EBM, and the importance of clinical trial findings to establishing treatment patterns, the impact of the ever larger proportion of industry-funded trials on doctors and patients is enormous. The straight line and arrow of influence—the chain of transformations that constitutes ordinary medicine—is not seen, however, by most sick people. They are simply trying to make choices among the options offered and the recommendations made to them. An increase in clinical trials designed to evaluate the safety and effectiveness of a drug or device eventually results in more drugs and devices on the market, more patient groups for whom they are prescribed, and more apparent choices for doctors and patients to make. And the growth in the clinical trials business has been nothing short of astounding over the past fifteen years.

The Clinical Trials Phenomenon: A New Component of American Culture

I hope I am eligible for the clinical trial.
—Seventy-six-year-old patient with metastatic prostate cancer

The idea of clinical trial participation as both treatment and an individual right emerged in the early stages of the AIDS epidemic in the 1980s, when desperate, politically sophisticated patients realized that their only chance for longer life was to have access to experimental drugs, then in various stages of slow development and testing. They could not afford to wait a decade or more for evaluation and FDA approval before a drug was marketable. With no other hope for survival, they wanted the opportunity to take untested drugs and wanted to serve as experimental subjects in research in order to get access to potentially life-extending therapies.[12] Beyond that, they wanted to participate in the organization of those trials in order to gain some control over who could access the new drugs and in order to influence the nature of the research enterprise, its funding, and especially the length of time it took to get new drugs approved and marketed.

AIDS activism during the 1980s changed forever the relationship of sick citizens with lives at stake to the biomedical research endeavor. In the United States that activism moved the clinical trial enterprise from the sequestered world of academic medical centers into the public domain of human rights in everyday affairs. Breast cancer activism quickly followed, and now there are hundreds of disease-based advocacy groups that are savvy about research and opportunities to access clinical trials for their conditions. Their collective goal is to ensure that experimental treatments not yet approved or rejected by the FDA are available to those people with serious and terminal illnesses who want to participate.

In response both to the importance of the clinical trials enterprise to medical practice and to growing patient sophistication about participation in those trials, the Food and Drug Administration, in collaboration with the National Institutes of Health, established a publicly available website, ClinicalTrials.gov, in 2000.[13] The website was designed to be an easily available data bank of clinical trials information. It serves as a "central resource, providing current information on clinical trials to individuals with serious or life-threatening diseases or conditions, to other members of the public, and to health care providers and researchers."[14] Both government and industry investigators are required to submit their experimental protocols for life-threatening disease to the data bank;[15] they may submit experimental protocols for other kinds of clinical trials as well.

The website serves several functions. It democratizes access to information about experimental research and, presumably, access to participation in that research. It enables the FDA to keep track of the burgeoning clinical trials industry since investigators must list their trials for serious diseases with the data bank. It standardizes the information that investigators must give to the public and to the FDA about experiments. In the year of its inception the website included about four thousand trials, most of which were sponsored by the NIH.[16] In 2002, 6,800 clinical trials sponsored by the NIH, other federal agencies, and private industry were listed; in 2008 the number rose to 65,755; in May 2014 the number was 167,034.[17] This growth illustrates that the politics of consumer demand for treatments is one of the forces perpetuating the structures and standards (clinical trials, evidence-based medicine) of ordinary medicine.

There is no doubt that the proliferation of the clinical trials enterprise expands the market for therapeutics.[18] For example, after new drugs are shown in clinical trials to be effective for specific populations with specific conditions, clinicians often use them and other technologies in populations outside the one on which they were originally tested. Unlike the ICD example, this later use is due not to trials having demonstrated expanded use for an existing product but to the assumption and hope of benefit on the part of physicians and sometimes patients as well. That hope may or may not be well grounded, but it nevertheless contributes to pharmaceutical companies' profits. Called "indication creep" and "off-label" use, this practice is exceedingly common.[19] Some drug firms have profited spectacularly from seeking FDA approval of a drug for a specific use and then marketing it for other uses off-label.[20] Many patients and families, seeking cures and hope, want access to the newest therapies that emerge from clinical trials. So there is also a certain amount of "folkloric creep," as one university-based clinical trials expert dubbed it. That is, some consumers ask about and demand therapies for conditions not tested in controlled research trials.

In addition to contributing to the evolving conceptions of what constitutes treatment benefit, the ubiquity of clinical trials has also led to an even greater shift in public expectations about what constitutes *treatment* in the first place. Patients have long misunderstood the difference between experimental interventions to test safety and effectiveness and approved, standard therapies;[21] nevertheless more patients today, including some older patients, want to be enrolled in clinical trials. In large part this is because, following on the experience of AIDS activism, they have learned that a clinical trial therapy or procedure may be their only hope for improvement, especially if they have advanced disease and no more standard therapies are available. As a result of the widely touted promises of experimental therapies and the popular perception that clinical trial participation can lead to a cure or remission, more and more individuals consider it their right to participate in those experimental studies.[22]

The Effects of Trials and Markets: Cancer Treatments

While the clinical trials phenomenon affects many therapies, its effects reverberate most keenly, perhaps, in the world of cancer research and treatment. In the United States more than ten thousand researchers at over three thousand institutions are registered with the NIH's National Cancer Institute.[23] In the first decade of the new millennium more than three thousand clinical trials were conducted for breast cancer alone, at a cost of over $1 billion.[24] As of 2014 approximately one-third of all the clinical trials listed at ClinicalTrials.gov were for cancer treatments, and industry funded twice as many of those studies as did the NIH.[25]

The pharmaceutical industry considers cancer drugs to be profit generators, and it has recently narrowed its focus from the quest for blockbuster drugs to treat a variety of ailments to a search for cancer drugs that attack specific mutations of cancer cells or that cut off the blood supply to those cells. In 2010 the industry poured money into clinical trials for cancer drugs, spending more than double the amount on cancer drug development and clinical research than it spent on development of treatments in nine other therapeutic areas (including central nervous system, cardiovascular, respiratory, and gastrointestinal diseases).[26] In its sponsorship of clinical trials to test the effectiveness of one cancer drug against others or to test drug combinations, Big Pharma contributes enormously to the expansion of the clinical trials enterprise and, through that enterprise, to more FDA-approved, Medicare-reimbursed drugs for expanding markets.[27] All clinical trials create markets, but cancer trials are especially adept at doing so.

All chemotherapy agents and the newer targeted therapies, their doses, and their schedules have been developed and approved through clinical trial protocols.[28] If trials show a benefit for the patient, the findings are evaluated by the FDA; then, following Medicare approval, the treatment becomes a new standard. The standard treatment regimens are constantly revised by consensus groups in light of new clinical trial findings (along with other forms of evidence). As was clear in my conversations with cancer patients, much of the work of today's oncologists is in fact to consider and then adapt those emerging guidelines for use with individual patients. For example, a primary goal of the National Comprehensive Cancer Network,[29] a not-for-profit alliance of twenty-one cancer centers worldwide, is to create practice guidelines and thus codify standards of care.

Unlike the implantable cardiac defibrillator, cancer drugs grew up in the context of clinical trials, and cancer trials owe their emergence and expansion to the development of chemotherapy drugs in the 1950s and 1960s.[30] From the 1950s on, efforts to increase the effectiveness of chemotherapy agents were linked with the development of large-scale clinical trials.[31] Beginning in the late 1960s new chemotherapy agents began to appear with some regularity, and a new generation of oncologist-chemotherapists emerged in the United States. Throughout the 1960s and into the early 1970s, when President Nixon announced his "war on cancer" (1971), oncologists struggled to find a common cure for what they imagined to be a "single, monolithic entity . . . *one* disease."[32] Chemotherapy was seen as the way to conquer it, and clinical trials were the pathway to testing those drugs.

The emerging practice of medical oncology was so intertwined with the expansion of cancer clinical trials from the 1950s to the 1970s that the medical historians Peter Keating and Alberto Cambrosio were led to remark, "Conventional wisdom would hold that cancer clinical trials are the by-product of medical oncologists. We argue, however, that it is the other way around: medical oncologists are a by-product of the emergence of clinical cancer trials."[33] (In addition the arrival of Medicare insurance in 1965 also contributed, along with private insurance, to the transformation of oncology from a moderately paid to a highly paid specialty. Insurance allowed oncologists to mark up the costs of drugs.[34])

In the United States the training of medical oncologists was closely associated with clinical research,[35] and in the clinic oncologists had become chemotherapists. Cancer therapy was inextricably organized around clinical trials, and through the mid-1990s there was a huge expansion of trials testing of chemotherapy agents.[36] Today combinations of chemotherapy, surgery and radiation, newer hormonal therapies, and the development of drugs with fewer side effects have led to more treatment options for doctors to consider. Now more can be done, and for longer periods of time, in the treatment of many cancers.[37] Immune system–based agents and drugs to inhibit the growth of specific cancer mutations are of interest to oncologists today. Yet cancer mortality in general has not been declining very much.[38] Overall the death rate from cancer in the United States fell only 5 percent between 1950 and 2005, whereas death rates from strokes and heart attacks fell dramatically.[39] Between 1990 and 2005 the cancer death rate fell nearly 15 percent, but those reductions were the result of discoveries made during the 1950s and 1960s and not the result of the explosion in research that has occurred since.[40] Much of therapeutic innovation today is aimed at tweaking cancer treatments by combining already standard drugs in new ways. The goal of the new approach is either to extend life by a few weeks or months, as evidenced in a clinical trial, or to lengthen the amount of "progression-free survival," that is, the time from the start of treatment to the recurrence of tumor growth.[41]

Regardless of the statistics on outcomes, everyone wants new cancer drugs, and, as a result, they sell. Medicare pays for cancer drugs, thus transforming them into therapies that physicians can offer patients and that patients learn to want. Medicare reimbursement for them feeds demand for them. By law, Medicare must pay for every cancer drug the FDA approves, and most private insurers follow Medicare in this regard.[42] Cancer is primarily a disease of later life: adults age fifty-five and over account for more than 75 percent of all cancers.[43] Of the 13,397,159 cases of invasive cancer in 2011, almost half involved patients over seventy.[44] In an aging population it is inevitable that more older persons are receiving cancer treatments than ever before. And because in the foreseeable future one out of two men and more than one out of three women will be diagnosed with some form of cancer,[45] and also because old age is not a reason to ignore disease or stop treatment, cancer drugs are an economic boon for the manufacturers.

The *Economist* reported in 2011 on income from cancer drugs: "Last year Gleevec grossed $4.3 billion. Roche's Herceptin (the HER2 drug) and Avastin did even better: $6 billion and $7.4 billion respectively. Cancer drugs could rescue big drugmakers from a tricky situation: more than $50 billion-worth of wares will lose patent protection in the next three years."[46] Provenge (sipuleucel-T), manufactured by Dendreon, a drug for prostate cancer that has spread beyond the prostate gland, costs $93,000 per treatment. In a clinical trial it was shown to increase survival by four months on average, compared with a placebo.[47] Avastin, (bevacizumab), created by Genentech (and now owned by Roche), costs about $88,000 a year for the treatment of metastatic breast cancer.[48] And Herceptin, made by Roche, costs about $40,000 per patient per year.[49] Cancer drugs are highly remunerative, and older patients are the growing market for them.

The Movable Goalposts of "Good Enough" Evidence and Benefit:
Avastin and the Politics of Access

The Food and Drug Administration is a crucial gatekeeper controlling access to the market for all drugs and devices. It sets the goalposts, and the stakes are extremely high for drug and device manufacturers. A complex politics of access is linked to their ability to show the FDA their "evidence of benefit." Yet, in the final analysis, it may be that the strongest player in this politics of access is the one that is masquerading as evidence: the ubiquitous ethical field. Where the goalposts end up is decided amid a cultural tension over how conflicting values are put into practice. This process is well illustrated by the Avastin case.

In 2010–11 the biotech company Genentech sought FDA approval to use the drug Avastin to treat metastatic breast cancer; what transpired shows how those high stakes play out when claims regarding a product's benefits are made in the interest of the corporate bottom line. Aggressive industry activism throughout the biomedical economy is not new, of course, and it has had far-reaching significance for what happens at the bedside—as a host of examples, from silicone breast implants to Vioxx, have shown.[50] The Avastin-FDA example centered on the question What constitutes scientific evidence for therapeutic benefit, and who decides?, and it reveals the tricky ethical terrain embedded in the science of determining "best evidence."

In the Avastin case Genentech attempted to renegotiate the ethical contours of scientific evidence and therapeutic benefit in its effort to get the drug approved for treatment of metastatic breast cancer. A furor erupted in the clinical science world in response. In a nutshell, years earlier Avastin had been approved for colon and lung cancer and then later (in 2008) for an expanded use to treat metastatic breast cancer. But conditions were attached to the expanded use: the FDA required additional clinical trials to clearly show treatment benefit. Not satisfied that those trials showed sufficient benefit, in 2010 the FDA withdrew the expanded use approval. Genentech appealed, arguing, in essence, that the goalposts for what constitutes good enough trials evidence should be moved.

The boundaries of what constitutes evidence are always being pushed, of course—by scientists, by government, by activists of all sorts, and today by industry. But the Avastin example is particularly illustrative of how market forces and political negotiations and choices can facilitate or prevent the conversion of research outcomes into scientific evidence for health care. It is important because the stakes are life.

The Avastin case demonstrates the joining of two major forces: the market and ordinary medicine's bureaucracy of control—in this case, the FDA. To be sure, AIDS activists had argued that drugs not yet FDA-approved (by the then-standard means of completed clinical trials) were good enough for them. Their efforts sparked a grassroots-initiated change in the organization of ordinary medicine—specifically in the value and meaning of evidence making, standard setting, and need—moving it toward what the activists considered to be the public good, that is, faster access to experimental therapies. There is no question that, in that example, the actions of sick people shaped our civic life, especially how we think about our relationship to scientific evidence and the right to treatment.

The Avastin-FDA encounter, however, was an *industry-initiated attempt* to use ordinary medicine to benefit the bottom line. AIDS patients wanted to try drugs that were still experimental. The makers of Avastin claimed their product offered *enough benefits* to be put on the market. At stake for Genentech (and by extension the industry as a whole) was the question of how *good enough* scientific evidence is determined. The FDA's response to Genentech's claims of benefit would affect future government rulings on and the public's perception of what constitutes good enough therapy for people's health.

The Food and Drug Administration has a conflicted mandate: it is entrusted by the public to get new, beneficial treatments to consumers as quickly as possible, while at the same time it is the authorized national gatekeeper mandated to thoroughly evaluate the safety of our food and medical interventions before they reach the market. AIDS activism complicated and blurred the boundary between those tasks by bringing new therapies to sick patients prior to completion of the traditional (at the time) evaluative process. The result was " 'confusion about what we, as a society use FDA approval for.' Was the purpose of the FDA . . . to *permit* access to a drug, or to *recommend* a drug as the standard of care?"[51] Today those gatekeeping and access roles remain intact, and they continue to be in tension and subject to new challenges, such as that posed by Avastin. The FDA must respond to emerging treatments by evaluating them, and those evaluations are entangled with the rising power of private industry (as well as with the ever-present pressures from taxpayers, the U.S. Congress, and many special interests groups).[52]

Over time the FDA has refined its criteria for considering what counts as beneficial treatment for patients, and thus, also over time, it has reconsidered and changed the rules for drug approval. It has "moved the goalposts," as one oncologist aptly characterized it to me. In 1991, in response to the fact that "one person dies of AIDS in the United States every 8 minutes" and to the unrelenting pressure from AIDS activists to speed up the approval process,[53] the FDA issued a new policy of *conditional* approval—conditional pending provision of additional required evidence that a drug was safe and beneficial. This new category of drug approval was a strategy for both managing the uncertainty inherent in new, untried drugs and giving a green light to certain promising interventions by letting patients have the use of them more quickly than the previous approval process was set up to allow. This new category of approval was lauded by AIDS patients and their supporters, but some observers expressed concern that conditional approval, in the words of Congressman Henry Waxman, "could allow promotion and sale of drugs that did not meet previous standards for safety and efficacy."[54]

At about the same time, the FDA endorsed the use of CD4 counts as a "surrogate" marker for demonstrating the effectiveness of new AIDS drugs.[55] A surrogate or substitute endpoint takes the place of one that is too difficult to measure routinely in a clinical trial, for example, overall survival in the case of AIDS, whereas in cancer studies survival time is the gold standard and primary endpoint. The need for surrogate endpoints was hotly debated in the AIDS research community in 1990–91 because there was stark evidence that "body count trials with survival as an endpoint simply were no longer *feasible*, regardless of whether they were desirable. 'Survival . . . studies with each passing day of this epidemic become less and less possible. As more data accumulate on each of these drugs, as we take more time to compare one to the next, fewer and fewer patients are willing to sit still in studies that take two to three years.' "[56] Debate ensued because some researchers and clinicians were concerned that approval of drugs on that basis would open the floodgates for drug companies to press the FDA for approval without adequate data to back up their studies.[57]

Yet because, as one activist noted, "scientific uncertainty is no excuse for inaction . . . we cannot wait for 'proof,' "[58] what had qualified as good enough evidence, good enough patient safety, and good enough U.S. government criteria for drug approval all became moving targets subject to ethical-political negotiation. In 1992 conditional approval was transformed into *accelerated* approval as FDA officials further acknowledged the impact of AIDS. This move was referred to (both positively and negatively) as marking the advent of the "new FDA."[59]

For cancer treatments in particular, the FDA has moved the goalposts in two ways in its effort to make cancer drugs more rapidly available to patients. First, accelerated approval became a new kind of regulatory action applicable to oncology drugs that seemed *likely* to provide benefit over existing therapies. Once pharmaceutical companies were given the okay for accelerated approval, they would be required to conduct additional, follow-up clinical trials to confirm that the drug indeed provided benefit. Regular approval would be granted, the FDA ruled in 1992, only if confirmatory studies proved benefit. From that year through 2010 the FDA granted accelerated approval of thirty-five cancer drugs designated for forty-seven new disease indications.[60]

In 2002 the FDA introduced the second goalpost move, a new endpoint for accelerated approval of oncology treatments: *progression free survival.*[61] This term designates the time from the start of treatment to the recurrence of tumor growth, and it was introduced as a surrogate endpoint in clinical trials in 2002 for the drug Gleevec (imatinib), used to treat chronic myelogenous leukemia. Progression-free survival (PFS) trials measure how long people survive without any worsening at all of the cancer (for example, growth of the tumor or worsening of other empirical measures of disease progression). As a *substitute* for actual, improved survival or for better quality of life,[62] PFS thus gained a foothold as a new "end" in the cancer clinical trials process. Regarding the decision to accept PFS as an endpoint, the director of the FDA's Office of Oncology Drug Products stated, "Although improvement in overall survival remains the gold standard . . . *delay in disease progression*" can be considered a "surrogate" for clinical benefit.[63] It was the advent of specifically targeted drugs (such as Gleevec) that fostered the search for alternative endpoints to replace overall survival and contributed to industry's need to find a means to speed up drug study reviews.[64]

Such goalpost moves occurred within a culture of experimentation that, since the 1970s, had become increasingly prominent in the world of oncology—a world in which growing numbers of physicians could participate in clinical trials and in which patients were beginning to learn (even before AIDS) that trials were "last chance" treatments.[65] At the same time, "advanced cancer" and "terminal cancer" started to be perceived as separate entities, first within the field of oncology and then in the minds of patients, to the point that "advanced cancer and the moment of dying came to be disconnected."[66] Moreover our understanding of the dividing line between the uses of chemotherapy and palliative care has shifted over the past half century. Often, perhaps mostly, today dying is not conceived of at the beginning of metastatic disease but much later in the trajectory of illness. That conceptual shift paved the way for the FDA moves in which the use of treatments, whether experimental or approved and reimbursed, approaches closer to the moment of death.[67]

Within these changing cultural parameters PFS was thus well positioned to be a categorical FDA response both to consumers' demand for access to potentially helpful drugs and to the pharmaceutical industry's pressure to shorten the amount of time (which had been growing ever longer) from a drug's discovery to getting it on the market. It was, in some respects, a radical move on the part of the FDA because, as some have argued, it allowed for a broader, or lower, standard for drug approval than evidence of overall survival. That is, it allowed goals other than the actual survival of a patient to represent *good enough science*.[68]

Genentech's push for Avastin's FDA approval explicitly connected the drive for good enough science to good enough and therefore acceptable, reimbursable, and needed therapy. Avastin got accelerated FDA approval in 2008 for use in treating metastatic breast cancer, following a Genentech-sponsored study showing that, given in combination with another chemotherapy agent, it extended the time from the start of treatment to disease recurrence by about five months. That is, it showed a modest amount of PFS, though it did not lengthen overall survival time for breast cancer patients with advanced disease.

But that same study also showed that Avastin was associated with life-threatening side effects, especially severe high blood pressure and hemorrhaging. That prompted the FDA to require Genentech to conduct two additional clinical trials in order to provide supplemental evidence of the therapy's safety record and its benefit to patients, whether in terms of overall survival, quality of life, or progression-free survival time. Those two additional trials did not show the same degree of PFS benefit demonstrated in the earlier study, and, in short, "patients didn't live longer, and they didn't live better."[69] The FDA withdrew Avastin's approval for advanced metastatic breast cancer.

In an unprecedented move Genentech contested the revocation by submitting an appeal to the FDA in late 2010. It argued that the benefits of even a small amount of PFS, even amid debate over the degree of its benefit, should be *good enough scientific evidence* for Avastin to be issued regular approval, regardless of the follow-up studies' significant negative findings. It wanted the FDA to review the studies again, specifically with this argument in mind.[70] Thus, in filing its appeal Genentech also introduced what it considered to be a new *good enough ethics* into the equation of drug policy review and the making of ordinary therapy; that is, evidence from the trials showing small or equivocal benefits and significant negative effects, including death, should be considered *enough* evidence. A great deal was at stake. Genentech was poised to lose $500 million to $1 billion a year in earnings if the FDA did not alter its decision.[71] In November 2011 the FDA confirmed its earlier decision, and the drug was not approved for use in metastatic breast cancer.

The result of Genentech's appeal has implications well beyond the company's loss of enormous profits. The appeal claimed that Avastin showed *enough* progression-free survival to be viewed as "an acceptable measure of direct, clinical benefit."[72] The potential ramifications of appealing an FDA decision on that basis—ramifications for the goals of cancer research and for the FDA's credibility as a means of upholding scientific standards and enhancing public health—are as yet unknown.

More broadly some observers noted (echoing the earlier criticism of substitute endpoints made during the AIDS crisis) that if the Genentech argument had persuaded the FDA to alter its approval policy for drug marketing by moving the goalposts yet again, then the agency would find it more difficult to require its higher standard—*overall survival*—as an endpoint in future study reviews. Such a decision would have opened the floodgates to putting more drugs on the market, drugs that had not been proven to increase quality of life or actual survival and that could have debilitating or lethal side effects.

Because all the drivers of ordinary medicine are interconnected, the outcome of the Avastin appeal is far from cut and dried. Avastin actually remains on the market for metastatic breast cancer and it is reimbursed by Medicare and some other insurers when doctors prescribe it for breast cancer patients off-label—that is, for conditions not approved by the FDA. This adds even more confusion to patients' understanding of the drug's life-prolonging value and confounds the final FDA decision to rescind approval. The drug's continued use for breast cancer is made possible by just one of myriad intricacies of Medicare reimbursement policy; in this matter, reimbursement is guided not by the FDA but, ultimately, by guidelines put out by the National Comprehensive Cancer Network, whose panel on Avastin "voted unanimously in favor of continuing to recommend it as a breast cancer therapy."[73]

The quandary of crossing the line that this book investigates weaves through the history of cancer treatments, especially chemotherapy, for that history is one of changing responses to the question: When facing near and certain death, where does one draw the line between prolonging life and prolonging death? Debates about the uses of chemotherapy have centered on that question since the 1950s.[74] While the issue of control over the right to live, the right to die, and the right to treatment remains contentious in the United States, the Genentech-FDA struggle over authority and control reveals that the politics of access has an impact on the work, the ethics, and the evaluation of clinical science itself. And the politics of access influences where doctors decide to draw the line and how patients and families respond.

Old Age, Trial Access, and Physicians' Postprogress Quandaries

Never before have so many people reached their seventies and eighties in such relatively good health. This is due primarily to two factors: first, the early and mid-twentieth-century development of childhood vaccination, antibiotics, and treatments for lethal cardiac disease and pneumonia; second, the promotions, especially later in the twentieth century, urging preventive activities (stop smoking, reduce fats, get more exercise, take statins, get screenings, etc.). Advanced age, however, is also accompanied by inevitable frailties—failing hearts, emerging cancers, other chronic illnesses, dementias, end-stage diseases of all sorts—and, significantly, by high expectations of medicine that are fueled by evidence that it can push away the symptoms of old age and death at ever older ages.[75]

Medicine is responding to all of this with high-tech and low-tech treatments, many of them life-prolonging, some potentially so. The burgeoning market for cancer treatments provides just one example of how the biomedical-cultural-economic behemoth is doing its work to offer treatments in a society whose most rapidly growing age group is over eighty. And it is difficult for doctors, patients, and families to say no to any treatment. The high stakes of life, the ethos of *more is better*, and the great success of life-extending treatments all ensure that difficulty stays robust.

Although great weight is given to scientific evidence in the treatment of later-life lethal conditions, ordinary medicine—the determinative standards and routines now set by clinical trials, the evidence they produce, and the politics inherent in both—erases a crucial, related fact: the burgeoning elderly population is itself mostly excluded from access to and participation in clinical trials. The status afforded the elderly *as research material* constitutes the prime exception to the medicocultural push for scientific evidence in medicine. Yet older persons have the most diseases, take the most drugs, and receive the most treatments in general. They exhibit great variation in their responses to diseases and interventions. They generally have more complex medical conditions than younger persons. They use the most health care resources; one geriatrician remarked to me that in his experience the frail elderly use about 90 percent of health care resources today. They account for more adverse drug events than do younger people, given that multiple drug interactions are not well understood, especially in older, frail bodies that experience more intense drug side effects.[76] "In an ideal world," one report stated, "data from clinical drug trials would describe how a given drug is likely to affect older patients differently from younger ones."[77] In that same ideal world that data would also explain the variances among older individuals in their response to treatments. Yet there is a big gap in such knowledge.

Both the FDA and the NIH have been slow to initiate reform in that regard. In 1989 the FDA issued a guideline to include older patients in clinical trials. Eight years later the agency stated in the Federal Register, "The medical community has become increasingly aware that prescription drugs can produce effects in elderly patients that are significantly different from those produced in younger patients. . . . People over 65 constitute only 12 percent of the U.S. population . . . [yet] they consume over 30 percent of the prescription drug products sold in this country."[78] A decade later those over sixty-five made up 13 percent of the U.S. population and were consuming more than 40 percent of prescription drugs.[79] By the late 1990s a number of studies showed that older persons were significantly underrepresented in clinical research.[80]

In response to this gap, the federal government under President Clinton directed Medicare to begin covering the costs of clinical trial participation for seniors in 2000.[81] Yet in 2002 Robert Butler, the founding director of the NIH's National Institute on Aging and (before his death in 2010) perhaps the most well-known advocate for older persons' participation in clinical trials, noted that there were still no requirements "to ensure that new drugs and treatment are tested in older people or that older people are represented in such research."[82] He and others suggested that the NIH establish formal guidelines for the inclusion of older persons in NIH-sponsored research. But no such formal guidelines yet exist, and, with few exceptions, the most recent studies also document the lack of representation of older persons in clinical trials of all sorts.[83]

Indeed the vast majority of clinical trials specifically exclude individuals over seventy-five, and most do not enroll anyone over seventy. There are several reasons for this. Clinical trials have specific inclusion criteria in order to be able to test the effects of the intervention under investigation with as little interference as possible from other treatments or diseases. Also the research subjects must be as similar to one another as possible in terms of their exact disease state. The multiple conditions and medications typical of many older people can confound research results, making it impossible to discern which outcomes result from the therapy being tested and which result from confounding factors introduced by the study subject. Older people may not tolerate intensive therapies as well as younger persons and thus may need to drop out of experiments before the research is completed. Or they may die before the end of a study. All in all, they present plenty of obstacles to the efficient conduct of research and to the interpretation of data about the benefits or harms of experimental therapies. Those factors make their participation in clinical trials more challenging and cumbersome for researchers and study sponsors, who want to enroll participants whose specific conditions will contribute clearly to knowledge about the efficacy of a treatment.

For their part, drug manufacturers do not want to fund studies (which cost millions of dollars and take years to complete) whose participants will not respond as positively as possible to experimental treatments.[84] The very old are less likely to be the vehicle for demonstrating "good" evidence for a treatment, and it is easier to obtain favorable study outcomes or unequivocally positive results from a trial that excludes older people. As a result, one oncologist noted, when people over seventy are included in clinical trials, research investigators sometimes make judgments about which older persons to enroll, preferring a very fit seventy-five-year-old to a frail person of that age.

Physicians in all specialties who treat the elderly are well aware of the lack of correspondence between clinical trial study populations and their own patients. One geriatrician summarized it thus:

Not many studies have been done on this population, and that's my concern. Those of us who take care of people in this age group, especially people over eighty, have to use data that was developed in studies in a younger population. We have to try to abstract it to the person in front of us. And it's hard.

Any new treatment, unless you test it with controls, is just your feeling. So, for instance, say you had a study that recruited a thousand people between the ages of eighty and eighty-five, and we treated one group with the usual medical treatment and the other group with stents, and they all had the same problem, same symptoms, and same follow-up. And then at the end of five years, the study showed that the people with stents lived longer, had fewer complications, had fewer days in the hospital, had less decline in function, then, yeah, it would help us a lot. But I can't use similar data taken from sixty- to sixty-five-year-olds, or sixty-five- to seventy-year-olds and translate that to an eighty- to eighty-five-year-old.

A cardiologist echoed that predicament:

In general the data that we use to make decisions on is only minimally age adjusted. There has been a trend to include some older people in some angioplasty studies, but in general, they are excluded from the studies that we use for decision making. And you can see immediately the fallacy of making decisions about someone who is twenty or twenty-five years older than the mean age of the group that has been in a research study. A lot of times studies are quoted which are not really appropriate to the patient that is being considered. . . . There's very little data on the over-eighty group.

For example, there are now studies that show very clearly that people who have rest angina [chest pain while at rest], particularly if they have some abnormality, will have, in general, their life prolonged, or a reduction in subsequent clinical events, if they have angioplasty. So even in elderly people who are very sick you're going to be considerably more aggressive. There is a greater tendency, even among conservative cardiologists, to be interventional, especially if the patient is literally suffering, having recurrent chest pain, not doing well.

So older patients are more likely to reap both benefits and harms from the many new therapies emerging from clinical trials, treatments not tested on members of their age cohort. They receive treatments proven to be effective yet not for those at higher ages. The generalizability of research findings, an important tenet of evidence-based medicine, simply does not hold in the case of the old. Nevertheless the value of generalizability is an essential ingredient in the making of ordinary medicine. It determines a great deal of medical practice and patient experience.

———

The increasing influence of industry in biomedical research, the importance of all the evidence-based research findings for patient care, and the explosion in the numbers of clinical trials conducted all contribute to the first transformation in the chain of health care drivers: the conversion of research outcomes into scientific evidence for best treatments. That evidence in turn determines Medicare insurance reimbursement policies, the second transformative link in the chain of logic by which effective therapies—however they are measured—become standard in the world of ordinary medicine.

4

"REIMBURSEMENT IS CRITICAL FOR EVERYTHING"

Medicare and the Ethics of Managing Life

_____

An accepted procedure really means that insurance
will pay for it.
—Physician's comment to author

For a growing segment of the U.S. population, older patients and their families, Medicare coverage and reimbursement policies have become fundamental to the way life is lived and can be lived. This is because life-threatening conditions are common among older individuals, because treatments for those conditions are now so ordinary, and because Medicare provides payment for so many of those treatments. Perhaps more than any other institution, Medicare, through its reimbursement guidelines, its mechanisms for organizing coverage, and its policymaking committees, is instrumental to the ways old age, medical treatment, and dying unfold in the United States. It guides how physicians practice medicine, and, more than ever before, it shapes a great deal about how people in the United States experience late life. Thus, at its core, Medicare plays a central role in the ethics of managing life because its coverage policies determine which potentially life-extending therapies become standard treatments for older citizens.

Simply put, older people see doctors, which in our aging society is why increasing numbers of us, patients, doctors, and families alike, are directly affected by the fee-for-service, procedure-driven reimbursement policies that reflect Medicare's approach to health care delivery. For decades many commentators have bemoaned this approach, noting that it emphasizes the use of technology to the detriment of caring practices, rewards medical specialists rather than general practitioners and internists, encourages doctors to focus on diseases and body parts rather than on whole persons, and is driving the rising cost of health care delivery. Yet while some among us might bemoan the plethora of diagnostic tests that are requested and routinely employed—what many have called the "overuse" of technologies—no one with Medicare insurance complains about the access it provides to potentially life-extending interventions, regardless of cost or the age and medical condition of the patient. Medicare's ethics of managing life is made concrete in the access it provides to life-extending treatments without cost or age limits.

Medicare insurance, then, is the next link in the powerful chain of health care drivers, and Medicare reimbursement policies highlight the next three transformations in the chain: how evidence becomes *reimbursable* and how reimbursed treatments then become *standard* medicine and *necessary* therapies.

From Trials Evidence to Reimbursable Treatment: The Second Transformation

Within the burgeoning medical marketplace, two phenomena strongly reinforce the commonly held view that death can always be averted and that the symptoms of disease in late life can be minimized or erased. The first is the vehicle through which new treatments reach doctors and patients, that is, the health insurance industry, but especially Medicare. Medicare reimbursement decisions—the next link after biomedical research in the chain of U.S. health care drivers—transform scientific evidence into therapies that are delivered to patients. They are the mechanism that makes treatments acceptable among doctors and available to patients and pave the way for widespread use of treatments.

The second phenomenon is the profound effect that the "technological imperative," as applied in medicine, has on the culture of medical practice. Coined by the health economist Victor Fuchs in 1968, the term *technological imperative* refers to the particularly American dependence on, lure of, and unwavering commitment to powerful new (and costly) medical technologies, a dependence shared by both the U.S. health care enterprise and the American public. Fuchs's term captures the way determinations about what is appropriate therapy—including for the very old—are driven by the availability of technological solutions (especially the newest and most advanced) and the value accorded to them.[1] (I describe the imperative's features and impact later.)

The two ethical decisions undergirding the Medicare program, which came into being in 1965, were, first, that "it was incumbent on government to guarantee health care for the elderly,"[2] and second, that the cost of drugs, devices, procedures, and all treatments would not determine how, when, and how much technology was used. In the industrialized world this ethical decision—to provide government payment for medical care to the elderly (and for the poor through Medicaid) with no cost limitations—was and remains unique in that if a treatment is deemed useful, Medicare has a moral imperative to pay for it. That mandate is the core value of the Medicare program.[3]

Together insurance reimbursement and the technological imperative have made possible an explosion in the number of available life-extending treatments and have added wanted years to millions of older people's lives.[4] Thus Medicare plays a dual role in shaping our thinking that death can be pushed away or even made obsolete; it brings us new treatments that quickly become standards of care, and it fosters the value and necessity of those treatments.

Because Medicare reimbursement policies also determine coverage decisions among private insurers, Medicare is the essential transformative link, the fulcrum point between the evidence created by research and what becomes standard, ordinary, and accessible medicine. Technologies of all sorts—from low-tech feeding tubes to the most expensive imaging machines and implantable devices—become widely employed by doctors *only if* insurance will pay for them. As a consequence many interventions are used *because* insurance will cover them. An oncologist described to me how this process works in his specialty:

> Insurers decide to cover the cost of drugs based on their algorithms, but things have gotten very complex and they can't read through all the studies. About twenty years ago the National Comprehensive Cancer Network was formed among twenty-one leading cancer centers. One reason for this was a concern that academic medical centers were becoming dinosaurs. A goal of the network was to create, based on panels of experts sifting through the research, guidelines for treatment, both to show that academic centers were and would continue to be the leading edge in cancer therapies and were not becoming irrelevant, and to codify standards of care. But really, the reason for the creation of guidelines is to get insurance coverage. The insurance companies follow the guidelines.

In this context "follow the guidelines" means that if a drug or procedure becomes part of a practice guideline, has been established as such by a panel of experts, it will be reimbursed by Medicare. Private insurance will follow Medicare's lead, thus providing coverage for Medicare-approved procedures for persons younger than sixty-five. Practicing oncologists base their choices of treatments for individual patients, regardless of age, on a number of factors, but the essential one is whether the drug or procedure is covered by insurance.

A liver specialist described to me the role insurance reimbursement played in the development of liver transplantation as a standard therapy for liver cancer:

> A procedure that expensive, well over $200,000, cannot be done in any routine way without the money behind it. In the 1980s one of the big reasons liver transplant became accepted as a therapeutic procedure is because insurance would pay for it. It was one of the most expensive procedures in medicine. Such a procedure needed insurance backup—otherwise, who was going to get it? And the insurance, of course, would not allow it unless the research evidence backed it up, it had FDA approval, and it was shown to be a lifesaving last resort.

Thus Medicare coverage decisions are the key to what becomes standard, appropriate, and, very quickly, *needed* medical intervention. Liver transplantation, similar to all other procedures, became accepted, routine, and necessary because Medicare and private insurance would pay for it. And Medicare pays for it because it clearly prolongs lives and the cultural value and societal demand that it be reimbursed is built into the very structure of the Medicare program. For all those reasons limitations on this and any other expensive intervention are, in today's political environment, unspeakable.

Payment policies not only establish what doctors do and do not recommend, but they are also the gatekeepers to life-extending interventions, and as such they inform our choices about what to do and our sensibilities about how to live, though most of us are completely unaware of that influence. That influence is strong, however, and the effects of Medicare coverage policies are actually even more far-ranging, in that they organize what patients and families come to want and to worry about. They frame our thinking about family responsibility and the "naturalness" of life-extending procedures for those already in later life. Because the policies guide us (or many of us) to reduce disease risks, they strengthen the value of risk reduction. They influence both physicians and consumers to minimize the risk of death—not only for those who smoke, are obese, or have high blood pressure, for example, but also for those who are frail, ill, very old, and would otherwise be near the end of a "natural" life. Medicare policies inspire the desire for more control over the last portion of the life span, and they allow us to pursue and choose "more" time as we grow old.

Mrs. Ames: From Evidence-Based Logic to Medicare Policy and Treatment Pathways

---

Four years after a series of interferon treatments cured her of the hepatitis C virus, Mrs. Doris Ames, age seventy-one, still had cirrhosis (scarring) of the liver, which was worsening, and she had liver cancer. Mrs. Ames had proactively started the interferon treatments. Now, she told the liver specialist in the exam room, she had come to the clinic because of the cancer, and she wanted a liver transplant. The liver specialist (hepatologist) explained, "You were very lucky to have gotten rid of the hepatitis C virus. It comes back after transplant if you haven't gotten rid of it completely, and there is still a small chance it could come back, even after transplant."[5] He continued, "Now you ask, 'Why do I have to wait for a transplant if I have cancer?' The answer is because we can treat the cancer with chemotherapy, keep it in check while you wait for a transplant according to UNOS criteria."

The physician was explaining that short term cancer treatments were necessary to keep the disease from spreading beyond the liver while the patient waited for her name to come to the top of the waiting list administered by the United Network for Organ Sharing (UNOS), the national pool for allocation and distribution of cadaveric donor organs.[6] The physician said, "You have to be monitored very carefully. CT scans every three months; chemoembolization if there are tumors. Our job is to put you in the best possible position for a transplant."

The chemoembolization (chemotherapy delivered by catheter directly into the liver tumors) is both a therapy to control the spread of cancer and an enabling technology. It can be used periodically to knock out the cancer tumors or reduce their size, and the aim is to keep the size and location of the cancer within the evidence-based criteria for a successful transplant, which Mrs. Ames hoped would cure her of the disease.

Liver cancer in which the tumors are beyond a certain size or are located outside of the liver is not curable with transplantation, according to contemporary research evidence, and in such cases transplantation would not be covered by Medicare. Thus the goal of the chemotherapy treatments is to prevent worsening disease in order to help ensure access to a scarce resource.

Mrs. Ames's physician continued, "If you're not in [UNOS and Medicare] criteria for transplant, we treat you until the tumors are knocked out, or reduced in size, so that you *are* in criteria. If you are in criteria, we put you on the waiting list for an organ." That rationale reflects the evidence-based criteria both for transplantation's being medically appropriate, thus establishing eligibility to receive and benefit from a new liver, and for its being within the Medicare reimbursement guidelines for the procedure.

In the ensuing months Mrs. Ames was listed for a transplant because she wanted one and because the size of her tumors was within Medicare coverage criteria for transplantation. She still had to wait for her name to come to the top of the regional waiting list. During that waiting period (frequently nine to twelve months in dense urban centers but a shorter time in less populated regions of the country) her cancer would have to be monitored and treated so that it did not spread beyond the liver. If she were to become sicker while she waited for a deceased donor organ, her daughter, whose offer to donate part of her own liver to her mother had been quickly accepted, would undergo testing for donor appropriateness. A living donation could take place much sooner, and Medicare covers costs for the donor.[7]

Medicare reimbursement rules organize access to organs, allow payment for surgery and follow-up treatment, and shape ideas among clinicians, patients, and families about the value of transplantation at older ages. By defining which procedures are eligible for reimbursement, Medicare policy transforms evidence-based logic into what doctors will undertake, recommend, and prescribe and what patients "choose," want, or reject. Thus, as an appropriate lifesaving therapy, transplantation could only come into existence, could only be perceived as *needed* when it became the state-of-the-art treatment for certain kinds of cancer and other liver diseases—*because* Medicare began to routinely pay for it.

Behind the Scenes: How Medicare Works

Medicare policy can be thought of as a legitimating tool, a means to rationalize and organize particular courses of action.[8] Here is how that tool works: The results of evidence-based clinical studies are continually reviewed by committees working through the Centers for Medicare and Medicaid Services (CMS), which administers the Medicare program. Those committees decide national Medicare payment policy. Yet many decisions are made at the regional level "by local carriers, the private companies that process Medicare claims. Thus it is entirely possible that a procedure will be paid for in one part of the country but not in another, even when used for the same reason. A national decision is made, which is binding on all carriers only if specifically requested" by the CMS, the pharmaceutical, device, or biotech company that is promoting the new therapy, or by physician groups.[9] Whether at the local or national level, the constantly emerging new evidence for beneficial therapies allows and encourages the Medicare program to expand the number and kind of interventions that it will cover. So when liver transplantation, cardiac devices, and new cancer drugs, for example, show evidence of benefit in studies, and if they are approved by the FDA,[10] the CMS allows payment and sets reimbursement rates for them.

Of course we want the insurance industry, both government and private, to respond to developments in research, to be guided by the scientific evidence. We want our doctors to use that evidence in determining our treatments. There simply is no alternative in a twenty-first-century democratic state. Yet the logic of using statistical evidence to determine treatment has significantly shaped the dysfunction, inequality, and no longer tenable financing of our health care delivery system. Relentlessly rising health care costs are due, in large part, to the fact that in its response to the first link in our chain—the all-encompassing, evidence-based apparatus of quantifiable truth making that the biomedical research industry has emphasized—Medicare is constantly expanding what it will pay for.[11] The organization of the biomedical economy, with its emphasis on new technologies and expanded patient populations, sets up the ethics of reimbursement and clinical practice and prioritizes the thinking of doctors and patients alike. It does not and cannot discriminate among kinds of evidence and kinds of patients. While there is no doubt that millions of patients benefit from the treatments Medicare covers, neither the research enterprise nor Medicare payment policies focuses on the implications for medical care and well-being in an aging society of the technology-oriented, technology-heavy trend in reimbursement decisions.

The CMS committees continually recalibrate the kinds of treatments Medicare will pay for and the types of diseases and conditions it will allow under its coverage umbrella.[12] Different kinds of factors contribute to the process through which payments for treatment are decided. New discoveries in the laboratory, clinical trial results, and data on additional evidence-based outcomes are all central to the making of reimbursement decisions, but pressures brought to bear by members of Congress, physician lobbying groups, proactive consumers, the device and pharmaceutical industries, and the private insurance industry also play their part. The materials scrutinized by the CMS committees include published and unpublished studies, clinical guidelines, clinical trials, technology assessments, and other sources of expert opinion.[13] They may also include technology assessments from the government's Agency for Healthcare Research and Quality and recommendations from the Medicare Coverage Advisory Committee. The latter is an independent committee of experts (scientists, physicians, ethicists, economists, and others) established in 1999 which meets in public to consider coverage criteria for treatments. The results of its proceedings are posted on the Internet.[14]

It remains true, however, that the CMS's evidence-based assessments of the overall risks and benefits of an intervention are the most important factor in determining reimbursement.[15] Importantly when industry accumulates quantifiable clinical trial evidence showing benefit for the use of a specific drug, procedure, or device, that increases the pressure on Medicare and other large payers to expand coverage. For example, although the cumulative results from a total of nine clinical trials of ICD use (conducted between 2002 and 2005) showed varying degrees of benefit among patient populations that had *not* experienced a life-threatening arrhythmia, when taken together those trials provided increasing evidence of benefit, and thus for ICD cost reimbursement. Pressure on the insurance industry also comes from physicians, along with the medical institutions in which they work, both of which want and need to respond to emerging evidence based research findings.[16] Finally, despite the elaborate process by which the CMS evaluates evidence, there are no criteria for what constitutes "reasonable and necessary" treatment—the wording used in the original 1965 Medicare statute.[17] According to some observers, private industry has blocked efforts by some health policy analysts to define that phrase. Others note that it is not necessary to define specific criteria as long as the reimbursement decision-making process is open and accountable.[18]

As already noted, private insurance schemes largely follow Medicare's lead.[19] Over time Medicare approves more disease treatments and more interventions for risk reduction to avoid or at least postpone death. In our aging society, as more people turn sixty-five and thus have the opportunity to access more therapeutic options for life extension, Medicare paves the way for more people to live longer. This, in short, is its culturally sacred value. At the same time, Medicare also paves the way for more family, physician, and societal concern about how much intervention is too much, and of course it paves the way for ever greater cost to the nation. These tensions are inherent in this second link in ordinary medicine's chain.

Payment Policies, "Choice," and the Ethics of Managing Life

Because Medicare reimburses doctors and hospitals for the services they provide, its coverage decisions have enabled intensive and aggressive therapies of all kinds to flourish. Those reimbursements have allowed and fostered the growth of specialties and subspecialties in medicine and all the support personnel and supportive programs in medical centers that those specialists require: nurses, social workers, technicians of all kinds, nutritionists, administrators and other office workers, physical and occupational therapy programs, cardiac rehabilitation programs, and so on. All this and more is what enables state-of-the-art, complex medical care to be undertaken in the first place and to be successful. Reimbursement policies make it possible for universities and hospitals to purchase expensive equipment so they can participate in state-of-the-art diagnosis and treatment and compete with other institutions, thereby attracting patients and referrals by doctors and garnering the huge sums required to operate complex treatment centers. For physicians that means offering and sometimes encouraging the use of life-sustaining treatments for patients at any age and any cost because evidence indicates that the treatments will prolong life and because Medicare sets no cost limitations on the treatments it will cover. Medicare does, however, set reimbursement rates and limits, and it does create rules for which kinds of centers and programs can perform certain complex procedures.

Medicare payment policies embody values and priorities about the kinds of structures of health care delivery that the government should support, such as cardiac, transplant, and cancer centers and the myriad research and clinical enterprises and attendant personnel that flow to and from them. Those policies also set priorities about which therapies are worth covering. Because Medicare reimbursement (and private insurance reimbursement) is organized by payment for specific procedures and therapies, doctors' day-to-day work is organized around offering and employing those interventions, more of which are always emerging.

INDIVIDUAL DECISION MAKING?

Because Medicare brings the logic of evidence-based therapeutics into its coverage policies, it creates both the infrastructure and the value for the linkage to occur among evidence, access, and standard making. The *individual* decision making by patients, families, and physicians that takes place downstream in clinics (and which has also been the focus of clinical bioethics) is thus already prefigured by Medicare's coverage policies and, crucially, by the kinds of technology-based evidence on which those policies rest. *Patient autonomy* invokes the importance of patient choice and participation in health care decision making, and in order to ensure that choice and participation the concept has been enshrined in a series of U.S. government reports that began in the 1970s and culminated in a 1990 federal law, the Patient Self-Determination Act.[20] But although it is given much weight in the public conversation about health care, patient autonomy does not really exist in some pure form in which patients can make treatment decisions uninfluenced by their degree of access to state-of-the-art medical care and unencumbered by social relationships, education, income, and other factors.

So, however much it is invoked, patient autonomy remains a misleading concept because it distracts from the fact that the "options" from which to "choose" are always already significantly determined by upstream choices, first by industry- and government-funded research and then by the production of evidence and by insurance reimbursement decisions. This is what my account of ordinary medicine aims to show. Medicare coverage policies themselves, based primarily on the latest scientific evidence and yet reflecting the circumstances and pressures described earlier, constitute an *ethical choice*. This feature of Medicare's decision making has been absent from public debate.

To see this decision making as ethical choice at work, take, for example, the recently approved, Medicare-covered, and very expensive cancer drugs that have been shown in some clinical trials to extend recipients' period of time without disease progression by weeks or months. Yet some approved expensive drugs have not been shown to lengthen life and frequently are accompanied by an array of toxic and even life-threatening side effects, as in the case of Avastin for metastatic breast cancer. For another example, consider the treatments (such as cardiac bypass surgery and ICD use) that have not been shown in research studies to benefit very elderly individuals yet continue to be covered by Medicare and thus are prescribed by doctors and wanted (or assented to) by elderly patients and their families.

THE IMPACTS OF SOCIETAL EXPECTATIONS
AND PHYSICIAN PRACTICE

The far-reaching effects of Medicare decision making are evident also in the relationship of Medicare-approved interventions to societal expectations. Many physicians have told me that patients and families influence or even dictate the treatments they receive by requesting interventions that they hope will thwart disease and death, regardless of whether the treatment has been proven in studies to be effective for their condition. Yet physicians also widely report that it is much easier and more "efficient" to give patients the treatments they ask for or seem to want—after all, the treatments are covered by Medicare and private insurance—than to hold the longer conversations that would be needed to explain that a requested intervention is not or may not be appropriate, that it carries serious risks and most likely will not lengthen life or cure disease. In this era of so-called patient autonomy, health care consumer awareness, and the ever-present specter of litigation, physicians learn to mention, and thus to offer, the treatments that are available—which means covered by insurance—even when they do not necessarily recommend some of them (for example, aggressive treatments for metastatic cancer in someone over eighty-five).

LONGEVITY AND MEDICARE'S BUILT-IN ETHICS

Because it includes more and more diseases and treatments under its reimbursement umbrella, Medicare makes it possible for more people to express the desire for longer life through their "choice" of interventions and to expect medicine to stave off death again and again. Medicare has enabled people to live longer and, as a result, to develop additional problems that later require more intervention, which Medicare will also pay for. Yet we can see the problematic ramifications of medicine's life-extending capabilities all around us: in the "epidemics" of Alzheimer's disease and heart failure that exist because medical interventions have enabled people to live long enough to suffer those consequences of old age; in the growing waiting lists for organs; in the profound responsibilities families shoulder for keeping patients alive and well after complex surgeries; in the ongoing care requirements, often lasting years, for the frail, dependent, and chronically ill elderly; in the growth of housing and support industries that offer assisted living, life care, long-term care, and memory care; and in the crisis of solvency that is facing the Medicare program itself because we spend too much money to prolong severe illness, end-stage disease, and dying. Such examples of medicine's limits as it comes up against Medicare's expansive reimbursement policies are all around us, yet we mostly prefer to ignore those realities and to think—still—of medicine as a series of progress-oriented "breakthroughs," with the next ones just around the corner. The coverage policies themselves, coupled with the media and our own expectations, feed that limiting perspective.

In essence Medicare brings into play values-based or moral decisions—by the government and by society—that have become normalized. Medicare's built-in ethics allows access to certain interventions in its payment policies. By means of its gatekeeping activities it legitimates certain life-extending treatments for certain groups. Medicare works as an instrument that (along with citizen interest groups and the U.S. Congress) facilitates the ever expanding use of life-extending procedures. Thus it also functions as a tool through which the U.S. government and taxpayers together shape the form and conduct of longevity making for themselves and their loved ones.

From Reimbursement to Standard and Necessary Treatment: The Third and Fourth Transformations

Following its transformation from evidence of benefit to reimbursable treatment, a reimbursable therapy almost instantly becomes the standard of care—which means that physicians and, immediately afterward, patients, will regard it as routine, appropriate, and state-of-the-art treatment.[21] That nearly instantaneous conceptual shift, from insurance pay-ment approval to standard, routine, and best intervention, is the third transformation in the chain of logic of health care delivery. Through this transformational move Medicare policy defines and continually re-defines both medical and popular thinking regarding which conditions are fatal, which are chronic, and which can be treated (as we have seen in the Dang, Carter, Tolleson, and Ames cases). Medicare's continual re-drawing of the boundary between treatable and fatal disease pushes that boundary line ever closer to the moment of death and makes the time for fighting disease and death last longer.

The fourth transformation occurs simultaneously, or nearly so, with the third: standard interventions immediately become *necessary treat-ments*. So not only does Medicare reimbursement policy define which conditions may be treated, thus making them standard-of-care practices, but it also defines which conditions *should* be treated. This latter shift creates the difficulty physicians, patients, and families face when consid-ering saying no to treatments because, once therapies are approved for use and are perceived as ordinary and routine, hope for survival and our deep-seated assumptions about medical progress adhere to those treat-ments. Patients and families think that if doctors (or the Internet or the media) mention a treatment, it must mean that it works to extend life.

BECOMING STANDARD AND NECESSARY:
STENTS FOR OLD HEARTS

For several decades the average age of persons who receive surgery and other aggressive interventions that extend life has been rising. The use of stents to open cardiac arteries is indicative of this trend and provides a clear example of the links connecting research on innovative technolo-gies to payment, standard use, and necessity. Stents are metal tubes or scaffold-like devices used to hold coronary arteries open so that blood can flow through them. Few consider it unusual to place stents (through a catheter inserted in the groin) in the coronary arteries of persons in their eighties, given that it is taking place in an environment in which more people than ever before are receiving them and cardiac interven-tions of all kinds have become so ordinary.[22] The more people in their eighties and nineties who receive stents, the more normal it becomes in the minds of doctors and older patients, and the less remarkable it seems to be for everyone in our aging society—as normal and standard as get-ting a flu shot. If stents are used routinely in late life to open cardiac vessels and thus, hopefully, to prevent heart attacks, if greater numbers of ever older adults are undergoing that procedure, then *not* having the procedure appears to be nonstandard, not rational, and an invitation to an "early" death. Who would condone that? Who would say no to the procedure?

Stents were first inserted into a human coronary artery in France in 1986. In 1994 they were approved for use in the United States and rapidly came into widespread use.[23] In the following decade new types of stent were developed, each more flexible and easier to insert into narrowed arteries than its predecessor. Drug-coated or medicated stents (called drug-eluting stents or DESS) were introduced in the United States in 2003. Coated with medication designed to prevent or slow the process of restenosis (the reclosing or reblocking of arteries over time), they were considered at the time of their introduction to be an advance over bare stents with no preventive medication. Debate has been lively and remains unresolved about the severity of the risk factors associated with medicated stents (in terms of causing blood clots or heart attacks) and whether DESS actually increase longevity compared to bare metal stents.[24]

The use of stents, drug-coated or not, provides a good example of the rapid and diffuse adoption of new technologies, from the creation of new devices and drugs to FDA and Medicare approval and widespread use as a standard therapy. In 2011 the cardiologist Rita Redberg, editor in chief of the *Archives of Internal Medicine*, described that transformational logic. She noted that it is only in retrospect, following at least several years of further studies, especially additional clinical trials, that therapies can be evaluated for their longer term negative effects and for their actual contribution to longevity:

> Since the Food and Drug Administration approved [in 2003] the use of DESS for discrete, new (i.e., previously untreated) partial blockages in patients' native coronary arteries (i.e., not in bypass grafts), and only in relatively large vessels, and the Centers for Medicare and Medicaid Services simultaneously approved payment, the increase in use of DESS has been meteoric. By 2005, DESS were over 90 percent of all first stents placed. It is estimated that more than 60 percent of DESS are placed for off-label indications and these patients have higher adverse event rates than on-label usage. . . . The cost of DESS is staggering, adding $1.57 billion to our national health care bill paid by taxpayers. It is time to clearly define what the value of this extraordinary

investment has been in terms of patient benefits and study the harms and determine if we are getting good value for this outlay.[25]

Writing in the *New York Times*, Redberg also noted:

> Multiple clinical trials have shown that cardiac stents are no more effective than drugs or lifestyle changes in preventing heart attacks or death. Although some studies have shown that stents provide short-term relief of chest pain, up to 30 percent of patients receiving stents have no chest pain to begin with, and thus derive no more benefit from this invasive procedure than from equally effective and far less expensive medicines. Risks associated with stent implantation, meanwhile, include exposure to radiation and to dyes that can damage the kidneys, and in rare cases, death from the stent itself. Yet one study estimated that Medicare spends $1.6 billion on drug-coated stents (the most common type of cardiac stents) annually.[26]

THE POWER—AND CONFUSION—OF EVIDENCE

Ordinary medicine is constituted and propelled by the production of evidence. Once produced, the use of that evidence is itself complicated by a number of features that are inherent in ordinary medicine and in the biomedical economy itself. For instance, negative findings from many studies are never reported (either on ClinicalTrials.gov or in scientific journals).[27] Even when negative findings are publicized, doctors still prescribe some drugs and devices despite their known lack of efficacy. Patients and families ask for treatments that have not been proven to show benefit. For its part, industry is slow to remove from the marketplace drugs and devices that lack benefit (or even prove to be harmful), and doctors may be slow to refuse to use them. Finally, once a treatment or procedure is reimbursed by Medicare, the dynamics of hospital and medical center economics, in addition to physician prescribing patterns, make it nearly impossible for all concerned to say no to it.

As already noted, Medicare is obligated to reimburse for interventions that its policy committees deem "reasonable and necessary." But that can be interpreted to easily include any new intervention shown to have benefit in a research study. Moreover the drafters of that language could not have taken into account the deepening effects that the clinical trials enterprise and the technological imperative would have on health care delivery, that is, that those two phenomena would make new interventions, regardless of their ultimate effectiveness following clinical trials, *seem* both reasonable and necessary—whatever the patient's age. And so, unless someone—doctor, patient, or family member—proactively opts out, elderly patients inevitably become the recipients of high-tech interventions.

In sum, the status quo has produced a gap, or a "shocking chasm," as Redberg put it,[28] between Medicare coverage and clinical evidence. That is, physicians are prescribing all kinds of interventions for patients whose diseases are not necessarily similar to those of the patients who benefited from the intervention in a controlled study. All the players are culpable here. Physicians employ treatments that are covered by insurance, and they are loath to say no to patients. Patients and families want and demand treatments. The Medicare program contains no administrative mechanisms to assess and track the appropriateness of interventions or to deny treatments for conditions for which the treatment has never shown benefit.

In the end the forces that coalesce to determine how evidence becomes reimbursable and how reimbursed interventions become standard do not discriminate between therapies that do what they promise to do—provide benefit—and those that do not.

The Technological Imperative and the Idea of Progress

The determinative link between Medicare approval and standard of care is the crux of the matter here because "standard of care" means *appropriate* practice, and that is difficult if not impossible for practitioners to ignore and for patients and families to turn down. And what has become standard is the use of new technologies.

Technological progress is an enduring feature and primary value in Western medicine, and its roots reach deep into Enlightenment philosophy, modern science, and contemporary life.[29] It underlies the technological imperative, which, along with reimbursement, organizes a great deal of health care delivery and shapes our expectations that medicine can avert death and erase the symptoms of disease. The technological imperative has been criticized by observers of U.S. medicine for at least four decades for being a means without an end, an activity carried out without consideration of its implications, especially regarding quality of life and, more recently, end-of-life care and cost controls.[30] Yet despite ongoing critiques, the technological imperative remains integral to medical practice (and to rising health care costs) in the United States.[31] This is because the notion of medical progress is inextricably tied to technological innovation (especially drugs and devices), because clinical medicine is mostly financed by and organized around the delivery of discrete procedures by specialists, and because the drug and device industries contribute so centrally to shaping standards of care in U.S. medical practice.

For clinicians the unavoidable technological imperative also becomes an ethical obligation and, as was evident in the accounts given by physicians who implant cardiac devices, a sometimes conflicted one. The anthropologist Barbara Koenig has described the ease, the seamlessness with which new therapies become routine *and* morally compelling. The shift in meaning—from new to standard and necessary—occurs because new technologies almost immediately "feel" routine to practitioners: "A new treatment may or may not be efficacious; it might be risky. The moral imperative for treatment overrides these concerns. It becomes unthinkable for the physicians not to perform the treatment. The social inevitability of therapy takes on a moral tone; the experience of a technological imperative becomes a moral imperative for action. Once a new therapy is available it becomes extremely difficult, if not impossible, to forego its use. . . . The standard of care becomes a moral, as well as technical, obligation."[32]

Once a technology is in use, it becomes ever more difficult to stop using it because, as observers have noted, resources are often poured into improving it and expectations for its success are high.[33] Cardiac stents offer just one example of device interventions that have come to be standard and necessary; others include the implantable cardioverter defibrillator, the cardiac resynchronizer device, which synchronizes the work of the heart's chambers, and the left ventricular assist device, which pumps blood through the heart.

When doctors and patients learn to think about interventions as appropriate and necessary, then *necessary* becomes the operative directive, the default that influences what they do and is difficult to challenge. That default is a value judgment influencing all of ordinary medicine. This is how it works: The success of certain interventions for *some* patients, as shown in research studies, becomes transformed into routine consideration of the intervention for a wider group of patients who learn, through their doctors, the media, and the Internet to think of the interventions as necessary for life.

I met Mr. Paul Fontini, a slight man, age eighty-eight, and his daughter in the waiting room of a busy cardiac clinic, where he had come for an examination and replacement of his old cardiac pacemaker and ICD. It would be his fourth. He had received his first ICD in 1998, following a hospitalization for severe fibrillation. A few years later the second one had to be removed when it was recalled by the manufacturer, Guidant. (When he related his medical history to me he noted, "Guidant paid for it. Medicare didn't pay a cent.") He has had the third device for five and a half years.

In the contemporary medicoethical environment Mr. Fontini's advanced heart failure was a condition that *needed* treatment in order to thwart death.[34] He fit the criteria for benefit shown in trials, and he had Medicare. That reasoning frames clinical medicine and patient desire, as Mr. Fontini's case makes clear. Not only do devices such as the ICD become appropriate therapy and satisfy *need*, but they also allow patients to think specifically about how many more years they want to live and how they want to live. (I explore this theme in chapters 5, 6, and 7.)

While he waited to be called to see the nurse practitioner and physician, Mr. Fontini told me, "I'm slowing down, wearing out. I've been in and out of the hospital a couple of times with heart failure." He had problems with his heart rhythm and relied on the pacemaker portion of the device, along with "lots of medications." "I know when the heart rhythm goes out of control and the defibrillator corrects it. That's a good thing." He recalled receiving only one "shock" from his first ICD and several "minor kicks" from the second and current devices. The devices had done what they were designed to do: return a life-threatening cardiac rhythm to normal. His daughter said, "We know full well that if he didn't have these devices he wouldn't be with us. Period. We also know this is a fairly expensive arrangement."

Mr. Fontini said, "I would like to live to be ninety-five—that's the age my mother lived to. But only if I can feel the way I feel now. I don't want to go downhill. As it is, it's getting harder to care for my wife, who had a stroke. I don't do too much anymore. I have shortness of breath. . . . I've had to give up my cabin, golf. But I'm satisfied with my condition, as it is now."

In the exam room the nurse practitioner reviewed his device history, his long medication list, his symptoms, and his waning energy level.

Mr. Fontini told her, "It's not good. It's kind of ridiculous to get up in the morning and then take a nap." The nurse practitioner talked about devices. He currently had a standard device; he could "upgrade" now, she explained, to the cardiac resynchronizer therapy device, which has three wires instead of two, to better coordinate the function of the two ventricles and thus relieve the symptoms of heart failure. But placement of those wires is a more complex procedure, entailing more risk. "I need your input, if you want one," she said.

Mr. Fontini asked if he still needed the defibrillator. The nurse answered, "We know that people who have an enlarged heart and ventricular arrhythmia are at greater risk for death, which is why it's a good idea to have a defibrillator." She continued, "The new device helps with heart failure. To get it, you have to meet the medical criteria, which you do. There is a 70 percent chance the device will make you feel better; 30 percent of patients say they don't feel better." Mr. Fontini's daughter asked, "So it's greater risk and cost and possibly no difference in how he feels?"

The nurse responded, "It's the same risk as the first implantation: infection, bleeding, stroke, poking holes in the heart. But because your kidney function is not that great, the contrast dye is a risk to the kidneys. We'll give you medicine for that. So I need your input. You can say, 'Just change what I've got' or that you'll take the risk and maybe feel better, do more at home. Maybe it will keep you out of the hospital with heart failure symptoms."

Mr. Fontini immediately replied, "I'll take the risk. I'm going to live to ninety-five. Whatever is necessary to keep me alive. Anything that has a chance to improve my condition, I'm interested. . . . But what does it cost? The old one, five years ago, cost $41,000." The nurse did not know, but she gave the routine answer, referring to the clinical trial evidence that established Medicare reimbursement criteria for the device. "If you meet criteria and we recommend it, Medicare will cover it."

She explained again the choices he faced and said, "While I'm reviewing this with the doctor, you need to decide if you want the procedure. We can do it tomorrow. If the doctor thinks you can benefit from this, and you need more time to think about it, we can work with you."

A few minutes later the physician arrived in the exam room and said, "We're planning to put in the extra lead. We think it will help with heart failure, so you can take fewer medications and do more around the house. We think it will help you." The nurse joined in, this time mentioning only the positive features of the device: "This will make you feel better, and you meet the criteria." The family scheduled the procedure for the following day.

BECOMING STANDARD AND NECESSARY:
THE EASY ACCEPTANCE OF THE HEART PUMP

Heart failure is a progressive and ultimately fatal disease, but death can be staved off for a long time by the use of incrementally more invasive devices. When heart failure is advanced and the pacemaker, ICD, and resynchronizer are no longer adequate to the task of maintaining cardiac function, the more powerful technology of the left ventricular assist device, the LVAD, now exists to do so. Mostly an age-related problem, heart failure has reached what some call epidemic proportions in the United States,[35] afflicting more than 5 million people, with 550,000 new cases diagnosed each year.[36] An aging population fuels these numbers, and improvements in cardiac medications, together with the implantable devices, enable people to continue living but with more advanced disease. Together demographics and the therapies that prevent death yet allow for more severe and chronic disease set the stage for the use of ever more aggressive, invasive, and expensive interventions. Those more intensive treatments then create more caregiving demands on health professionals and families to monitor physical health, respond to life-threatening problems that arise from both the technologies and the diseases, and do everything possible to ensure the patient's survival and well-being.

The evolution of the LVAD offers a classic example of the technological imperative and Medicare reimbursement in action. Perhaps the most technically advanced life-extending intervention to become standard in the first decade of this millennium, in 2005 the LVAD was considered one of the ten "most promising" technologies of the year.[37] The idea that a device should be created to provide partial circulatory support emerged in the 1970s, at a time when little progress was being made with either the artificial heart or cardiac transplantation.[38] Because of the disappointing progress on those fronts and because of "the magnitude of the problem of heart failure in the United States and its emotional valence,"[39] in the early years the NIH drove the research for some kind of device, an unusual departure from its normal practice of supporting only basic and not applied investigations. The left ventricular assist device was first approved by the FDA in 1994 for short-term use only, to keep people alive while they waited for a heart transplant.[40] It was truly a "half way technology,"[41] not a fully artificial heart but a partial, temporary, artificial assistant for cardiac function. The NIH wanted to further develop the LVAD as a permanent therapy, and scientific evidence was needed to do so. The first clinical trial was sponsored by the NIH in collaboration with Thoratec, the manufacturer of the HeartMate device, and carried out between 1998 and 2001. It was designed specifically to assess the efficacy of a permanent device.[42]

In 2003, first the FDA and then Medicare approved the LVAD for two applications: as a temporary fix while a patient waited for a suitable heart for transplant, that is, as a "bridge" to transplant, and for permanent use, that is, as "destination therapy."[43] The creation of practice guidelines by medical experts followed, establishing the LVAD as standard of care for advanced heart failure and further solidifying the rationale for insurance payment for the very expensive procedure. As we have seen, insurers tend to pay for procedures that are recommended by specialty experts in clinical guidelines. The guidelines issued in 2005 by the American College of Cardiology and the American Heart Association cited the LVAD's clinical trial data as the basis for the statement: "Presently, destination device therapy is anticipated to benefit those patients predicted to have a 1-year [chance of] survival of less than 50%."[44] The Heart Failure Society guidelines, developed in 2006, stated, "Permanent mechanical assistance using an implantable assist device may be considered in highly selected patients with severe heart failure refractory to conventional therapy."[45]

The LVAD costs at least ten times more than the ICD, approximately $250,000 for the device, surgical implantation, and intensive care and rehabilitation follow-up, as of this writing.[46] Between 2007 and 2009 I asked several people age seventy or older how they came to receive the LVAD, and they all offered a version of this interchange: "My doctor said, 'You will probably die in the next few months from your heart disease, and this device could give you up to five years.'" The logical response, the only possible response, as one seventy-one-year-old man reported four weeks after receiving his device, was to say, "I'll take five years, no doubt about it." Who wouldn't? Especially if Medicare is footing the bill.

A social worker at one of the more than one hundred centers that implant the LVAD described the ease with which acceptance of the device usually occurs, though she tells patients, "The device can keep you alive while the rest of your body may be dying." She went on, "Most people who come this far already have a pacemaker and an ICD. They are already on the road to an LVAD, socialized to it. The LVAD is the next step." Though it involves major surgery, intensive care follow-up, and a period of rehabilitation, it seems to some patients only incrementally more invasive than the pacemaker, resynchronizer, and defibrillator that they have already.

The LVAD is implanted just below the heart by means of open heart surgery. A cannula connects the device to the heart.[47] A tube passes from the device through the patient's skin at about waist level, connecting the pump to an external computer controller and battery-operated power pack; these are carried on a belt or vest. The power pack has to be recharged at night, and extra batteries must be available at all times during the day. The external pump enables blood to be moved through the heart vessels. Importantly the effects of this newest kind of cardiac device have proven to be highly variable in practice.

I met a seventy-one-year-old, fit and energetic gentleman who walked into the room for our interview in 2009 and announced, "I love my device." He had received it only two months before we met. I asked about any decision making beforehand and he replied, "The doctor said, 'Your heart is real bad. I think we want to put a heart pump into you.' I didn't know what it was. He said, 'Well, you're going to have to wear a battery pack for the rest of your life.' And I said, 'Hmmm. How big is it?' And he said, 'Pretty big.' Just like that. And I asked him, 'If I don't get this done, what's gonna happen?' He said, 'You won't live a year. You may not live two months, really. Your heart is that bad.' So I said, 'Well, when do you want to do it? Let's get it over with!' So that was pretty much it. A ten-minute conversation."

He carried all the active equipment in the pockets of a fishing jacket and slung the second set of batteries, along with the recharger, over his shoulder in a tote bag. Together the equipment weighed more than ten pounds.[48] He was not going to let this device slow him down. He cooked, drove, traveled; he had plans to go out fishing in a boat, which his doctor had advised against because if he fell into the water that extra ten pounds could drown him. I asked how he felt about his life expectancy now that he had the device. "Oh, I've heard that people have lived up to eight years with it, but I think this will give me at least ten years. And they'll probably have a better unit out within the next ten years, and I can go through another heart surgery. It's no fun, but I would go through another one to get a better unit, a smaller unit, maybe with the implanted controller, and I know they've already come up with smaller batteries. . . . So I look to get twenty more years out of life. I'd like to get more than that, to be real honest."

At the other end of the health continuum, I observed and spoke briefly with a man, age seventy-five, who had been hospitalized ever since he received the device six months before our meeting. His kidneys had failed during the placement of the device and he was on dialysis, shifting in and out of conscious awareness in his hospital bed. He had recurring, serious infections that were being treated, though some of his infections were resistant to the drugs available. No one expected him to live to leave the hospital, and he did not. He died there two months after I met him.

Between those two poles was another man, age eighty, who had been living with the LVAD for a year and a half. He told me he felt burdened by his disease and by the device. He and his wife worried a great deal about whether he could get to a hospital if something went wrong; he had already been hospitalized a couple of times. But he also traveled and enjoyed life, including traveling by plane so that he could fish and hunt.

The clearly apparent ease with which physicians have accepted this device illustrates that regardless of the extent of its benefits, it has become a feature of ordinary medicine. A national study reported in 2008 that the devices were being used too often in patients too sick to benefit from them and were being implanted at hospitals that lacked the experience to give the expert care the recipients needed. Prolonged hospitalizations and a high rate of early mortality with the device were lead findings. Among patients sixty-five and over, the one-year survival rates declined over a seven-year period, from 41 percent in 2000 to 21 percent in 2006. A possible explanation is that the eligibility criteria for implanting the device were loosened during that period, allowing patients too sick to benefit to receive the device. The study concluded, "Among Medicare beneficiaries receiving a ventricular assist device, early mortality, morbidity and costs remain high. Improving patient selection and reducing perioperative mortality are critical for improving overall outcomes."[49] But the fact is that the evidence, reimbursement, and standard setting for devices such as the LVAD and the drug-eluting stents occur seamlessly. Only after the fact, in the commentaries and studies that review the use of particular devices, do reports reveal the fault lines of ordinary medicine: overuse, exorbitant cost, less benefit than predicted, individual patient burden, and more. But by then the forces determining treatment are frequently too powerful to shift the default setting to ensure a more measured approach to the potential benefits and harms of the intervention.

The medical indications for the uses of this complex, expensive device are only one piece of the story. One social worker told me in 2009 that when patients are medically eligible for the LVAD according to Medicare reimbursement criteria, surgeons want to implant it because they believe in its life-extending capabilities. Yet those surgeons, she noted, ignore the elements of social support, personal commitment, and financial means that are necessary if people are to stay alive with the device. She said that when the LVAD was first used, "they were throwing these devices in any one, regardless of social support." She gave the example of an older man who received an LVAD and was discharged to his home. "Patients say they have social support so that they can get the device," she explained. "This guy was a loner, and he managed to get two people to take him home from the hospital. But afterward no one was around to check on him. He lived alone, had no family. He died within months. His body was not discovered for three days. We learned a lot from that." Since then, she reported, in several cases nurses and social workers at her center have put the brakes on surgeons, preventing them from implanting such a complex device in patients who were "good candidates physiologically, but psychosocial train wrecks," meaning that they could not care for themselves and had no network of social support.

Reimbursement Criteria and the Promise of Technology: Shaping Our Expectations

The lure of technology is powerful indeed—for hospitals to bring in income, for doctors, who want to try anything to extend patients' lives, and for patients, who want to live. Medicare reimbursement policies enhance that power. The broadening of its criteria for payment for (potentially) life-extending procedures can be considered from at least two perspectives. The first is that, most simply and positively, the broadening is a testament to the idea of medical progress. Previously fatal diseases have slowly given way to treatments that save and prolong life. No one wants it to be otherwise. Implantable devices and many other procedures have become so ordinary and are so often successful in extending lives that we cannot think of them as anything other than lifesavers.

The idea that our bodies are *fixable* at any age is reinforced by medical technology's many success stories. I met one seventy-one-year-old man who for years had been extremely debilitated by heart disease and was near death shortly before he received an LVAD a year before our encounter. He told me, "I feel ten or fifteen years younger than before I got the device. I can walk without a cane. Walk upstairs. Work on the farm. My blood sugar is normal. I don't take any medications. My appetite is back."

The ordinariness of life-extending therapies for those in later life has deepened our conceptions of the body's resilience, the open-ended quality of the life span, and the powers of clinical interventions. It has led to the widespread assumption that greater longevity is nearly always possible. These perceptions have become part of the fabric of social life in the United States.

Yet seen from another, second, perspective, the broadening of Medicare reimbursement criteria signifies a much more complex cultural arrangement because those criteria are the *vehicle* that links clinical technologies to necessary interventions and, by extension, to notions of personal choice and individual rights. By valuing new technologies above all else, by legitimating more life-extending procedures for those in later life through payment for them, by joining clinical trial evidence with standardization and ethical necessity, Medicare coverage policies expand our sense of entitlement, of the right to a therapy. They do so without regard for the myriad social repercussions of that therapy for patients, families, and the nation.

Thus for patients and families the world of longevity making is prefigured by the ethical field and the political choices that drive the health care chain. Their entry into that clinical world carries with it the responsibility for settling on the right amount of treatment—that is, for walking the personally perilous line between doing too much (thus prolonging suffering and dying) and not doing enough to extend life. Hope, guilt, love, and obligation are central to both patient and family calculations, as I highlight in the following chapters.

For our society the most visible and touted result of the deep connection between payment policy and technology-driven clinical practice is that increasing numbers of older people are alive and thriving following cardiac, cancer, and other interventions. There is another profound result, however, which is that a great deal of medicine today serves to prolong the very end stage of a disease process, and that has complex repercussions, not the least of which is cost.

There is no doubt that many people today have come to understand their body, life, and future—including the idea of what constitutes a normal life span and ordinary treatments—in terms of the options for medical intervention that Medicare provides.[50] The difficulty of saying no to treatments that Medicare will pay for and that are considered standard—which means appropriate and necessary—illustrates how deeply entangled the progress narrative and longevity making have become.

PART III

MEDICINE'S CHANGING MEANS AND ENDS

5

STANDARD AND NECESSARY TREATMENTS
The Changing Means and Ends of Technology

Can new technologies relieve us of the burden
of choosing our own fate?
—Michael Jackson, *Existential Anthropology*

Doing nothing is non-standard.
—Doctor to patient

The specific tools of the clinic, medicine's means, are the drugs, devices, and procedures that we hope will do the tasks they were designed to do, thus achieving medicine's ends and fulfilling its mandate to reduce symptoms, improve chances of survival, and prevent the spread of disease. Broadly put, medicine's ends have always been to promote health and prolong life. Yet because medicine could cure little until the mid-twentieth century, those two ends were mostly subordinate to another: to provide comfort.[1] Over time, however, medicine's ends have been further complicated as its technological means have evolved and have themselves come to be seen as standard and necessary.

Evolving Means and Ends: The Technological Imperative
and the Creation of New Needs

This chapter highlights four points about the path of that evolution. The first three focus broadly on the technology itself and how we interact with it. First, medicine's ends were redefined and grew increasingly complex as effective treatments became routine and expected by doctors and patients alike and as the rapidly emerging tools of the biotechnology revolution changed the landscape of research, promising even more effective treatments. The complicating factor was and remains the perfect storm of ordinary medicine—the confluence of greater numbers of old people, more chronic diseases, more diseases made chronic by more treatments, more treatments made possible by the avalanche of evidence and then reimbursement, higher patient expectations for interventions, and more pressure from the market to make therapies available to doctors and patients.

The second point is that the technological imperative has now become an end in itself, further confounding both doctors and patients as they pursue their treatment goals, contributing further to the quandary of crossing the line. Thus while doctors and patients like to think that the tools of the clinic are theirs to choose or reject, it is the foundational chain that drives U.S. health care delivery that shapes those choices. The technological imperative is one of the forces guiding the scope of our treatment choices and even how we regard "choice" itself. This is because, once technological solutions become standard therapies, they become necessary as well. Thus the technological imperative is a major player in the contemporary predicament that is ordinary medicine.

My third point is that any innovative procedure or practice that has been created with one specific goal in mind spurs us to think also about other potential uses, uses not previously imaginable. In that context clinical technologies are not merely means to specific ends, and ends are not static and already known. Rather a technological society changes the ends as new means emerge and develop.[2] So interventions in medicine are interventions into ideas as well as into the body;[3] they expand our thinking about what to want from them.

For example, from the moment the mechanical ventilator became standard hospital equipment and use of the dialysis machine became routine (both in the 1970s), one predominant end of medicine has been to use noncurative technologies to stave off death, regardless of what postponing death may mean for older patients, families, and the practice of medicine. The ICD is a recent example of a tool that became standard and has led physicians and patients alike to think it is *necessary* for people in late life to avoid the risk of sudden death. None of these three interventions promises a cure for underlying disease, and patients (those who are realistic) know that. Yet each of these therapies contributes to our societal condition of postprogress, which is why they serve throughout this book as examples of ordinary medicine.

The Mechanical Ventilator: From Operating Room Tool to Standard Care

The mechanical ventilator, or breathing machine, which is standard equipment in every hospital intensive care unit today, provides perhaps the most well-known (and often most feared) example of how a medical tool, designed originally with one purpose in mind, easily invited and paved the way for other uses. The mechanical ventilator was developed over a fifty-year period in response to the demands of surgeons, who needed to maintain patients' respiratory function, that is, keep them alive, while they operated on hearts, lungs, and other vital organs. While the ventilator's original intention was to keep patients breathing during surgery, by the mid-1970s it had become standard equipment in intensive care units. Within a few years its use expanded again. Physicians quickly discovered that the device could be used for a long list of diseases and problems beyond those originally targeted; it could achieve other ends. Recovery from life-threatening pneumonia or chronic obstructive lung disease became possible with the ventilator, enabling many to get better. It saved lives. Because that technology can also keep the organs of the dead oxygenated, it opened up the realm of organ transplantation beyond anything previously imaginable: "brain-dead" persons (without brain function) maintained on a ventilator became the most important resource for organs for the transplantation industry, enabling that practice to expand and flourish.[4]

Another use of the ventilator also quickly came into play: it could keep "alive" people who were in a vegetative or deeply comatose state. This function came to illustrate what many think of as the dark side of medical technology, and Karen Ann Quinlan was its first publicly acknowledged and quintessential example. Her case made headlines in 1975, not long after the machine came into widespread use in American hospitals, and she exemplified, as no person or situation had before, the condition of postprogress.

After a bout of drinking and taking prescription drugs, Quinlan lay comatose for months in a hospital bed while her parents sought to have her removed from the mechanical ventilator that kept only her body alive. When her physician and the hospital administration refused to allow it because they feared criminal prosecution, her parents petitioned first the Superior Court of New Jersey and then the state's supreme court, seeking permission to let her die. During the months of court deliberations the case was debated on the public stage, bringing with it what generally was seen as a new awareness of the troubled and troubling means and ends of medicine. The case made it widely apparent that new technologies could create, unintentionally, a gray zone between life and death that no one wanted. The state supreme court eventually ruled in favor of the Quinlans.

The Quinlan case was arguably the pivotal event that triggered the ensuing public debate in the United States about what kind of life has value and how we deliberate the worth of new treatments in relation to the hope for recovery and the idea of medical progress. It contributed to health care consumer activism, especially regarding the desire to control one's own end of life without the use of technologies that prolong dying. It opened the way for the hospice movement to gain support in the United States and gave momentum to the use of the living will and advance directives. It also publicly brought medicine together with the language of rights, ethics, and public policy.

Since the 1970s the fact that thousands of people have been enabled by the ventilator to hover in a persistent vegetative state has provoked endless conversation within and outside of medicine—conversation about the goals of medicine, what degree of "life" equals being alive, and what the role of the law, the family, and the profession of medicine should be in fostering or ending that "life" for any one person.[5] In addition, when frail elderly patients with pneumonia or other lung problems cannot be removed from the ventilator because they are not able to breathe on their own, someone has to make a decision about what to do—either to keep the patient on the breathing machine in a specialized hospital unit indefinitely or to authorize an end to life. That particular dilemma, now occurring for families routinely in hospitals across the country, is one pervasive and wrenching result of the changing means and ends of ventilator technology specifically.

The quandary the ventilator presents illustrates a development that was not—and could not be—anticipated during the seventy-five years of the machine's evolution prior to its contemporary, ordinary hospital use.[6] To many minds the mechanical ventilator remains the most glaring example of the mutable nature of the goals of medical technologies and of the troubled relationship that has developed among life-sustaining interventions, the desire for them, and the changing uses of them. The sociologists of science Bruno Latour and Couze Venn have articulated this development: "If we fail to recognize how much the use of a technique, however simple, has displaced, translated, modified, or inflected the initial intention, it is simply because we have changed the end in changing the means, and because, through a slipping of the will, we have begun to wish something quite else from what we at first desired."[7]

So technologies are never merely passive instruments, utensils that fulfill a predetermined function. They are tools adopted because they fill (and then may create) a need. In that way they are active agents and a form of mediation either between possibility and intention or among competing goals. Thus while specific tools may in fact fulfill one intended, preconceived purpose, they also, and perhaps more importantly, incite new ways of thinking about what to expect, what to hope for, and what is appropriate to do and trigger new kinds of problems for patients, health care workers, and society as well.

A New Cultural Perspective: "Most Deaths Are Premature"

The fourth and final point this chapter highlights about evolving means and ends is that we, patients and physicians, are changed by the way medical technologies come to be used. When certain interventions become normal, routine, standard, and, importantly, life-prolonging for some older patients, their potential and actual uses (which are always evolving) become intertwined with our longings, our perceived opportunities, and, in the United States especially, our sense of individual and citizen rights. So not only do the ends of a technology change (the ventilator moves out of the operating room), but the ways technologies come to be used change us as well—researchers, clinicians, and health care consumers alike. And this happens without much public reflection. All in all, the drugs, devices, and surgical procedures now available to treat what used to be end-stage diseases have altered and continue to change our ideas about premature death and the appropriate time for death. Medicine's tools allow us, indeed invite us, to recalibrate what ordinary medical treatment consists of and what "health," that elusive notion, should feel like at age eighty, ninety, and one hundred.

In sum, the changing means and ends of technology have enabled today's dominant cultural tendency: to think, to act as if most deaths are premature. Because the tools of medicine can seemingly "add" time, the value of life has come to be measured, in large part, by its length. Thus medicine is implicated in how we value life and how we attempt to control the time that is "left."

In addition I have heard many people in their eighties and nineties express some variation of the following sentiments when discussing treatment options with their doctors: *I want to be back to where I was before (the heart attack, cancer, renal dialysis). I think I should have this treatment because I expect—and want and hope—it will help me feel and be the way I used to be.* For their part physicians and families commonly (though not exclusively) support older patients in their expectation that some previous state of better function, better health *will return*, that medical treatment has a clear end—reduced symptoms, greater energy, longer survival—that is possible and attainable, regardless of age and severity of disease.

For example, in the oncology clinic, an eighty-eight-year-old man with prostate cancer and many complaints—hip pain, low energy, weakness, problems with urination—is told by his oncologist:

> *We need to get you back where you were. . . .* Yes, the hormone shots can take a lot out of you. Have you had a bone scan? It's not in the file. We should check on that. You should be taking extra Vitamin D and calcium pills because you really need to keep up these nutritional supplements, especially when you're on Lupron [the hormone] because Lupron leads to the risk of breaking hips or the spine. It's very important to protect the bones. . . . I would suggest no more Lupron, and then we'll watch your PSA and testosterone levels, and if the PSA goes up, what we worry about is cancer going out of the prostate. But the risk of that is low.[8]

Physicians who have been practicing for many years note that their expectations regarding the treatment of ever older patients have shifted over time in response to the changing uses of medicine's tools. We saw in chapter 2 how physicians' responses to clinical trial evidence for the expanded use of the ICD shifted the ends for that particular device from a tool for those who already had experienced a potentially lethal heart rhythm to a tool to prevent the risk of sudden death among older persons. Societal expectations made that shift one that is easy to accomplish.

There is no doubt that the tools of medicine have enabled doctors and patients to formulate new ways of thinking about the life span. Both physicians' and patients' hopes and expectations about the promise of medical intervention now merge with the outer reaches of the commonly achieved life span: the late eighties and beyond. It is there, at those ages and at that joining, that our troubles mostly lie.

Prolonging Life, Complicating Medicine's Relationship to Age:
Three Paradigmatic Interventions

The three examples of life-prolonging interventions this chapter investigates—the ICD, kidney dialysis, and liver transplantation—reveal how the changing means and ends of technologies impact the goals of medical practice and patient sensibilities. Each illustrates features of ordinary medicine in a different way, shows how doctors and patients have learned to respond to each intervention, and illustrates ways our aging population is driving much of health care.

The ICD and kidney dialysis are interventions that have become routine, standard, and necessary. They keep people alive and thus are difficult for anyone to refuse when life is at stake. Both of them complicate the relationship of medicine to age because they stave off death but do not improve health. They do not necessarily make patients feel better. They turn treatments into death prevention but allow for the body's slowed-down slide toward death. Both got their start as a tool for a specific purpose that over time expanded to use by a wider variety of patients, generating greater need for the intervention. Both therapies illustrate how doctors and patients confront (or dismiss) the risk of dying.

The ICD and kidney dialysis turn life-threatening diseases into chronic conditions, enabling people to grow older in need of more intervention, more risk awareness, and more prevention—all at the same time. Those demands bring with them uncertainties about crossing the line that become the norm: for patients the uncertainties are about whether they want the interventions at their age and then how long to continue with them; for physicians they are about prognosis and how aggressively to fight end-stage disease in later life. In this uneasy meeting of age and technology, a key question of postprogress ordinary medicine often looms large: How is "successful treatment" to be defined? What is to be measured and against what standard?[9] And from whose perspective? The standard use of the term *successful treatment* denotes life prolongation (regardless of the age, frailty, and specific condition of the patient). Today the term's meaning is tempered by the fact that thousands of patients, families, and doctors grapple with whether prolonging the life of someone who is extremely frail and ill really constitutes "successful" medicine.

In contrast, liver transplantation does cure disease and make patients feel better. It has become the logical endpoint for treating primary liver cancer and other fatal liver conditions. The procedure has become standard and unremarkable (similar to kidney transplants, which I discuss later), even though it is one of the most complex and expensive surgical procedures, is not performed in all hospitals, and requires a scarce resource in order to extend life. Its expanded use and success and its acquired ordinariness as a means to save life and restore better health have fostered more need for it and more medical and societal dilemmas about how to satisfy that need in an aging country. For some it has also fostered a sense of entitlement, as we saw in the cases of Mr. Carter and Mrs. Ames.

Each of these technologies extends wanted life for many people; that is, of course, the bottom line. Each has also opened up an ever-expanding market for devices, dialysis centers, and organs, respectively. And each triggers quandaries about how one can or should live in relation to medical treatment, perhaps especially when one becomes old. I am not seeking to make a case for or against the use of these or any other therapies by patients of any particular age. Rather the issue for me is how life-extending therapies in an aging society have been caught up in the perfect storm of ordinary medicine; how and why they bring increasing numbers of patients and families, indeed our entire society to face the quandary of the line; how, as more elderly people come to need these treatments in the future, we must understand the forces that constitute ordinary medicine in order to better confront the consequences of our postprogress predicament.

Ironic Technology: Heart Disease and the Implantable Cardiac Defibrillator

Today the implantable cardiac defibrillator, ICD, often is part of a multipurpose device that, in addition to shocking a potentially lethal rhythm into returning to a normal one, can also correct the pacing of the heart beat (as a pacemaker) and resynchronize the functions of the heart's two chambers (as a resynchronizer, or CRT). Multipurpose devices exemplify the constant reinvention of medical means and ends and the corresponding evolution of our sensibilities about old age and what to want. As Mr. Fontini's case demonstrated (chapter 4), the development of these all-in-one devices makes it easy for physicians to suggest to patients being offered (or advised to get) a pacemaker that they consider adding the defibrillator (or "shock") function as well, and patients who are told they need the defibrillator often are asked to think about adding the resynchronizer.

As a technological actor on the stage of life-extending treatments, the ICD, with or without the resynchronizer, confronts especially older patients and their families with the demand that they think about "successful treatment" in relation to the "need" to thwart death and stay alive. It demands as well that patients imagine and choose between two *future* scenarios: on the one hand, the risk of death, maybe imminent death, without the device and, on the other hand, potentially "more" life with it. But that additional life will also include more eventual debility and possible suffering, as the case of Mr. Tolleson (chapter 1) and recent medical literature show.[10]

Two additional stories, of Mr. Jones and Mr. Albert, further illustrate those elements in play.

Weighing Risks—Imminent Death versus Prolonged Dying: Mr. Jones

---

At age eighty-four Mr. Claude Jones was struggling with congestive heart failure and had had several emergency hospitalizations within a few months. (The pattern of repeated hospitalization for increasing heart failure in late life is common. Health professionals refer to those kinds of patients as "revolving-door patients" because they return to the hospital so frequently.)[11] Because his cardiac function was monitored closely during the hospitalizations, the medical staff was able to observe some episodes of ventricular tachycardia, a potentially life-threatening rhythm.

When the physician confronted Mr. Jones with the need for the ICD device in order to avert death *now*, his strong recommendation of that choice pushed Mr. Jones to acknowledge the ICD's ironic feature: *it can thwart death at the same time that it prolongs the amount of time it takes before one eventually dies from the heart disease being treated.* Those dual possibilities, when understood by frail elderly patients, force them to consider the worth of a (potentially) extended life *but with worsening heart disease.*[12]

Mr. Jones took his age into consideration as he decided. His daughter, a nurse, recounted what ensued:

> My dad's cardiologist, who had been treating him for a long time, became concerned about the documented runs of ventricular tachycardia and said to him, "I want you to have an ICD." And so, my dad said to me, "What do you think I should do?" And I think he wanted

me to make the decision for him. So I gave him a list of questions to ask the cardiologist: What's the intended outcome? Will it really make a difference to the state of the heart failure? What's it going to feel like when it defibrillates? I felt I knew the answers to those questions, but I wanted the cardiologist to address the pros and cons with my father. That it would, very simplistically, prevent a ventricular tachycardia that could possibly cause sudden death, but that it would not cure the heart failure. I phoned my dad after the cardiologist had been in to see him. I asked, "What did he tell you?" My dad started sobbing on the phone and replied, "He told me I need to have one right away or I will die."

I went to the hospital with an internal struggle. As a daughter I wanted him to have it. I didn't want him to die. On the other hand, I didn't want him to suffer. And how much will he suffer when he's kicked in the chest [by the defibrillator]? How many episodes [of ventricular tachycardia] is he going to have anyway? He may have been having them for five years. We don't know. It just happened that he was monitored in the hospital and they happened to see it. So, if he's been having episodes for years and hasn't died, why put in an expensive device? He already has a pacemaker. The heart failure is the debilitating part, and treating that is the hard part.

When I got to the bedside he was still sobbing, telling me how frightened he had been, that he thought he might die immediately. I told him that the defibrillator would protect him against the likelihood of sudden death, but it would not cure the heart failure. He asked me a few questions. And it didn't take very long for him to say, "Well, I'm not going to have it." He said that the heart failure is bad enough. "Why would I want to keep from dying from that? If the heart failure is going to get worse and worse, wouldn't it be merciful if I would have a sudden death, instead of a long suffering?"

Mr. Jones's daughter articulated what his physician had failed to describe: that the ICD, if it responded to a lethal rhythm, would prolong his life *with* end-stage heart failure. As she recounted it, the doctor's approach to her father's treatment was in the service of the device. He was, in a certain respect, led to recommend it for the patient by virtue of his understanding of the device's capability. It was *through the physician's urging* that the device elicited for Mr. Jones a confrontation with the need to choose between two options. On the one hand, he could live with increasingly uncomfortable symptoms into a dreaded, open-ended future because the device could create that kind of future. On the other hand, he must (it seemed to him) assume full responsibility for dying soon yet perhaps unnecessarily because the device could prevent death for a time. For Mr. Jones the device raised thoughts about what constitutes value in living and suffering. For his daughter it created tension between wanting her father to live longer and wanting his suffering to end.

Mr. Jones lived another three years without an ICD in his own home.

Two factors make the now standard ICD difficult to refuse. First, it seems to be against medical progress and common sense to say no to it. Second, medicine emphasizes that refusing an ICD puts one at risk for death—as if one (and certainly Mr. Jones) were not already at risk for death simply by having advanced heart failure in old age. As we saw in chapter 2, for physicians the device has become a tool to treat the *risk of death*, changing it into a medical condition that implantation can thwart. Like Mr. Jones, patients in a study of the experience of living with the device also reported being told they needed the ICD in order to live. That study found that "choice"— especially the choice to accept death—was actually preempted by the technological imperative. "It was not acceptable not to want the device implanted," the author of the study reported.[13]

The Lure of Eligibility: Mr. Albert

Mr. Joe Albert's physician made a strong case for his eighty-one-year-old patient's eligibility for the ICD. Mr. Albert was eligible because his condition was similar to that of patients enrolled in clinical trials, the results of which showed the benefit of the device, and he was eligible because he had Medicare insurance. Clinical trials findings and Medicare reimbursement criteria are persuasive reasons for physicians to offer and for patients and families to choose the full range of capabilities that a device currently has. As we have seen, new technologies often are extended far beyond the populations on which they were originally tested, and an assumption of benefit usually prevails until proven otherwise. In clinic discussions the "value question"— What is the actual existential worth of these technologies to persons in later life?—is muted or erased entirely by the presentation of clinical trial evidence and by the fact of the device's standardization.

In the outpatient clinic Mr. Albert was urged to consider getting an ICD. He was told there was no emergency and was also given information about the possible complications of implanting the device in the first place and about the negative consequences that may result from living with it. Yet the power of the device to thwart death is compelling. The physician offered him the ICD as part of a multifunction device that could reduce his symptoms of ill health and restore the well-being he associated with his younger self. At eighty-one, who would say no to that? Mr. Albert's story illustrates that the way doctors recount evidence-based findings and the standards that emerge from them shapes patients' consideration of what to do. In Mr. Jones's case, the standardization of ICD use was translated into necessity by the physician, who felt strongly that Mr. Jones should have it implanted. Mr. Albert's case shows the way evidence is transformed into standard of care and how standardization becomes necessity for the patient.

After greeting Mr. and Mrs. Albert, the cardiologist at a major medical clinic said, "I want to talk to you about a defibrillator and a pacemaker. The question is whether you might benefit from an ICD with or without pacing of the heart all the time. The defibrillator is a special pacemaker that has the ability to shock the heart if it is in a rhythm that would lead to death. It can be thought of as an insurance policy to prevent that kind of arrhythmia. Do we want to incur the cost for something we may not need? It's a balance that needs to be thought of in that way because it's hard to predict which individuals will actually benefit from the device."

"Really," he continued, "that's all the defibrillator is. It's not going to make you feel better. In fact sometimes it gives inappropriate shocks when it doesn't need to. It's extremely painful. Also there's risk of infection. So it's that type of decision."

The physician then offered an additional procedure, the resynchronizer pacer (CRT), newer technology that could improve the symptoms of Mr. Albert's advancing heart failure. The doctor continued, "If we decide to do the ICD, should we do a more extensive procedure at the same time, putting in an extra lead in the heart to better synchronize the two chambers? It is a more complex procedure. We have to inject dye in the heart, go into a small vein. The cardiac resynchronizer is designed to make you feel better. The problem is we don't know who will feel better. About two-thirds of patients will feel better, but one-third won't. So you could undergo the surgery and not feel better." Though the doctor clearly invoked the range of technological options and the different kinds of evidence in play, he did not paint an unduly rosy picture.

The patient and his wife asked a common question: Is it worth it when you're in your eighties? What would you do? And of course it was impossible for the doctor to answer definitively. After more discussion the physician summarized the rather complex decision-making tree the patient now faced: "There are two possibilities. First, the defibrillator—you do *qualify* for it. You are *eligible*." This familiar language is used repeatedly in clinic encounters and it is important. To the patient, however, such language sounded as if he had won a lottery. "Second," the doctor noted, "we could go for the ICD and the resynchronizer in hopes of making you feel better in terms of symptoms. But this is an unknown."

He concluded, "Considering your risk, it would be appropriate to buy the insurance. It's not black and white. I'm not the one who is paying the premium, having to live with infections, shocks, et cetera. I do think it might benefit you; that's why we are offering it."

Mr. Albert replied, "I'm wearing out. Things are degenerating, deteriorating. That's why I'm here. I think I should have it." The patient gave his consent, and the doctor scheduled the procedure for the next day.

Similar conversations with a similar outcome take place daily throughout the United States. Mr. Albert's final reply is a common one. It is based on the clinical expectation that the symptoms of heart failure in later life can be reduced, and on the societal expectation that the signs of aging can be pushed further away (or even made to disappear) by medical technique. This physician's offer and recommendation reinforced Mr. Albert's desire and influenced his choice.

Although the evidence points in more than one direction, the cardiac devices, similar to other technologies, enable many patients to hope and to assume, like Mr. Albert, that "growing older without aging" is possible,[14] indeed normal, as long as the right tools are available. Because medicine has contributed so powerfully to better health into late life, and because it *promises* better health through its technological offerings, patients expect technologies to make them "feel like themselves," that is, feel the way they did prior to the worsening of their disease.[15] Given the current ethical and political underpinnings and the organization of our health care enterprise, there is no natural cutoff point for patients' expectations regarding medical technologies or for physicians' use of them.

Mr. Albert was not (yet) aware of what Mr. Tolleson learned and research has revealed:[16] some persons with ICDs become acutely aware of how they will *not* die. A kind of angst and even terror is sometimes associated with anticipating a shock from the device, and some patients experience fear of receiving multiple shocks and then dying. Because I had no further encounters with Mr. Albert, I do not know if he also would experience a foreshadowing of death and whether the fact that he was over eighty mattered to him in that regard.

The doctors emphasized to both Mr. Albert and Mr. Jones that the device can reduce the risk of death—a powerful reason to want one. The other potential consequences of the device—its contribution to prolonged dying from heart failure and the chance of shocks during the dying transition itself—were not made apparent to either man. Those negative consequences are rarely mentioned by doctors to patients.[17]

EXPANDING THE PARAMETERS OF RISK AND NEED:
THE EVOLUTION OF THE IMPLANTABLE DEFIBRILLATOR'S
MEANS AND ENDS

As a result of the surge in ICD trials between 2002 and 2005, both the means and ends of the device changed. It became a tool to reduce the risk of death from a *potentially* lethal cardiac event for those with underlying heart disease, even for persons who have never had an arrhythmia. Similar to other technologies, the ICD has been subject to "indication creep," the inevitable extension of its use to more and more persons, the vast majority of whom are over sixty-five. In a survey of a random national sample of 9,960 physician members of the American College of Cardiology, nearly 90 percent of respondents rated patient "preference" regarding the ICD as less important than their own favorable attitudes toward that device. Those attitudes were based on the strong evidence of benefit from clinical trials, which compelled physicians to support ICD implantation, to "do the right thing" regardless of patient preference.[18]

The simpler cardiac pacemaker, approved by Medicare for reimbursement in 1966, provides another example of the changing means and ends of cardiac devices. Originally created as an external device "the size of a breadbox that stood on a hospital cart and plugged into a wall socket,"[19] it was shown in 1952 to enable patients to survive an acute medical crisis. It became transformed over the years into a battery-operated implantable machine, with the early implants occurring between 1958 and 1960. With Medicare paying the bill beginning in 1966, the market for it grew enormously and the age of patients receiving it increased. The pacemaker's expanded use was supported by treatment guidelines, written by expert consensus panels from the American College of Cardiology in 1984 and based primarily on retrospective studies and case reports.

Those guidelines recommended that the pacemaker be used for fifty-six types of heart conditions; by 2008 the list of indications, again based on reviews of reports by experts in consensus meetings, had grown to eighty-eight conditions. The device industry influenced that expansion, and the entanglement of the expert physicians who sat on those guideline panels with industry is apparent—another feature of ordinary medicine. "Of the 17 cardiologists who wrote the 2008 guidelines, 11 received financing from cardiac-device makers or worked at institutions receiving it. Seven, due to the extent of their financial connections, were recused from voting on the guidelines they helped write."[20] Today many of the pacemakers that patients receive also include the ICD function.

Meanwhile Medicare coverage criteria for the ICD (with or without a pacemaker) broadened considerably. In 2000 only thirty-four thousand Americans received the device; by 2010 approximately 600,000 persons annually, most of them Medicare beneficiaries, were considered by doctors to be appropriate ICD candidates.[21]

As the U.S. population ages and Medicare and other insurance reimbursement criteria for ICD use continues to expand, the number of older persons receiving the device will increase—and, importantly, the proportion of devices going to the very elderly probably will increase as well. In 2010 one-fifth of the combination ICD and resynchronizing devices implanted went into persons eighty and older.[22] No longer rare among the very old, these cardiac devices have become the standard of care for patients with moderate to severe heart disease.[23] One study notes that ICDs have become so commonplace that in one clinical trial patients randomized to the non-ICD group withdrew from the study in order to have the ICD implanted.[24]

Even as use of the ICD has burgeoned, since 2004 there have been lively discussions and debates in the medical literature pondering which patients, and especially which elderly patients, might benefit the most from ICD implantation and which are unlikely to benefit.[25] In a 2009 study, the first to focus on older patients, the device was shown to be effective in reducing mortality only in certain specific groups of patients over seventy-five.[26] Yet few patients eighty and older were enrolled in that study. A 2004 study considered the value of an ICD in patients eighty-five and older; that is, it considered the likelihood that the recipient would survive long enough to have an arrhythmic event and receive the ICD's "shock" therapy.[27] It found that the benefit would most often be much smaller than for younger patients.[28] The Harvard Medical School

Newsletter reported in 2011, "More than 80% of sudden cardiac deaths occur in people who are 65 and older. Yet an analysis of five studies found that ICDs did not improve survival more than drugs or other treatments in participants in this age group. While there are no hard-and-fast rules regarding age, *Heart Letter* editorial board . . . counsels people ages 80 and older to consider an alternative to an ICD whenever possible."[29]

THE PROBLEM OF "PREMATURE" DEATHS

The ICD complicates the quest for control over the experience of aging and dying, and it creates quandaries that are distinct in at least three ways from those raised by other therapies. First, most patients are unaware that the ICD can be deactivated at any time (Mr. Tolleson's decision to do so was unusual), and reports show that physicians do not generally discuss that option with them.[30] Despite this lack of routine discussion with patients, the ethics of deactivating cardiac devices looms large in the medical literature and the popular press.[31] For older patients with heart failure and other ailments, and for those already near the end of life, this situation has significant implications. Toward the end of life ICD shocks can occur repeatedly as a patient's condition deteriorates, and shocks can occur while the patient is dying.[32] Since 20 percent of the patient population for implantable cardiac devices is now over eighty,[33] the ICD is actually reshaping the dying transition for significant numbers of people because the shocks that occur to correct a lethal rhythm may reverberate throughout the body and cause pain.

Second, as the cases of Mr. Jones and Mr. Albert reflect, increased usage of the ICD reinforces the powerful societal assumption that sudden death is *premature* death and is a failure of medicine *regardless of the patient's age.*[34]

Third, because "ICD therapy transforms sudden death risk to a subsequent heart failure risk," it may simply prolong living in a state of dying from heart failure,[35] thus creating a need for more intensive interventions. Ordinary medicine's organizational pathways move patients along to the sub-specialists who implant devices, and as a result, they and their families face the quandary of choosing one (potential) sort of death over another.

This is where choice has come to rest in the context of the implantable cardiac devices: in the kind of death we prefer. The ICD device thus contributes to a new engagement with one's own role in the *timing* (amid uncertainty) of one's own or a loved one's death. Mr. Jones's story illustrates this dilemma, as do the stories of other patients and families I will introduce later. Families especially feel ethically responsible for the kind of death that occurs, and the question of timing weighs heavily on them. Should one advocate for death sooner or hope that prolonged life will not be accompanied by suffering? The burden they bear regarding the personal ethics of caregiving is rarely acknowledged within the medical community.[36] That burden, experienced privately within families, is now widespread in the United States.

This is not to imply that the ICD is widely *viewed* as a burden—far from it. I spoke with dozens of individuals over eighty who were glad they had received an ICD because whenever they experienced painful or startling shocks, they knew the device was indeed keeping them alive. They were grateful to have it and were not bothered by it. None were concerned (yet) with its role in the dying transition, and when I asked them whether their doctors had mentioned deactivating the device in the future, all said no, that they did not know anything about deactivation.

And yet the device made the silent, fatal heart attack in the night—which many claim to want eventually because it would be quick and presumably painless—more difficult to achieve.

Once the idea of extending even the oldest lives with the ICD had been conceived and made widely available, it became an ordinary, normal part of the medical-cultural landscape. Progress and postprogress, combined in one small device. Ordinary medicine at work.

"Halfway Technology" and "Forever Disease": Kidney Failure and Dialysis

Kidney dialysis for those who are already old seems, at first glance, to have nothing in common with the ICD.[37] Yet the dialysis procedure and the cardiac device share the same ironic quality. Dialysis too is designed to prevent death. But it is a therapy whose ends—simply to prolong life—have not changed significantly since it was first introduced, even while the population receiving the therapy has grown much older and sicker. Nephrologists are aware of how advanced age and associated infirmity have changed the benefit–no benefit balance. The authors of a 2011 article noted, "For more than 20 years, nephrologists have been reporting that they are increasingly being expected to dialyze patients whom they believe may receive little benefit from dialysis therapy."[38] Nevertheless those specialists have the obligation to prolong life. Thus, within the world of dialysis, they face cultural expectations to continue therapy regardless of how the patient population has aged because dialysis is reimbursed by Medicare and it is standard care. Those factors have created a predicament for some older patients who feel they are being kept alive by the dialysis machine while their bodies deteriorate from other conditions. For while it keeps older persons with multiple diseases alive, kidney dialysis permits the ongoing breakdown of other bodily processes. In our ordinary medicine environment, patients expect therapy as intensive as dialysis to result, if not in a cure, at least in some obvious improvement in their condition. This is not what older people on dialysis experience.[39]

What, then, does it mean for these elderly patients to live outside the notion of medical progress? The lack of improvement after lengthy therapy can be a source of great distress. "It's the 'no progress' that I can't stand," one patient complained, speaking also for many others.

DIALYSIS BECOMES ORDINARY WITH "ORDINARY" EFFECTS

Fifty years ago, when the procedure was new, few predicted that kidney dialysis for those with end-stage renal disease (ESRD) would confront old age. But now the sick and frail elderly constitute the fastest growing segment of the more than 400,000 patients receiving long-term dialysis therapy. By the end of 2010 more than 147,000 ESRD patients were seventy and over; more than twenty thousand were eighty-five and older.[40] The number of patients seventy-five and older who are beginning dialysis has nearly tripled in the past two decades.[41] Because the therapy is so well established, it has remained under the radar of public scrutiny in our aging society. While a number of medical studies and reports since the turn of the millennium note that dialysis does not offer life-prolonging benefits to many sick elderly patients and that it may instead increase suffering among them, it remains the default treatment for those with ESRD.[42] And because many, if not most, physicians do not discuss with elderly patients the symptoms that the therapy causes or propose turning instead to hospice and palliative care (though this is beginning to change), older patients and their families generally are not aware of the effects of maintenance dialysis therapy.

The emergence of dialysis as a common therapy followed a path unlike that taken by any other treatment in American medicine. Never subjected to rigorous clinical trials and scrutiny of trial evidence, dialysis therapy was first funded by Medicare in 1972 due to both advocacy by middle-class patients for government intervention and pressure on Congress by health professionals who had stakes in the dialysis machine.[43] End-stage renal disease became, and remains today, the only medical condition for which treatment for all patients, regardless of age, is subsidized by the U.S. government.[44] It began as a therapy to enable small numbers of patients with permanent kidney failure to return to work. Most patients were wage-earning men who were in the middle of their working lives. One year after the therapy became available to all through Medicare funding, approximately ten thousand patients were receiving dialysis, and apparently few observers of health care thought the numbers would increase.[45] But over the years the population receiving dialysis has not only mushroomed but has also grown older and sicker.

Renal dialysis first emerged in the 1940s and 1950s as a short-term, intermittent procedure for persons suffering from acute, life-threatening kidney failure. It was among the first of the post–World War II treatments that transformed and complicated the relationship of doctors and patients to complex life support systems that do not cure disease. (It became available for routine use a decade and a half before the mechanical ventilator arrived.)

Maintenance hemodialysis for the continuous, long-term treatment of individuals with irreversible loss of kidney function came on the scene in 1960, and with it the realization of an emerging medical goal: lethal kidney disease could be treated, seemingly indefinitely. No longer a death sentence, ESRD became a chronic condition for patients to live with in an open-ended way. Life could be sustained but without curing the underlying disease. Today, however, experts note that ESRD "has practically become synonymous with geriatric medicine."[46]

The dialysis technology cycles blood out of the body and filters it through a machine that removes the waste and excess fluids that the patient's kidneys can no longer process. Without functioning kidneys, or without a machine capable of taking over for them, one dies within days to a few weeks. Most patients in the United States undergo hemodialysis in clinics, spending several hours there three days a week undergoing a treatment that many find exhausting, painful, and debilitating. The result for older patients is often a mixture of feelings—of the avoidance of death yet also of anxiety because continued life depends on continual connection to the dialysis machine. For persons in later life the burden of undergoing treatment to remain alive can rival the burden of living with multiple illnesses, and many are forced to confront the value of persisting on dialysis. Dialysis as routine therapy for an ever older population both reinforces and raises questions about the obligation to longevity.

The sociologists Renée Fox and Judith Swazey were the first to study the interpersonal and societal effects of this treatment when it was new, and in the early 1970s they questioned whether long-term support on dialysis would constitute a blessing or "merely a labored and painful hanging onto life."[47] They were aware of the ambivalence expressed by some of the physicians involved in the first U.S. dialysis program, during the 1960s, when it was referred to as a "half-way technology,"[48] the only means of coping until better cures for kidney disease could be found. Those early critics expressed qualms that the therapy simply prolonged the process of dying and that therefore its use should be restricted from the very start, as it was in Britain.[49] They worried too about costs if it were to become open to all. Yet Congress and Medicare agreed to underwrite those costs and, importantly, to guarantee access to all who suffered permanent kidney failure.[50]

The question about prolonging dying that a number of observers posed in the early 1970s would not occur to a broader public until fifteen years later, when Karen Ann Quinlan, unconscious and maintained on a ventilator, captured the collective imagination. Today, with so much attention focused on control of the dying process and the desire for a dying not prolonged by technologies, it is perhaps surprising that the questions about dialysis that were posed a generation ago are not widely discussed today. Dialysis seems to be invisible to those beyond the realm of the health professionals, patients, and families who live with it, thus keeping its inherent irony in an aging society well below the radar.

THE GRAYING OF DIALYSIS

The graying of the dialysis population over the past several decades reveals how the original end of the therapy during the 1960s and 1970s (to keep people in youth and midlife alive as long as possible to work, raise families, and function in society) no longer fits the kind of patients who so routinely receive the therapy today: sick older people, many of whom have multiple debilitating and end-stage health problems. The problem for medicine and for society is that the goals of treatment from a half century ago have not changed to reflect that demographic shift. When the new therapy was focused on younger people, the idea of kidney failure as an end-stage disease was pushed aside, and it mostly continues to be ignored in today's day-to-day treatment routines. Yet many older dialysis patients have other end-stage conditions in addition to kidney failure, and the lack of acknowledgment that the end of life is approaching creates a state of psychic disquiet in some patients, and in dialysis clinics it creates a situation best described as being out of sync. Indeed, with a few early twenty-first-century exceptions, the medical literature is only just now beginning to acknowledge the nearness of the end of life in dialysis settings.[51] That avoidance shows that clinicians are uncomfortable with and thus shy away from discussing death with patients in dialysis as in other medical settings.

The result of this discomfort is that many older patients are left feeling stranded. They are not getting better, are hoping not to get worse, yet are aware of their increasing infirmity and deterioration. They don't fit into the ethos of treatment, which stresses that dialysis allows and extends life, but they are not yet within the ethos of hospice, which acknowledges the acceptance of death. Although the vast majority of dialysis patients are not ready to "choose" death, many older patients are ambivalent about continuing treatment. In settings in which end-stage and end-of-life discussions are not part of the therapeutic enterprise, having more older patients in dialysis therapy means the treatment suspends more lives in a state that patients have described as "between life and death" and "already promised to death." For those who are already old, the therapy raises anew, and more urgently, the question Fox and Swazey posed in the 1970s: Is this a good thing for patients or not?

Between 1960 and 1972 the story of dialysis revolved around a growing demand for the therapy amid a scarcity of dialysis machines. Maintenance dialysis simply was not allowed for anyone over forty-five.[52] Selection decisions—who was worthy of access to the machine and thus to life—plagued health professionals and dominated the media and at times an outraged public, which angrily referred to selection committees as "god committees."[53] Working white men with families were given preference over, for example, single women, minorities, and the unemployed. Churchgoers were chosen before atheists. The selection criteria were criticized for being based on social values that the white middle class held dear: marriage, employment, civic engagement, family orientation, and so on. And the selection process, instituted in response to the scarcity of machines, was the most ethically fraught topic in health care delivery during those years.

In 1972 Congress extended Medicare benefits for dialysis to all individuals with end-stage renal disease, regardless of age, ethnicity, or any other characteristic, and it guaranteed access to everyone who needed the machine. Overnight the selection criteria became irrelevant. For all those who needed it, dialysis was now understood to be the means to survival.

ACCESS, OBLIGATION, AND PARADOX:
THE CHANGING CULTURE OF DIALYSIS

Today's culture of dialysis strongly emphasizes access to the therapy for all, the right to pursue the therapy, and the obligation of health professionals to make it available to patients regardless of age or medical condition. A social worker described the dramatic change:

> Everyone has the right to dialyze today. Nothing disqualifies patients. When dialysis first started in the 1960s it was selective medicine. Not everyone with kidney failure was placed on dialysis. Older people were looked at carefully, very carefully—their life span was looked at. If they only had a few years to live, they probably didn't get dialysis because it was so expensive to run the machines. Now there is a drive to keep people alive longer. Period. We look toward prolonging life a lot longer these days. Patients are just placed on dialysis and told that this is what we need to do. . . . If a patient has cancer, or another progressive medical condition, then sometimes the doctors will advise him not to start dialysis because it would be one more thing to have to deal with. However, the lack of dialysis would lead to the patient's demise, so it would be discussed. And mostly it is automatically assumed that a patient wants dialysis. "No" is never presented as an option. It should be, but it's not.

Physicians state that advanced age alone is no longer a limiting factor in evaluating patients for dialysis, and advances in dialysis care over the past thirty years allow physicians to dialyze patients with complex chronic diseases. Dementia or life-threatening conditions sometimes do emerge as eliminating criteria, but not always. Most often any questions about the therapy's appropriateness and duration for older patients, who typically have more medical problems and poorer prognoses than younger patients, lurk under the surface of the practice of ordinary medicine.

Because the therapy's goals have not shifted with the changing patient population, dialysis treatment is a poor fit for many elderly patients. The means and ends of dialysis are cast in an entirely positive, curative light, stressing compliance with the regimens of the therapy and activism in the pursuit of life (and for some in the hope of staying healthy enough to receive an eventual kidney transplant). Yet this emphasis is ill suited to most elderly patients, who are concerned neither with compliance and future-oriented activism nor, for that matter, with anticipating the end (as in hospice). Rather their focus is on some kind of negotiation in and with the present in order to make life on dialysis acceptable.

Speaking about this state of affairs, a dialysis center technician noted that many older patients on dialysis are "in one of two places." At the beginning of treatment, he said, they have "not adjusted" and they do not see dialysis "as their life, how they want or need to live." For those patients treatment is a "vicious circle." (He drew a circle composed of three separate arrows.) But some patients, typically those with "more schooling" or "with a family," "can find acceptance," making dialysis "part of their life, not an obstacle." (He drew a complete, closed circle.) "Most don't reach that stage," he said. "They die earlier." At some point, of course, one can no longer negotiate or finds oneself in an increasingly poor negotiating position, and, conceivably, at this point one must prepare for life's end. But this point is something for which the culture and structure of dialysis treatment rarely prepare patients.[54]

Dialysis units thus are paradoxical spaces for elderly persons. The overall trajectory and ethos of the treatment (framed as *life*saving and *life*-prolonging) operate to deny and conceal its complicated effects on older persons. The focus is instead on patients' pragmatic and, over time, habituated efforts simply to arrive at the unit every other day. The physical symptoms of dying are therapeutically masked by dialysis—thus effectively delaying the onset of dying—and there is a shared reluctance of patients and providers to acknowledge the impending decline to death.[55] Because, like other therapies, dialysis can be employed up until the moment of death, dying is often acknowledged only in its most final stages;[56] thus in dialysis units the foreshortening of the time for dying is further intensified.

THE LIVED EXPERIENCE OF POSTPROGRESS MEDICINE:
A "HOLDING PATTERN" AND "SLOW DEATH"

Older patients' accounts of their experience of dialysis highlight some of the existential quandaries the therapy poses among the elderly and show that the goal of life extension with this particular therapy is complicated and not an unequivocal good when one is already old and sick. "You'd kinda like to see some progress as you go along," said a ninety-year-old woman who had been on dialysis for six months. "I might feel I was making some progress if I only had to come two days a week instead of three, but that's impossible. It's not a cure—there's no cure for what I have. It's just treatment. I have to come here. I'm not here by choice."

Choice is complicated for those on dialysis. Most patients do not regard having started dialysis as a proactive matter. "I just wound up here" and "I have no choice" are common remarks. Patients assent to the therapy in order to stay alive. Older, sick dialysis patients can find their situation—being in treatment to prolong a life of perpetually increasing illness—disquieting. One woman reported, "The only choice you make is accepting the need for dialysis." A seventy-eight-year-old man who had been on dialysis for ten years aptly noted, "You make the decision to go on dialysis and then you live with it. Those are two very different things." "And then," he added, "whatever they told me to do, I had to accept, whatever it was." He described the start of his treatment in the context of this constrained sense of choice: "I had seen the doctor twice, I think, before that. When he said, 'Are you ready for dialysis?' and I said, 'Is that what I'm supposed to do now?,' he said, 'Yes.' And so he had me come over and look at the unit. And I went over and looked at it; and I had to have the surgery, to put the graft in my arm. . . . I don't think I really questioned anything, I mean, what would that do?" An eighty-two-year-old man reported, "Your creatinine level keeps going up. You don't have a choice. That's how you start." He spoke of choice starkly, saying, "You don't want to accept anything like that until you finally have to. And then they give you a choice—you can die now or die later. . . . You get used to it. That's all."

Many expressed not wanting to know or to be made to understand the complex issues around, for instance, their creatinine levels or why potassium in their diet is bad for them. "I try not to think about it" and "I try not to dwell" were typical responses to interview questions. One man stated emphatically, "I don't want to talk about it. I don't even want to think about it. It's difficult enough that I have to be here."

In addition to the lack of choice and absence of progress while in therapy, there is the impact of the ambiance of the hemodialysis unit, where most Americans receive the therapy. A seventy-three-year-old woman described her feelings about it: "When you come into a situation like this, it's horrifying. And then you have to see other people go through pain. All the time. Like Maria. She cried out today [when they inserted the needles]. And I know Rosa is having a hard time. And it breaks my heart. And you get close to all these people. And you're exposed to all this death."

Cumulatively the testimony of older patients is that dialysis takes time but does not substantially fill it, that it drains their energy and capacity for life both inside the unit and outside. Patients (and sometimes their families) therefore remain ambivalent about dialysis therapy. On the one hand, it may extend life and allow older individuals to persist. On the other, it is, as some patients remarked, a "slow death." Dialysis patients live, as several of them put it, in a "holding pattern."

Most older patients on dialysis are not expecting a kidney transplant, nor are they on the waiting list for one. There is thus no projected end to dialysis treatment for them. They do not have the same incentive as do younger patients to demonstrate compliance or activism around their kidney disease. Instead most can expect to be on dialysis until they die. Although many patients express the feeling that the treatment has a *forever* quality to it, it often dawns on them only slowly that this therapy will proceed up until death. A frail ninety-year-old woman said, "There are times when I start thinking about how I'd like to not come here. Then when I think about stopping, I guess I decide to continue. I don't know whether I will quit voluntarily or not."

"I want to get off dialysis," an eighty-three-year-old woman who had started dialysis two months before stated emphatically. "At the very least, I want to shorten it. I know I'm probably in denial thinking either of those will happen. But they don't tell you how long to expect! Do you know how long [one] can go on like this?"

The existential ramifications of chronic life support for elderly patients are therefore different from those for younger patients. Patients struggle to discern an end or outer limit to their situation. For example, they routinely asked how long older people can "last" on dialysis, what kinds of conditions or events lead to eventual decline on the procedure, and whether or not people who decreased their time or discontinued treatment stayed alive.[57]

The question of progress comes up often: "I don't know if I'm progressing or not. It's unclear. I know that I don't want to come here anymore, but I can't get a direct answer about that. The doctor shakes his head when I say it, but he doesn't say anything. I just want to know, based on my blood tests, am I progressing? Do they see a change? Any movement at all? A shift in those [results]? That's what I don't understand. Is there *any* change?" Yet another patient said, "With most other maladies "one has some reasonable expectation of being cured or at least of some progress, but not with this one—so dialysis *is* a treatment, you see, but one with no cure, and no real tangible evidence of progress." He described a meeting he'd had with his physician:

> The doctor said to me, "You're doing so good." But there was no progress! No change in my condition for the better! I can see now that the best that I can hope for is for things to remain the same, . . . that dialysis is about struggling to stand still, to stay exactly where you are—as the most that one can wish for. It was then that I realized I was going to have to give up on the dream of leaving here, of getting out of here. So that's that. I can live with this. I have no other choice. But let me tell you, I love walking out this door on Saturdays knowing that I'm sprung for two days.

"In many ways," this patient concluded, "dialysis is the end of hope."

The tension between dialysis and the life it extends finds expression in patients' claims that dialysis is "no way to live." Clinicians tell patients that dialysis is intended to assist and support life but not to *be* life. They appeal to patients to make dialysis "part of life, but not all of it." "Think of it as your part-time job," a physician said to a patient who was complaining about the negative features of the therapy. This call to action and responsibility for maintaining one's own life outside of the unit can be a tall order even for younger patients and the most fit and motivated of the older patients as they confront the challenge of how to remain vital in this situation of chronic passivity and enforced dependency. The challenge is uniquely difficult for most older people for several reasons. Many have outlived their peers, even their children. Their world is further diminished as some lose their mobility, sight, fingers, toes, or limbs to disease. "I'm dying in pieces," one patient stated emphatically, revealing her dead fingernail and then noting the lost function of two of her fingers and mentioning the toes she had lost before the below-knee amputation of both legs. "I have everything wrong with me," she said, "but I keep going." She compared her experience of illness and treatment, in dialysis and through her successive amputations, to that of a plant that must be pruned, the dead or dying parts excised in order to maintain the parts that are living.

Some patients feel that they are in a truly desperate situation. They question why and to what end they are still alive. A distressed eighty-four-year-old woman cried out one day, "I look at the other old people here [gesturing to the unit], and I ask, 'Why are we here?' I guess it's not our time yet, but . . . [crying, shaking her head] I don't know why I'm here. I wish I could go. My husband doesn't like it when I talk like this, but I think, why? What good am I? I can't do anything. I can't even pee! I pee mud. My hair is gone and I can't get out by myself to get a wig. I look in the mirror, I don't recognize myself. I itch all the time, I can't sleep. . . . Why, why am I still here?"

Others feel that in significant respects they are already departed, irrevocably altered, or at a remove from life. "I wake at night and say out loud, 'I'm gone, I'm dead,'" said another patient, a double amputee who in previous conversations had expressed feeling "stranded alive," without family, without legs, with overwhelming debt, and without any sense of possibility for the future. "It takes you away from life for so much of the time," commented another patient.

Over the course of a therapy that can go on for years, death occupies progressively greater experiential space for older patients. In addition to "standing still," many patients characterize life on dialysis as "slipping." "Nothing gets any better, there's never any improvement," cried one eighty-six-year-old patient just returned from months of rehabilitation following a double amputation, "and now, I'm losing ground." When patients become more debilitated and dialysis more clearly is their central preoccupation, when the question of life's value is gradually and then more powerfully raised, patients are sometimes forced to confront the issue of their continued participation in treatment. A seventy-three-year-old patient evoked the paradoxical circumstance many older patients face: not wanting to be kept alive (and dependent) yet not wanting to die:

Dr.———told me straight, "You're in an environment of death." I have to accept that. But I didn't like hearing it. Now with death, there's something you don't talk about, you don't want to think about, and we don't know how to prepare or handle it. So when you come into a situation like this, it's horrifying. And then you have to see other people go through the pain. *All* the time. And it breaks your heart. And you get close to these people. So dialysis is treatment, but just to prolong your life. And it's giving, I think, false hope. Because you think you won't die on it, but that's not true. Things can happen at any time to anybody. When your blood pressure goes down, you can go into a coma just like that. And they wouldn't catch it right away.

I've seen that happen many times, that they weren't able to revive the patient. If that were to happen to me, if I get to the point where I'm so incapacitated—in my living will, and my girlfriends know this, I don't want to be kept alive. I don't. But I don't want to die. But I definitely . . . I don't know how you do it, though. I talked to the doctor about it and said very clearly what my wishes were. He said that I was the first [of his patients] to bring that up on my own.

People receiving routine maintenance dialysis do not necessarily want to talk or think about the end of life. A seventy-three-year-old patient in the final stages of lung cancer chose to leave one dialysis center and dialyze at a different facility when she suspected that her nephrologist might have raised the possibility of dialysis discontinuation with her oncologist. The oncologist had encouraged her to consider whether the procedure, which she found draining, was still providing the benefits and quality of life she wanted. Her response reveals some of why discontinuation, and ends in general, are so exceedingly difficult to bring up with patients: "My doctor wants me to commit suicide! I can't do that. I can't take life, only God can take life. And I'm putting my faith in Him up there. Black people don't commit suicide! Why couldn't they give me [a little] longer? I'm not an animal, I'm a human. Would the doctor recommend this to his wife, to his children? And then he asked if I were to have a heart attack and I was on dialysis, would I want them to revive me? What's this about a heart attack?! [She begins crying.] I'm very hurt, very hurt."

Indeed most patients express the desire to remain alive. During the period of researching this book, health professionals at one dialysis unit conducted a "quality of life" study. Patients there were asked to consider, hypothetically, whether they would choose one year of good health without dialysis or five years as they are now, on dialysis. Everyone who discussed this—including patients who had complained vehemently about the treatment, about their life and loss of quality of life on dialysis, and about their inability to see any end to it all—chose the five years, though not without some deliberation. "I really had to think about it," said one elderly woman, "and I pictured myself with legs and able to walk—and oh [dreamily], it was so wonderful." "Why do I want to live so long?" she wondered. She then answered her own question: "I guess I want to see what's going to happen." "That's right," contributed another patient. "We want to see what happens." Yet another patient, commenting on the same study, insisted that it was precisely through his feeling of being "removed from life" on dialysis treatment that he was made aware of his own strong "attachment to living." As his quality of life diminished, his attachment to life grew. These patients offer both a powerful reminder of why it is impossible, in the abstract, to be for or against life-prolonging therapies for older individuals and a glaring example of the quandary about where to locate the line.

An eighty-six-year-old woman, frail and wheelchair-bound, when asked what quality of life meant to her, responded, "I do get frustrated that I can't do what I want to do, like go to the grocery store and that kind of stuff. But I have a good husband, I have good children and grandchildren, and my great job now is my six-month-old great-grandchild. When I'm around her, it's all worth it. We have a family dinner every Sunday night, with twelve people around the table, so it's really about as good as it can get." Yet she also said, "I've been in this state so long that I'm more or less used to it. Now I just take what comes. I don't even think about quality of life—it's not really the point."

The relationship between age and quality of life on dialysis is not simple. Early accounts of the treatment suggested that older patients adjusted more readily to dialysis and its associated restrictions than did younger patients.[58] Dialysis was seen as simply an extension of what was already happening to older patients—that they were becoming weaker, less active, more tired—as opposed to the sea change in identity and daily life the therapy was thought to produce for younger patients. Some studies are more equivocal about the relatively unproblematic adjustment of older individuals, and the most recent studies note that there is no evidence showing that there is a quality-of-life benefit for the elderly on dialysis.[59]

LOOMING MORTALITY AND THE QUANDARY
OF TREATMENT BENEFIT

During the early 1970s, when the legislation that would provide Medicare payment for maintenance dialysis was being debated, physicians and other advocates of dialysis for all predicted that the U.S. dialysis population would "stabilize somewhere around 20,000 patients."[60] They had absolutely no idea what lay ahead, either in numbers of patients or the upper limits of their age range.[61]

Today, because most older dialysis patients have other serious diseases, including diabetes, stroke, heart failure, and dementia,[62] their life expectancy is poor—the average survival time for patients eighty-five and over is less than one year—and may not be much longer than for those who receive medical management of their end-stage disease without dialysis.[63] Yet even so doctors recommend the therapy, and some patients insist on it.[64] One survey of nephrologists discovered that nearly half would be willing to continue the therapy for a patient who had permanent, severe dementia.[65]

The graying of dialysis has come at considerable cost in Medicare dollars—$40 billion to $50 billion in 2011[66]—prompting some physicians and other observers to question its suitability for older patients whose lives may be only marginally lengthened and possibly with added suffering. Those costs are augmented by another recent trend: the timing of the start of dialysis therapy inched forward over the course of the decade from 1997 to 2007. That is, patients are beginning therapy with relatively better kidney function than previously. This trend is most pronounced for patients over seventy-five,[67] yet no evidence shows that it prolongs life or contributes to its quality. In fact at least one study suggests that an earlier start of hemodialysis may hasten rather than postpone mortality.[68] The costs of this trend are enormous, estimated in 2011 at more than $1.5 billion for the population that began dialysis (regardless of age) in 2007. One study notes that Medicare provides less oversight now than it did a decade ago regarding the level of kidney function a patient must have lost before it will pay for the therapy.[69]

The Quinlan case forced medicine, the law, and government policies to consider in a new way the twinned problems of in-between-ness and continued therapy but without a cure. Though dialysis shares those problems, it never had an equivalent eye-opening effect on the public. Rather for the past forty years those problems have remained sequestered among ever older dialysis patients, their families, and some who treat them. Few foresaw the dilemmas that would result from the expansion of a population that would exist in a condition some of them describe as being between life and death, tethered to a therapy without progress. Few who work in that realm of medicine are outspoken about those dilemmas. But although the consequences of dialysis therapy in late life have remained invisible outside that circumscribed world, dialysis nevertheless complicates the relationship of medicine to age, for the treatment elicits the following questions: How long should we treat disease? What constitutes treatment benefit? The ethics of access to dialysis technology coupled with the medical mandate to prolong life has come to rest today in the lives and sensibilities of old patients. Their poignant response to the seemingly endless treatment and the existential predicament it creates is one result, sequestered in dialysis units, of ordinary medicine.

The "Best Option" for Life-Threatening Liver Disease: Liver Transplantation

Just like the ICD, the LVAD, and the ubiquity of dialysis treatment, liver transplantation was "unthinkable" several decades ago,[70] yet it has become the most effective treatment for liver cancers and other end-stage liver diseases. Though far less common than cardiac device implantation and dialysis, liver transplantation too provides a telling example of how developments in research and clinical practice pave the way for broadened Medicare payment coverage. That coverage, as already noted, is interwoven with the ethics of managing life, especially at older ages, and if current disease and treatment trends persist, by 2020 the majority of patients being evaluated for liver transplantation in the United States will be over the age of seventy.[71]

In this context Medicare itself can be understood to function as a technology, for it provides the *means* through which we rethink what is possible, appropriate, and successful therapy. It is a tool that legitimates and rationalizes all these treatments at older ages. Its *end*, to fund treatments shown to be "reasonable and necessary," remains unchanged at the same time that its reimbursement responsibilities continually expand in response to new evidence. The example of liver transplantation highlights the work of Medicare reimbursement as an enabling technology and illustrates the relationship among emerging evidence, expanding payment, increasing need, and the ethics of managing life.

The example of kidney dialysis for those in late life offers a version of Medicare-enabled life management in which there is no socially acceptable, agreed-upon reason to stop treatment, and doctors and patients are loath to say no to it. Liver transplantation, as practiced in the United States, provides an even more dramatic example of ordinary medicine, showing how Medicare reimbursement, in combination with individual rights, increasing demand, and the medical obligation to save lives, makes a complex and costly treatment seem routine. As with other technologies, the means and ends of liver transplantation shifted over time as research and clinical evidence accumulated to show that the procedure saved lives and Medicare was led to expand its reimbursement criteria. That development, wanted by all, of course, then fostered more need and demand for the procedure. The drama of liver transplantation, in addition to the complexity of the procedure, attaches to the fact that the cure for fatal liver disease requires a scarce human organ, and, in addition, the surgery and the lifelong follow-up drug regimen are so very expensive.

FROM EXTRAORDINARY TO ORDINARY

The first human liver transplants were carried out in the 1960s, but without the immunosuppressive drugs developed in the early 1980s, the surgery was not a viable treatment. With improvements in immunosuppression, liver transplantation gained widespread acceptance among doctors and patients and became the only curative treatment for certain liver diseases. A recent review of the history of liver disease treatment summarizes the changed thinking about the intervention: "By 1983, results were sufficiently convincing for a National Institutes of Health Consensus Development Conference to conclude that liver transplantation should be considered an acceptable, clinically applicable, lifesaving procedure."[72] By the end of that decade liver transplantation was no longer considered "so drastic that it was used only as a last resort."[73]

Though only for a limited number of diagnoses, payments to hospitals for liver transplants for Medicare beneficiaries began in 1991,[74] and 2,953 were performed that year, 144 among older adults. Broader Medicare coverage for transplantation as the appropriate treatment of end-stage liver disease became available in 1996, following more research that provided evidence of positive outcomes. That year 4,087 liver transplants were performed, 275 among patients sixty-five and over.

Initially hepatitis B (HBV) and liver cancer were excluded from coverage because of the unresolved medical problem that those diseases recurred following transplantation. But by 1999 developments in molecular diagnostic and antiviral therapies had dramatically improved medicine's ability to prevent recurrent HBV infection after liver transplantation, so Medicare expanded coverage to include transplants for patients with HBV.[75]

By 2001 the evidence base from research studies was strong enough to indicate that, when specific medical conditions were met, transplants prolonged life for patients with cancer that originated in the liver (hepatocellular carcinoma).[76] That year Medicare began to cover transplantation for eligible patients with certain liver cancers, and thus the total number of liver transplants among persons sixty-five and over grew to 339.[77] Transplantation numbers have grown steadily ever since.

Today livers are the second most commonly transplanted organ (after kidneys) in the United States; according to the Organ Procurement and Transplantation Network website, twenty-one American centers performed liver transplants in 2011–12. A total of 6,256 individuals received liver transplants in 2012; 835 of those transplants (over 13 percent) were performed on persons sixty-five and over (up from 10 percent in 2008).[78] Though those numbers are not large, the percentage of liver transplants for older persons is increasing.

EXPANDING ELIGIBILITY

Who gets liver transplants today, and why? Approximately 1.3 percent (some 3.2 million persons) of the total U.S. population is chronically infected with the hepatitis c virus (HCV), and the number of cases has increased among those over forty. In addition approximately 800,000 to 1.4 million people are living with chronic hepatitis B, about half of whom are Asian or Asian American. These statistics have made hepatitis c and B the leading causes of chronic liver disease and liver cancer in the United States.[79] The hepatitis c virus is the leading cause of liver disease in transplant recipients,[80] and 1 to 5 percent of persons with HCV will go on to develop cancer of the liver. Improved medical management of cirrhosis (death of cells and scarring of the liver) resulting from both HBV and HCV has led to increased numbers of individuals living *longer* with chronic liver disease.[81]

While the hepatitis B and c viruses themselves do not directly cause cancer, they do cause liver inflammation and scarring, which, when chronic, can and often does lead to liver cancer.[82] The average time it takes to develop primary liver cancer after initial exposure to the hepatitis c virus, for example, is about twenty-eight years; after the development of liver cirrhosis it is usually about eight to ten years. Importantly for the Medicare program, the time from initial viral infection to complications from the virus, including cancer, is about twenty to thirty years.

In clinics I observed two ways this long gestation period can play out for patients. Some older patients have known about their hepatitis B or c for many years, and they go to a specialized liver clinic periodically to have their condition monitored and treated. Others learned that they have hepatitis or liver cancer from recent symptoms or blood work their primary care physician carried out for some unrelated reason. Physicians attribute many hepatitis C infections to blood products patients received for surgeries performed before HCV was well understood and before the first blood screening for the virus was developed in 1992. Generally the surgeries were twenty to thirty years prior to HCV diagnosis.

As with other therapies, the shift in medical practice and consciousness regarding transplantation as an appropriate intervention—from the unthinkable to the standard treatment—was facilitated by insurance payment. Even in the case of this medically dramatic example, it was reimbursement that ushered in the *need* for liver transplantation as a means to rid the body of cancer, and thus stave off death, and fostered the expectation that the treatment represents what is normal, as the stories of Mrs. Dang and Mr. Carter (chapter 1) illustrated. Both the need and the expectation have increased dramatically over the past decade, along with the aging of the American population.

DEVELOPING NEW MEANS FOR STAYING ELIGIBLE

Also now standard, because they too are reimbursed by Medicare, are all the supportive interventions—the ancillary means—that have emerged to enable patients with primary liver cancer to continue to stay eligible, according to Medicare payment criteria, for transplant surgery while they wait for a donor organ. Those standard, reimbursed, supportive interventions serve to increase the size of the population that is appropriate for and needs a transplant. The interventions include the various radiofrequency and chemotherapy techniques used to reduce the size of tumors while waiting for an available organ so that a successful transplant, without disease recurrence, can best be achieved and, crucially, so that the transplant surgery itself will qualify for Medicare reimbursement.[83]

An interventional radiologist who performs one such procedure, chemoembolization, at a busy center noted, "It's big business. We meet weekly with the imaging people and the hepatologists to decide who should get it—can we knock the tumors out? . . . We are one of the pillars of the whole liver transplant enterprise. Chemoembolization has been great for patients. It's bridged them from being untransplantable to being transplantable. The transplant is the key to life. So [chemoembolization is] the bridge to life." In 2009 he reported that his center was completing all the regulatory paperwork so that it could acquire a newer technology, radioembolization, which other centers were already using.[84] "It's very expensive," he said, "and it's more effective than chemoembolization and with fewer side effects. It inserts beads of radioactive material into the tumor, which are released there, cutting off the blood supply to the tumor."

These embolization procedures, involving several medical specialties and multiple technologies, are one more example of how Medicare reimbursement enables the myriad enterprises surrounding a major intervention such as transplantation. By enabling more patients to be eligible for, to need, to want, and to expect a transplant, it exerts a direct influence on both the means and ends of that technology. Added to the mix is the fact that medical centers compete for patients and for excellent clinicians, and in order to do so they must acquire and use the latest tools. Institutions must consider, however, whether use of those expensive technologies will be reimbursed by Medicare. If so, the tests and therapies they can perform are recommended to patients and used without considering the cost. If not, doctors will not employ them.

"If a Transplant Is Necessary, I'll Go with That": Mr. Chin

For more than twenty-five years physicians monitored the hepatitis B virus in Mr. Ming Chin through repeated blood tests. He had no symptoms and received no treatment, a common approach if no cancer is present. When his doctors thought he might have developed liver cancer at age seventy-five, they referred him to a major center where the medical staff did indeed find one small cancer tumor. At the clinic appointment to discuss the new diagnosis, the surgeon told Mr. Chin and his wife, son, and daughter, who had accompanied him, that hepatitis B affects the entire liver. Even if the cancer is treated, he said, about 60 percent of patients will get tumors again in a couple of years. "We have no way to prevent other tumors," he said. "We can only watch for them with CT scans." He noted that there was quite a bit of debate in medicine about "what to do with a person of his age. Should we do repetitive ablations, if tumors keep appearing? Chemoembolizations? No transplant? If there are a lot of tumors, we might not be able to do anything. There is added risk because of his age. In China and Korea they would just ablate him."

Mr. Chin responded, "If there are other treatment options better than transplant, I'd rather go that way, but if transplant is better, if it's necessary, I'll go with that." His wife said hesitantly that if transplant proves to be the best treatment, she would support it. The son and daughter agreed. The doctor pointed out that it is hard to make that determination. "If all tests are okay, the risks of transplant surgery are low. His life expectancy is about ten years or so. If he were younger we'd say transplant is best. At his age, it's difficult to say if transplant is best. If he only has one small tumor, probably transplant is not best. If it grows, ablation is good. If another tumor grows, then he's a transplant candidate. But if there are four or five tumors, then he's not a candidate. So it's trading risks. It is controversial. That is, everyone will have an opinion about it."

The liver specialist came into the exam room after the surgeon left and confirmed the cancer diagnosis. "It looks as if he may have more than one lesion," he told the family. "If the lesions are within the limits set by the United Network for Organ Sharing, I anticipate we'll put him on the [waiting] list for a liver. The caveat is age. But he seems pretty vigorous. We could potentially go forward with transplant. But it could be a wait of many months." He asked Mr. Chin, "Do you want a transplant if we find you eligible?" Mr. Chin responded, "If that's the best option, of course."

The physician recommended chemoembolization or radiotherapy ablation as the next step. "Both of these treatments are not curative," the doctor pointed out. "They are used to buy time. They can be used alone or together, to bridge someone to transplant, to keep tumors from progressing. For some who do not want transplant, these are effective palliation."

Five months after that diagnostic clinic visit, a chemoembolization treatment "knocked out" the cancer completely, Mr. Chin reported, at least for the time being. The treatment was harder on him than he or the family had expected. He was hospitalized for a week, significantly longer than the usual single night the physicians anticipated. He remained open-minded about considering a transplant if it was needed, but he was ambivalent as well. Nonetheless he remained on the waiting list, though he hoped he would not be offered a donor liver; he hoped the doctors would not call. After all, he wasn't feeling sick.

Mr. Chin received a phone call a few months before his seventy-eighth birthday. His name had come to the top of the waiting list, and he was offered a liver from a seventy-two-year-old donor. The surgeon described the liver to him, and Mr. Chin decided against it. His family was impressed with the doctor; he neither encouraged nor pressured Mr. Chin or the family to accept that organ. The rejected liver was "used" (meaning it had lived in an older patient who had had some disease, such as hypertension or diabetes), but the clinic staff noted that one reason Mr. Chin decided against it was because he felt healthy and had no symptoms. He wasn't sure he needed a transplant at all. Several months later he was offered a second organ, this one from a forty-year-old donor, and, though still feeling no symptoms, he accepted it. He had remained ambivalent while waiting to be offered an organ he would accept, but during that period one of his children had said, "Dad, everything is a gamble. It would be a gamble not to have a transplant, especially if the cancer returned. It could spread, and then you wouldn't be eligible for a transplant anymore."

At age seventy-eight, two years after his cancer was diagnosed, Mr. Chin had transplant surgery. Three months later and experiencing no complications, he was grateful to be rid of the cancer and was relieved that the surgery was behind him. But, he noted, he would be okay going forward at his age with "letting go," if that was what was next. For now he only needed to return to the clinic for CT scans every six months to make sure the cancer did not reappear.

A PROGNOSIS FOR LIVER TRANSPLANTATION

The demographics of the hepatitis B and C viruses, together with those for obesity, alcoholic cirrhosis, and other conditions that affect liver health, forecast an explosion in the number of older patients who will need liver transplants in the future.[85] Older persons who went to liver clinics for evaluation in the first decade of the new millennium, some of whom I met, constitute the leading edge of this trend. Need expands and will continue to do so because HBV and HCV can be diagnosed and monitored before patients become too sick to undergo transplant surgery, because primary care physicians refer patients with liver disease to major centers for transplant evaluation, and because the size of cancer tumors can be controlled prior to transplantation, thus keeping the disease "in criteria" to receive an organ and Medicare reimbursement. Transplantation becomes the logical medical endpoint for liver cancer and other end-stage liver diseases. As a result liver transplantation is an increasingly desired enterprise, *especially* among older persons.[86]

There is no doubt that liver diseases have slowly succumbed to treatments that save and prolong life. Yet the taxpayer and government carry the cost burden of these treatments—one ramification of the success of transplantation as standard therapy for liver cancer. A patient I followed from 2007 to 2009 told me that his liver transplant in 2008, at age seventy-eight, cost nearly $300,000. He reported that it was fully covered by Medicare. Taken together the aging of the population, disease patterns, and greater need and desire forecast an ever-increasing cost burden. The government could potentially choose not to fund liver transplants (and other procedures), but desire and expectation (long nurtured by the links among research, reimbursement, standard making, and necessity) cannot easily be altered by rescinding a reimbursement decision. Again the burden of costs actually rests within the sociocultural foundation and the drivers of ordinary medicine.

Embracing New Means, but to What Ends?

Each of these three technologies has changed the idea of what constitutes therapeutic benefit for older people in our society. In doing so each also raises questions about "successful treatment"—questions about whether success is to be measured by resource use and the goals of medicine in an aging society in addition to the staving off of death for individual patients. But who is to do the measuring? And to what ends? The constellation of forces of ordinary medicine works against a thorough accounting and re-visioning of what successful treatment means, and could mean, in the contemporary context.

Medicine's changing means and ends can be motivated and organized by the conduct of a series of clinical trials and the evidence they produce, by Medicare payment decisions, by patient activism, and by industry's efforts to ensure Medicare reimbursement of its products. The technologies of medicine that are employed to extend older lives—regardless of the extent of disease, frailty, or age, regardless of cost, and regardless of the implications for more illness, more surveillance, and prolonged dying—have become difficult to refuse. This is because Medicare pays for them, escalating expectations demand them, and treatments often do extend wanted life. Within this ethical field of imperatives, shifting goals, and emerging standards ("Doing nothing is non-standard"), and because desire for life and for *more* life is so fundamental, the value of life has become strongly linked to the *amount* of it. Thus *the technical ability to intercede becomes the moral reason to proceed*. We must because we can. The chapters that follow address this point in greater detail.

6

FAMILY MATTERS
Kidneys and New Forms of Care

————

Renal transplantation has emerged as the treatment of choice
for medically suitable patients with end-stage renal disease.
More than 60,000 patients await kidney transplantation and
are listed on the United Network for Organ Sharing (UNOS)
recipient registry. Live donor renal transplantation represents
the most promising solution for closing the gap between
organ supply and demand.
—Dorry L. Segev and others, "Kidney Paired Donation
and Optimizing the Use of Live Donor Organs"

We're always victims of our success. The numbers
on the waiting list are rising.
—Transplant surgeon, 2011

The final development in this story of ordinary medicine lies in how its
drivers organize our judgments and frame our experiences. The first
four links in the chain of drivers—leading from scientific innovation
to testing in studies, then to the evaluation of research evidence, and
finally to insurance reimbursement, the setting of standards, and the
creation of necessity—actively shape what we think about and choose. In
the clinic ordinary medicine is what frames our deliberations, including
how we express love and caring, especially when it comes to the value of
more life in relation to the qualms of crossing the line.

The care that families feel, give, and deliberate about—that is, the
way they *practice* concern, love, and obligation in their actions—is not
to be confused with *health care*, the umbrella term commonly used to
refer to our fragmented, dysfunctional delivery system of medical services. While there is no doubt that individual practitioners strive to offer

their patients empathy, compassion, and comfort, the health care system works against their ability to do so, as many complain.

Perhaps nowhere are the demands on families about obligation, love, and the meaning of care expressed as starkly as they are in the example of living donor kidney transplantation. Clinical evidence shows that kidney transplantation is now the most effective treatment for end-stage renal disease, and given the apparent ease of living donor transplants, sharing body parts has become implicated in perceptions of love, generosity, and family responsibility. The technical success and normalcy of living donor kidney transplantation reinforces the unquestioned good of this practice and in doing so offers another example of ordinary medicine at work. (Living partial liver transplantation provides another, though far less common example.)

Our society has reached a point where we now assume that we have extra organs to give away. We cannot avoid contemplating this fact; it is another example of how medical interventions are also interventions into ideas. The language of the "spare" or "extra" kidney circulates widely now in popular discourse around the world. As the sonogram opened ways of seeing the fetus and the idea of prebirth intervention, as surrogacy opened up the idea of motherhood and family, and as cardiac surgery, the implantable defibrillator, the mechanical ventilator, and emergency CPR all changed ways of thinking about the risk of death, so too did the idea of organs moving among family members, friends, or even strangers open up social and familial obligations to being expressed via emerging medical-technical means. The idea of living kidney donation, especially from an adult child to a parent, is now a routine feature of the clinical landscape and a routine social fact. It is also an ordinary dimension of individual responsibility and love.

The "Available" Organ: Greater Demand, Older Patients, New Obligations

What are the consequences of a clinical and cultural practice that normalizes "extra" kidneys and kidney transplantation to older persons? Demand for organ transplants, kidneys especially, is growing worldwide, and in the United States demand is growing in great part because of the aging of the population. Similar to dialysis, few predicted that transplantation would come up against age.[1] Antirejection medications, which came into use in the 1980s, relaxed the biological rules about donor-recipient compatibility, thereby creating more desire for transplants and turning maintenance dialysis into a potential bridge to transplant surgery. More recently the surge in diabetes, the most common single cause of renal failure, has added people of all ages to the waiting list. The increased incidence of obesity and hypertension, with or without diabetes, also contributes to higher rates of end-stage renal disease.[2]

More people living longer with conditions that can lead to end-stage renal disease means that more want and are medically eligible for a transplant, according to the scientific evidence and Medicare reimbursement criteria. They go onto the United Network for Organ Sharing (UNOS) waiting list, but its supply of deceased donor organs simply cannot keep up with escalating demand. Since Dorry L. Segev et al. asserted in the *Journal of the American Medical Association* in 2005 that transplantation is the "treatment of choice" for those with end-stage renal disease,[3] the gap between supply and demand has grown ever wider. As of August 2014 there were more than 100,000 people waiting on the national list for kidney transplantation. Yet the number of available deceased donor kidneys has remained nearly static for about a decade. In 2012 only 13,040 kidneys were available for transplantation (from a total of 7,421 deceased donors).[4]

The number of kidneys transplanted to people over sixty-five from either living or deceased donors has increased steadily in the past two decades in the United States.[5] In 1988 less than 3 percent of the UNOS kidney supply went to persons sixty-five and older. By 2010 those over sixty-five constituted 15 percent of recipients from the national pool. In the past few years transplants have become routine in the seventh decade of life and sometimes are performed into the recipients' early eighties. Recently cadaveric kidneys from donors over fifty have been sought and used specifically to ease the shortage of transplantable kidneys for older recipients.

The inadequate supply of deceased donor organs increases the pressure on family members, friends, and acquaintances of persons with end-stage kidney disease to become living donors. Because kidney transplantation has become an ordinary medical procedure and because the supply of cadaveric organs cannot meet demand, almost everyone between eighteen and eighty who is healthy enough has the potential to be a living donor. There is no escaping this fact; indeed living kidney donation is on the rise for all age groups. In 1988 the ratio of living to deceased donors, for all age groups, was 32 to 68 percent. In 2001 living donation exceeded cadaver donation for the first (but, to date, the only) time in the United States.[6] In 2011 there were approximately eight thousand deceased kidney donors and nearly six thousand living donors. Among the 2,950 kidneys transplanted to people sixty-five and over in 2011, 753 came from living donors, 43 percent (324) of those from adult children of the recipients.[7]

New kinds of obligations emerge and are at stake when the age for transplant moves up into later life and especially when living donors come from a younger generation. A new moral order comes into being, and new questions are being raised: How far does responsibility for longevity making go? How and how much does age matter?

These questions emerged for me when I walked into a kidney transplantation clinic for the first time in 2002. The medical director there asked me a direct and personal question: "What would you do if your father needed a kidney?" My father was eighty-five at the time, and my first thought was not about his age but rather what would happen if I give a kidney to him, and then one of my children needed one. The medical director's question caught me in the multigenerational tangle of love, responsibility, need, and deliberation that kidney transplantation triggers.

The Ethics of Appropriateness

The standardization of organ transplantation in the context of shortage and expanding need is the basis on which we have come to understand the routineness of *living* donation and, along with it, our obligations to relatives and friends in later life. Biological relatedness is no longer a clinical imperative due to improved immunosuppressive drugs (which kidney and all other organ recipients must take for life), and the greatest increase in living donations has been from donors not biologically related to the recipients,[8] but relatedness is nevertheless a matter of enormous importance in terms of donors' sense of duty and responsibility for the health and longevity of a family member (or friend) with end-stage renal disease.

Spouses, siblings, and adult children are generally the first to volunteer to donate when they learn of the need for a kidney, and they represent the vast majority of living donors in the United States. Adult children in their twenties, thirties, and forties are donating kidneys to their parents, who are usually in their sixties and seventies. Nephews and nieces, spouses, other relatives, and friends are also donating kidneys to older persons. Grandchildren sometimes offer to donate to their grandparents, and sometimes the offer is accepted. While solicitation of organs from strangers and donation to strangers has become ordinary and seemingly unremarkable in recent years (I explore this phenomenon in chapter 8), and though the global traffic in illegal organ sales has been widely reported,[9] there is little public knowledge or discussion of the transfer of organs from younger to older people. Yet that latter phenomenon is affecting ever greater numbers of families.[10] Families have always been responsible for supporting a member's medical treatment through the duty of follow-up care and attention. But today the ability to offer and give an organ extends that caregiving to include the *obligation of donating a piece of one's own body for the continued existence of another.*

Each patient in need must decide on the limits to his or her demands. Each family member or friend who is a potential living donor must work out a personal ethic of care, self-interest, and obligation in relation to the worsening disease or impending death of the patient and in relation to medical recommendations for a transplant. Mr. Carter's desperation put pressure on his family to consider living liver donation and who among them might donate, and put pressure on Mr. Carter to decide whether he would actually accept part of his daughter's liver. What is eventually decided emerges both as medical events unfold and through the emotional webs of relations that already exist. How care is practiced is also shaped by the ways doctors and families influence each other. All those transactions—of kidneys, emotional commitments, and doctor-patient talk—are framed by the apparent mechanical ease with which body parts can be transferred from one person to another.[11] "I thought it was going to be like going to the dentist," several prospective kidney recipients have told me.

Expectations for ever longer lives join expectations that routine medical treatment can extend a good life. One patient's daughter spoke for others when she said, "It's a shock to learn that a parent has a terminal illness, no matter what their age." Her father was seventy-five at the time. A kidney can be given to extend a parent's life. That is how love is expressed. The question of age does not arise as a limiting factor when love, family obligation, and need are at stake and in play.

Sitting in Tension: Responsibilities, Rights, and Obligations

> The theme of the gift, of freedom and obligation in the gift, of generosity
> and self-interest in giving reappear in our society like the resurrection
> of a dominant motif long forgotten.
> —Marcel Mauss, *The Gift*

The prospect of living donation sometimes (though not always) generates a tension between responsibility to oneself and individual rights on the one hand and, on the other, responsibility to social connection and social obligation. Patients and those who care about them experience this tension. When the potential recipient of an organ from a living donor is in the later part of his or her life span, the tension acquires additional dimensions as concerns emerge about the worth of more later life (and more *good* life) as measured against the potential risk to the donor and, in some instances, against the greater need for that organ by a younger person.

On one side of the tension equation are the perceived right to open-ended choice about life-extending medical treatments and the responsibility to take care of one's own health. These are enabled by the fact that Medicare creates the possibility for transplant medicine in the United States, adding yet another sphere in which Medicare is deeply implicated in the ethics of managing life. It pays most of the cost of kidney transplants. When it funded dialysis, it also funded the cost of procurement for kidney transplantation and funded the surgery for those sixty-five and over and for those at any age with permanent disability and dialysis dependence.[12] Fixed-income and low-income individuals often receive transplants; this is not a procedure only for the affluent. In addition the donors' surgery and postsurgical costs are covered by Medicare. While rationing has always been a part of the transplantation story because demand is always greater than supply, there is no question that federal reimbursement for transplantation and dialysis, together with the success of kidney transplantation and immunosuppressive drugs, has paved the way for more transplantation and thus for more scarcity.[13] Thus Medicare reimbursement policies organize the right to a transplant and the right to greater longevity in the later years, as they organize the demand and need for other interventions.

On the other side of the equation is one's obligation (whether as donor or recipient) to loved ones across generations, and this is affected more and more by biological knowledge and medical evidence. The obligations inherent in family relationships are what enabled living donor transplantation to be accomplished in the first place; the first successful living donor kidney transplant, in 1954, was between twin brothers. That donation proved that when the immunological rejection response was minimized, *and when one family member was committed to saving another through the use of his own body,* this kind of surgery could succeed. Since then the normalcy and appropriateness of transplantation has had profound interpersonal effects; in the case of kidneys, thousands of people are deeply implicated in sick patients' desire and responsibility to remain alive and to be as healthy as possible.[14]

Older potential kidney recipients sometimes told me and their health care team that they felt an obligation to stay alive for their family members, a characteristic they share with some older dialysis patients.[15] If taken up by the patient—and some do say no—that obligation is a pledge (as well as a burden) to others that he or she will follow the logic of medical intervention wherever it leads and will continue with treatment in order to prolong life. The growing normalization of kidney transplantation at older ages highlights how we "make the ties that bind" between and among family members and generations.[16]

The "Tyranny of the Gift"

The clinical world and the bureaucratically crafted infrastructure have created the need that compels us to consider giving and receiving and to choose how, when, and to whom. It sets up the terms for the ethics of appropriateness between individual donors and recipients, and, as we will see, those terms are constantly shifting and expanding.

For nearly forty years the sociologists Renée Fox and Judith Swazey have documented the impacts of organ transplantation on patients, families, medical practice, and American society.[17] Their work draws attention to the parallels between contemporary organ transfer and the "symmetrical and reciprocal" obligations of traditional gift exchange long studied by anthropologists—to offer and give, to receive and accept, and to repay.[18] Fox and Swazey describe (now famously) the way a transplanted organ carries with it a "tyranny of the gift"—the imperative to offer and give, accept and receive the gift of an organ and the gift of a longer life, regardless of health or suffering, guilt or desire. Often, they found, a painful "creditor-debtor vise" also envelops givers, receivers, and families alike.[19]

In the 1990s they and others described the "tyranny of the gift" as being located in relationships,[20] and it resides there still, gaining additional moral and social ramifications, I found, when the direction of organ transfer is from younger to older persons. That younger-to-older tyranny is marked by a sense among some recipients that this direction of transfer is unnatural, and among some health professionals and others that it is inappropriate from the standpoint of medical goals and use of resources. Nonetheless health professionals want to extend life, patients want life-extending treatments—whether by desire or obligation—and donors feel responsible to facilitate that.

Two relatively new evidence-based facts underlie this interpersonal obligation and also form the basis for the tyranny of the gift—that tyranny being our contemporary way of understanding need and the obligations it instigates. First, a transplant from a living donor has a comparatively high success rate and offers a better prognosis than the continuation of renal dialysis.[21] Recipients also live slightly longer (on average) than those who get kidneys from deceased donors.[22] A transplant professional made that evidence clear to me in a conversation:

> Let me ask you, would you rather have a kidney that was harvested in one part of the country, put on a plane, and brought to you here? Or would you like to have one from your full-blood sibling, who's in excellent condition and would take no impact. It's the gift of love from a family member. You both have the same parents, the same genetic makeup. Probably less immunosuppressive problems. And there's hardly any clamp time on that—it's from one operating room to the one next door. So in the best interest of that human being who needs a transplant, a living donor is your best bet, for the longest outcome you possibly could have.

Second, transplantation among older persons is successful,[23] thereby driving demand and strengthening the ordinariness of older patients receiving kidneys. Combined, these two facts put enormous pressure on family members, especially adult children, to offer and to donate. Old and young are also deeply committed to one another, often beyond the realm of making a genuinely deliberative choice. I was told repeatedly by donors, "It's just something you do, no question about it," and "It's the natural thing to do." Many prospective and actual donors view donation as simply "giving back" for all a parent or other relative or friend has done for them. And because medical technique has made kidney donation ordinary and of negligible physical risk to the donor, many donors told me after the fact that giving the gift was "not a big deal."

Physicians state that the gift is simply the best way to extend one life while not placing another at great risk.[24] Yet it is fundamentally a sacrifice of the wholeness of the body and a nonreciprocal bargain.[25] Recipients express much more ambivalence about the exchange, as many of the comments below illustrate. Often recipients would like to refuse the gift, but this desire is muted, and usually overwhelmed, by a series of factors: the routineness of accepting; the discomfort of dialysis or of having refused dialysis; increasing serious illness; the willingness, enthusiasm, and persuasiveness of a donor; and the medical truth that a living donor's kidney will provide the best health outcome. These are powerful influences on what happens in the clinic. Though disquieting for some, the giving by younger donors and accepting by older recipients has become simply one more expression of care in a society in which more older members need more kinds of assistance and nurture.

So, in addition to the interpersonal effects of the tyranny of the gift, there is now also a diffuse tyranny, one that is located in clinical evidence and routine treatment pathways and woven into the disposition of the entire transplant enterprise. And that enterprise creates the shortage and the demand.

The Added Pressures of Time and Age

Greater scarcity also contributes to the tyranny by putting the additional pressure of time on potential living donors because the waiting time for an organ from the pool has increased tremendously in the past decade. A person with type o blood living in a densely populated urban area, for example, will probably have to wait seven to ten years for a matching organ from UNOS—an untenable amount of time for someone who is, say, seventy or older when end-stage renal disease develops. By the time a kidney is available, it is unlikely that the patient's cardiac function or overall health will support transplant surgery and recovery. Moreover clinical evidence now shows that the more time one spends on dialysis waiting for a transplant, the less likely one is to be a good candidate for retaining and living with the new organ.[26]

Doctors pass on this information to their patients so that they can make evidence-based decisions. For example, I listened as one nephrologist said to a patient, "Data show that six months or less of dialysis gives the best transplant outcomes." Another summarized the driving medical logic of kidney transplantation by saying, "We take an evidence-based approach. We look at life on dialysis. The biggest issue is the organ shortage." When physicians express evidence-based findings like these in the context of organ shortage, the information becomes a ticking bomb spurring decision making and action. Time becomes part of patient and family deliberations about what to do, and it guides younger persons to offer organs to older relatives.

Decision making is complicated by another variable that has come into play in the past decade: the expansion of the medical criteria under which a transplantable organ is considered "good enough." Faced with more people, including older patients, wanting organs, with the number of organs in the national pool (primarily from young, healthy accident victims) not being able to meet demand, and with the "utility" of younger organs placed in older patients not being "maximized," something had to be done to ease the shortage and extend the useful life of more organs.[27] Medicine decided to expand the definition of a "transplantable" organ to include those from older persons (mostly over fifty) with a variety of medical conditions, including hypertension, diabetes, and stroke. Organs from 'expanded criteria donors,' as they are called, became available in 2002 and now make up about 20 percent of donated kidneys.[28] Kidneys donated after cardiac death are now being used in addition to kidneys from donors who suffered brain death (accepted since 1968).[29]

When physicians stress the time sensitivity of the transplant decision they are shaping the options for older patients and their families and are thus encouraging living donation (whether explicitly or implicitly). The waiting time for an expanded criteria donor kidney is perhaps only a few years, much shorter than the wait for a younger, healthier cadaveric kidney. But an organ that has lived longer and may have other medical conditions is not "perfect," and certainly is not preferred by patients. In contrast, there is virtually no waiting time for a kidney from a living donor.

So patients and families quickly learn that their choice about the source of a new kidney must take into consideration time and age. Consider, for instance, this statement by a physician to a seventy-seven-year-old man with heart disease: "Realistically, you'll have to have someone donate you a kidney if you have a chance of getting one." And this to a seventy-one-year-old woman: "I think getting you a kidney would be a great thing. But the sooner the better. It could be five to seven years if you wait for a cadaver donor, especially because of your blood type."

Though health professionals tell patients that a kidney transplant carries some risk and that living with a transplant will not eliminate all health problems or the lifelong need for medications, they also stress that a transplant will free them—as nothing else can—from the physical side effects and functional limitations of dialysis. If physicians consider a seventy- or eighty-year-old patient to be a good candidate for transplant, it is because life extension and better quality of life are possible for that patient.[30] I heard a transplant team member tell a seventy-five-year-old patient, "It depends on how active you are and want to be. Transplant frees you. . . . People who want to be active want the added years. It all depends on what you want. It's a personal choice."

The choices presented to older patients and their families, or that emerge for them during conversations with nurses and doctors in the clinic, often boil down to two: either accept a longer waiting period for a deceased donor kidney—and possible death or greater infirmity while waiting—or seek a living donor, "someone you know," transplant professionals say. Although starting or remaining on dialysis is always an option, when health professionals consider patients to be good candidates for a transplant, the patients are encouraged to proceed because the health outcomes are better with a transplant.[31] The vast majority of patients choose not to remain on dialysis if they can receive an organ. One seventy-one-year-old patient echoed others when she said, "Now that dialysis has started, I feel I'm in a holding pattern, a waiting pen. I could never stay on it for years. I see transplant as my liberator, the light at the end of the tunnel."

The shadow of death, the last and often unstated choice in these conversations, along with the negligible risk to living donors, informs what gets decided, and that shadow mostly tilts the patient toward moving forward with transplant surgery.

In large measure, then, if the patient wants a transplant and has Medicare or other financial access to transplantation medicine, it is up to him or her to decide where the new kidney will come from: "It's a personal choice." This fact marks a new kind of weighing of rights and obligations.

Claims on One Another: The Tasks and Sensibilities
of Patients and Families

Explicit features of the ethics of appropriateness became apparent to me after speaking at length with scores of kidney recipients and prospective recipients (all over seventy) and with donors and prospective donors.[32] As I've emphasized, the ordinariness of living donor transplantation encompasses the ways people think about how the body can be used as well as the time sensitivity of decision making about what kind of donor one will accept. This generates complex questions and choices for those involved. Prospective recipients may ask: Will I accept a living donor kidney? Where will I draw the line for acceptance: spouse and siblings? children? coworkers? friends? strangers? How hard should I push for a living donor? How willing am I to begin renal dialysis at all, stay on dialysis for an unknown duration, or use dialysis as a short-term stop-gap measure only? Donors may grapple with questions such as: How willing am I to donate? And to whom? What would persuade me to offer to donate sooner rather than later? Both parties face questions such as: How urgent is any of this? What is the worth and value of my own life, age, and need in relation to another's? These questions require deliberation about the order of things: seeking a living donor first (and among whom) and viewing cadaveric donation as a last resort, or first deciding to wait for a cadaveric organ and turning to a living donor only when one's health deteriorates significantly.

The ways patients and families work out these choices vary greatly. Need, eligibility, willingness, ambivalence, and obligation form the basis for what potential donors and recipients do and what they feel, whether one offers and gives an organ ("It was just the thing to do, to donate— no question about it"; "This is the way it should be"), accepts an organ ("I didn't want to accept, but they talked me into it"), or refuses to accept it ("I will never accept a kidney from a living person. I would rather die than accept that responsibility").

Such questions are ways of calculating the tyranny of the gift, and they could not have been conceptualized before living kidney transplantation became doable, before control over more time was normalized, and before end-stage kidney disease was routinely treatable this way. The work done by all the players involved is to rationalize and come to terms emotionally with the prospects of offering and giving, accepting and receiving, and, importantly, deciding where to draw the line in networks of family (however construed) and friends and across relationships that are defined by protection, love, obligation, and indebtedness. (Lines also need to be drawn in the case of strangers or casual acquaintances, and these relate to apparent altruism and its acceptance, as I explore in chapter 8.) For adult children, offering is a sign of thanks and payback for all the protection and nurturance a parent has given over a lifetime. Between spouses, offering reflects mutual care, support, sacrifice, and its acceptance. For recipients, taking the gift is the sign of thanks for love and mutual obligation, or it may simply be a sign that they are receiving what they think is owed to them.[33] Or it may be both.

The Recipients' Perspective

When someone needs a kidney transplant, a perception of excess and deficit comes into play: one person has an "extra"; the other has an absence. In light of that perception, an ordering takes place within the social worlds of potential recipients and potential donors of what kinds of relationships, if any, will be recognized as socially and emotionally eligible and appropriate for offering and giving, accepting and receiving. Kinship bonds rank the highest, but offers from other sources— friends, acquaintances, church members, coworkers, and, most recently, strangers—appear to be a growing phenomenon in the United States, as does acceptance of those offers.[34]

Recipients and prospective recipients express a broad range of opinions about their need and the urgency to ask for and accept an organ, their obligation not to ask and not to take, and their responsibility either to wait years for a cadaveric donor or to quickly solicit their own potential living donors. Many styles of engagement with transplant medicine exist, from proactive self-education about transplantation and strategic avoidance of dialysis to passive acceptance of whatever treatment a physician recommends. Neither ethnicity, immigration status, nor gender necessarily determines the values and practice of seeking or accepting an organ.[35]

Each person contemplating a kidney transplant weighs the pursuit of better health against personal measures of selfishness and irresponsibility. As with other interventions, the difficulty of saying no organizes almost everyone's terms of engagement with transplant medicine. Patients know that longer life is possible with medical intervention, but they do not always know immediately how to ethically rank their options for achieving longer life.

Some people want a kidney transplant as soon as (or even before) they learn that they have end-stage disease, and they actively solicit and line up prospective donors even before their first visit to the transplant evaluation clinic, that is, before talking with health professionals about transplantation. Some in this group organize a list of potential living donors in order to avoid starting dialysis at all, regardless of whether their physicians suggest or offer transplantation as a treatment. Some patients report that although their doctors told them to begin or remain on dialysis, they were adamant about receiving a transplant and ignored that medical advice.

For others, the possibility of a transplant (whether from a living or a deceased donor) dawns slowly, over a period of weeks, months, or years after dialysis has begun. Those in this group often go to a transplant clinic for a workup and evaluation, not necessarily because they feel ill or are seeking a transplant but because their primary care doctor or renal specialist suggests that they do so. If they are found eligible following a thorough evaluation, and if they agree, they are put on the UNOS waiting list. They may or may not also consider a living donor; some latecomers remain ambivalent about the prospect of a transplant. For example, a woman who was seventy at the time of her cadaveric transplant recalled:

> From reading all the literature they gave me, I knew that family could be possible donors. . . . Right away, my doctor set it up for testing the family, whoever was willing. . . . Six people volunteered—even my mother, who is twenty-six years older than I am. Only one sister matched, and she was too squeamish to go through with it. I had a few other friends over sixty, sixty-five, but I turned them down, thinking [the clinicians] wouldn't really consider them at that age. But I stayed on the list a long time, until they found a cadaver donation. . . . I felt at the time that I was getting old, and my life wasn't as important as some young person who needed the kidney. You would think that they needed it more than I did. And I was not even considering the transplant too seriously. Especially when I'd been on the list for over five years, and nothing had come of it, and most of my family had been eliminated or refused to do it. It just didn't seem like a very important possibility. Or it just seemed too removed an idea. So I was just gettin' set to go ahead with dialysis for the rest of my life.

The fact that no medically acceptable family member volunteered, coupled with the patient's assumptions about who outside the family would be eligible, shaped her ambivalence about receiving a transplant at all. Over time she conceived a hierarchy of worthiness based on the fact that kidneys are scarce resources, and she decided that younger people are more deserving. Transplantation as a solution to her health problem waned as a priority, yet she accepted a cadaveric kidney when her name came to the top of the waiting list.

The most passive actors are those who never even entertain the possibility of a living donor, wait for years, and eventually receive a deceased donor kidney. For example, a seventy-year-old scientist with a wife and six children said:

> When I was diagnosed with kidney failure, the nephrologist decided to put my name on the transplant list, even though I didn't really have any intention of having a transplant at that time. I was quite hesitant about it, really. Then, as long as the hemodialysis was working out, and I had accepted that as an alternative to transplant, I really didn't think much about having the transplant. And it was never clear to me where I stood on the list, either. I just accepted going through the routine of having these things done, in preparation for a possible transplant, but still, never with the idea of undergoing the procedure myself. . . . But the reason I went ahead with it was because it was available, it was an option.

Because the clinical pathway is set up to move them in that direction, even the most passive, ambivalent patients may eventually receive a transplant simply by staying on the list and waiting for one (provided they continue to be medically eligible). In those cases it requires more proactive engagement on the part of sick patients to reject a cadaveric kidney than to accept one because people want to live, and they want to live without dialysis treatments.

People seventy and over who have actively made decisions of some kind regarding whether or not to seek or accept a kidney from a living donor describe a range of ethical imperatives that guided their thinking. From among those who refused to accept a living donation, a seventy-five-year-old woman told me:

> The only thing they asked me was, did I have anyone in the family who was willing to donate a kidney for the transplant. And I flat out told them no. My nephew was willing to donate, and I said no way, I wouldn't do it. . . . If his other kidney failed, he would have been in

trouble, and I couldn't give him back the kidney. I even asked that question to others: Can I pass this kidney on after I pass on? Can they reuse it for somebody else? And they said no. . . . I morally would not accept a live donor. It is not worth saving my own life to take on that moral burden. I waited for a cadaver kidney and I waited five years.

A man in his late seventies said, "I did not want a living donor. If something happened, I wouldn't like it, whether it's a relative or not. Let's face it. I'm not that young. I only have so much to go. I don't want to enjoy it at someone else's expense. I don't want to put someone else in jeopardy. I've got to go sometime. If I've got to go, I've got to go." A seventy-four-year-old woman said, "I got a cadaver transplant after a three-year wait. I would never ask my son. I had three years of peritoneal dialysis. I had to." I heard the most extreme version of this stance from a seventy-six-year-old man with a wife and five children:

I had at least two people offer to donate me a kidney, if they were matches. I never had them go through the workup procedures because I took the initial position that I would never take a living kidney from anyone else. And if a cadaver kidney had not become available [after five years on hemodialysis] I would just have gone through the regular dialysis until the end. . . . And it was beginning to be a little more problematic near the time I was called for the transplant. . . . If this fistula were to fail,[36] I had come to the conclusion that I would just let it go and let nature take its course. I was just prepared to go ahead and expire.

Those who refused a living donation, a small proportion of the recipients I spoke with, could not reconcile the potential risk of death or debility for a donor with the gift of a longer life for themselves, regardless of how and whether they were biologically related to the prospective donor. In these patients' decision-making criteria, the prospect of inflicting bodily harm on another person loomed larger and weighed more heavily than the desire or need to extend their own lives, and their judgments in this matter were unequivocal, regardless of who made an offer to them. Each took his or her chances on waiting for a UNOS donor.

In contrast, I heard a variety of responses from individuals over seventy who actively sought living donors, among them these three examples:

I was willing to be on dialysis. I didn't know anything about it. . . . But then I hated it and wanted to get off it. In the beginning my doctors did not offer or discuss transplant. When I learned, two years later, that I wouldn't have to wait around on dialysis if I had a live donor, my wife lined up fourteen people who would donate. One of the transplant nurses told me that that was nothing. She's seen people who have lined up a hundred prospective donors. You have to be proactive. You can't just sit around or you'll die waiting.

————

When the team said, "We'll put you on the list for a cadaver transplant," my granddaughter brought up live donors and said, "We're ready." We had the forms filled out by seven people in twenty-four hours. I didn't consider anything else—I never went on dialysis.

————

My doctor said I would need a transplant when the creatinine got high enough.[37] So I said, "How about if I line up some donors, or try to?" And he said, "It's kind of early for that. Let's wait a while." When he decided it's time, I never hesitated. I knew I needed a kidney. I was real sick. . . . With so much help from my wife, my kids—they're emailing everybody—I mean, it was a full court press to find donors. Talk about lucky. I never went on dialysis. I missed it by probably about a month. I had twenty-five volunteers to give me a kidney, and ten matched—they had type o blood. . . . Of them, I had never met one, and one or two I knew casually, and the rest of them were close—two granddaughters, my daughter, and friends. Six women, four men. The hospital chose two who scored the highest, and amazingly the two happened to be friends. And they were kinda arguing about who was gonna give me the kidney. They both wanted to do it. And I wasn't gonna get into that. The doctors made the decision. . . . My secretary gave me a kidney. I just felt the luckiest guy in the world.[38]

For these three patients the naturalness and value of transplantation as standard medical treatment muted or made irrelevant any personal deliberation about their own relative worthiness or about what they understood to be the relatively minimal potential negative health consequence to a donor. Though talk of sacrifice or risk to the donor sometimes emerged as one element in these patients' moral decision-making process, those factors did not tip the balance away from a proactive search for and then acceptance of the gift. Moreover these patients had a great deal of family support in mobilizing potential donors from within and beyond family networks. The last of these three examples shows that kinship (however defined) is not necessarily a quality that patients require when they accept an offer, even if both kin and nonkin are medical matches.

Solicitation of a living organ, regardless of how widely the patient casts the net or how the donor is categorized by the patient, occurs when patients, along with their support systems (which includes health care professionals), understand transplantation first and foremost as a right and, along with donation, as an *ordinary* medical practice. "I wanted to get back to a normal life. Dialysis was just not acceptable. We are too active," said a seventy-six-year-old man who easily accepted his daughter's kidney. His stance is possible because contemporary clinical medicine hands older patients the opportunity to continue living well despite end-stage disease and also because of widespread expectation that one can strive to grow older without feeling older, without an embodied sense of aging.[39]

Of course there are also intermediate sensibilities that fall between outright refusal to accept a living donor organ and proactive solicitation of one. The criteria for accepting the prospect of a kidney from a living donor, and then choosing who will be considered, are idiosyncratic and often change as the patient gets sicker, adjusts (or not) to the routine of dialysis, or receives an unanticipated offer of a kidney. A seventy-seven-year-old man said, "I have seven kids, but I don't think I want to ask one of my kids. If they volunteer, that's one thing. But I'm not going to ask. Who can take off from work? No one." A woman who received a kidney transplant at seventy-nine noted:

> My sister knew I needed a kidney, and I was tellin' her, "I sure wish somebody would come up with something." So my nephew called me out of the blue—I hadn't seen him since he was a young boy—and he said, "Aunty, I hear that you are sick." And I said, "Yes, I need a kidney." And he said, "I'm willing if you are." I said, "Are you serious?," and I explained how serious this was and how I wouldn't ask anyone to do this. I said, "Well, I don't know. You better think it over and call me up some other day." And he did just that, called me up another day. And they found out from the very first testing that we were com-

patible. . . . And I said, "God, what if it doesn't work because of my age and I have to go back on dialysis?" But the doctor gave me a lot of confidence and said I had a strong heart. And I felt kinda funny, you know, about my nephew—suppose something happened to him? Or something should happen to him more than me? And he was young. But, no, it was something he was gonna do. So here we are. I think it was meant to be.

Thus some patients will not ask for a kidney but will accept one if it is offered by someone they know. They draw the moral line at the place where unprompted, insistent generosity meets a request that could seem coercive because of the significance of the bond. For them an unsolicited and insistent offer of donation is evidence enough of genuine altruism, and they thankfully accept. Others do not accept. Regardless, insistence and persistence on the part of the donor seem to be crucial to prospective recipients' judgments. That is one form that the ethics of appropriateness takes.

For some, accepting a kidney from a younger family member is not objectionable per se. Rather the issue is the life circumstances of the one who offers. A woman who was on dialysis for five years until she received a cadaver kidney at age seventy said:

The doctors talked to me about a live donor, but there were only three that were a perfect match in my family: my oldest daughter and two grandchildren. My oldest daughter has the same problem I have, and eventually she's gonna go on dialysis too. The other one is her son, my oldest grandson. He was in the military. And when he found out about it, he went and got tested and he was a perfect match. And he came home to do it. I didn't know about it. And the [transplant clinic] coordinator called to tell me they had a match for me. My grandson was coming home to give me a kidney. That's how I found out. But she said, "I just got a call from his commanding officer and they're not clearing it. If he gives you a kidney, he's gonna be discharged. And your grandson says he doesn't care." I said to him, "No, you're not giving me a kidney. I'm not taking it. Because you're in the military, and if you give me one, they'll pull you out. I'm not at a life-threatening time now, so I'm not taking it. . . . When I reach a life-threatening time, I'll put it in the newspaper. I would advertise. I'll put it out on the Internet, everywhere. So, until I reach that point, forget it."

People who will accept an organ from a living person ultimately establish a hierarchy of potential donors that is based on any combination of the following characteristics (and not in any particular order): biological relatedness, the strength and length of tie to the prospective gift-giver, the degree of enthusiasm or hesitation that person expresses about donation, and whether that prospective donor has responsibilities for other lives. That list reflects the qualities that the patient considers appropriate for donation. For example: The son is running a business; he has four employees who rely on him. The daughter has two young children. But another daughter is not married, does not have children and does not have the financial responsibilities of the son; she is the ideal candidate. Or the daughter with two children believes she is the most physically fit member of the family; she offers and is adamant about it. Or, as one patient said, "the children have their lives ahead of them. I wouldn't accept from them because they may need their kidneys later on. But I will take a kidney from someone else, someone not as young as my children."

One daughter donor explained, "My parents considered having my dad stay on dialysis, considered waiting for a cadaver, considered other potential donors who were nonfamily, at first. The reason is because family comes first, and you don't want to put your kids at risk." Patients organize a ranking system not only of who they will put at risk but also of whose commitment to them they will honor by acceptance. That ordering is made in a pragmatic context of who volunteers with the greatest persistence and who embodies the strongest dedication to their well-being. Thus adult children arrive often, but not always, at the top of the list.

Sometimes patients have strong feelings against asking family members to donate. Those who say "I'll never take an organ from one of my children" are generally resigned to and accepting of the fact that the end of life—a long life—is near and, maybe, is appropriate. As one man told me, "My wife wants to be my donor, but I don't want to take from her. We've been married fifty years. I don't want to bring her into this. This is end-stage." The daughter of a seventy-five-year-old patient said, "He has a sister and me to donate, but he's not accepting it. He's very close to his sister and doesn't want anything to hurt her. . . . He says he's at the end of his age. But I say, 'No, that's not true, you're not at the end of your life.'"

An initial refusal to consider donation from one's family members frequently gives way to acceptance after weeks or months, whether because some patients feel extremely ill on dialysis or because they want the freedom and better health that a transplant promises: "The dialysis was killing me. I wanted to get off it as quickly as possible. I didn't want to wait that long for a cadaver"; "I was getting sicker and my daughter kept offering"; "She was saying, 'Come on, Dad. My kidney isn't getting any younger.'"

Pressure on patients to accept a living donation is applied both by prospective donors and by the structure of transplant financing, which makes surgery and medications affordable for large numbers of people. While health professionals consider personal choice to be paramount for patients when deciding whether to have a transplant in the first place, there is relatively less choice about accepting a living donation if someone offers unequivocally. This is because, together, enthusiastic prospective donors and the transplant team support moving forward with transplantation. Standard treatment, prospects of better health, and the fact that love is expressed through clinical intervention are compelling reasons to offer and accept. In the example of living kidney donation, the family—and friends, acquaintances, and, most recently, strangers—serve as agents, or extensions, of medicine and its goals.[40]

In addition patients' feelings of responsibility to pursue greater health and longer life often merge with the obligations they, their families, and doctors have toward one another. To paraphrase the line of reasoning that stood out among the patients who ultimately accepted a kidney from a spouse or adult child: My family needs and wants me to live because it is possible for me to do so, and I want to live. Therefore I need to live, and so they (or some of them) will offer to donate a kidney for me, and (though it may not seem right) I must accept it. One seventy-four-year-old recipient recalled his clinic evaluation:

> We were sitting there and the nurse said, "Do you know anyone who would be a potential donor?" And my wife, for years before, had said to me that she would be willing to donate a kidney, and I said, "No, you're not gonna do that." I really didn't want her to donate. That's way too much to ask of anybody. And this lady [the transplant coordinator] asked, "Is there anybody in the family?" And I said, "No, they all have polycystic kidneys." And my wife said she wants to be the donor. And I said, "No, I don't want you to be a donor." And they said, "Well, you don't really have anything to say about it. If she wants to be a donor, she can." And they did a workup and she was a match, very, very close. . . .

And then as things got worse and there was no possibility of being on the [deceased waiting] list. I guess I kind of caved in and said, "Well, if the match is that good and it will work, let's do that." I could have adamantly refused, but I didn't.

Another man, age seventy-five, recalled:

The children talked me into it. I said, "I'm not taking my daughter's kidney!" But other family members persuaded me. You know, I kind of went along with my older daughter's insistence, and we didn't say too much one way or another, whether I wanted to or not. But I was hopeful that I could get a cadaver—right up to the night I was hospitalized. My point was I didn't want to take an organ from my child. If it were the other way around, I would have gladly given my kidney to one of them, but because it was coming, as a hand-me-up sort of thing, I thought about it a lot. It didn't feel like it was the right thing to do. Help should go the other way, from parent to child. I, really, there were periods of time I just really didn't want to do it. There was no real point in time where I decided I wanted to have it done. I just went along with the flow. I was going along for the ride because things were being arranged for me.

Saying yes to life-prolonging treatments also represents acceptance of the obligation to remain alive. Several people said they were enduring, seeking, or continuing treatment (whether dialysis or for transplantation) for the sake of their children, some of whom were their prospective donors. A seventy-one-year-old woman described how obligation overrode her own desires: "The huge decision was starting dialysis. That was a major decision, beginning dialysis at all. I knew it would impact my life. I did it for my son, for my family. I realized I needed to stay alive for my family. They needed me. I have an obligation to remain here for them. If I had no family to persuade me to go forward with dialysis, I would not have done it. I would have chosen death instead."

The woman who was seventy-nine when she received a kidney from her nephew had lost a daughter to cancer years before. Her sense of obligation to remain alive predated her need for a kidney. She said, "I was determined to take care of her five kids. I promised my daughter on her deathbed that I would take care of them. My husband and I, we told her that. That's why I went through this. . . . When the doctors told me that I was good enough to have a transplant, that I was still in good shape, then I knew that I could do it, that I could deal with it. And that's when I decided."

For those patients who do not embrace all the available sources of donation, one can summarize their choices around two themes. First, choice is most clearly expressed in instances of refusal of a living but not of a deceased donor kidney. Those who refuse living donation do not exclusively refuse offers from family members and ultimately do not point to the bonds of kin relations as the reason for that refusal. Rather as reasons to say no they name unacceptable risk to all potential living donors or their own relative worthiness in terms of age and nearness of the end of a "natural" life. Second, refusal often gives way to acceptance as health deteriorates or as donors persist in offering. This is because the stakes of life and relative health, the encouragement and guidance of the health care team and family, and the routine success of kidney transplantation together act as imperatives to go ahead with living donation, regardless of the recipient's sensibilities.

The Donors' Perspective

Donors' and prospective donors' side of the story of obligation, gift-giving, choice, and no choice is reflected in how they understand issues of urgency and necessity in the life-and-death matter of kidney disease and its treatments. They mostly express a sensibility, a clarity about their responsibility. From a daughter: "There was no choice, no decision making. This was simply the thing to do—to donate a kidney. He needed one. I could save his life." From a friend: "I don't think of it as a great thing. I just think of it as a normal thing that people you know would do. . . . I just think it's a natural thing." From a daughter: "Saving the life of my parent outweighed any other future consideration. There's nothing more important than family—it's just that simple."

I heard many variations on this theme, including the widely shared assessment that long-term dialysis is not a viable option. Dialysis is characterized as hopeless, a slow death, the cause of problems, something that restricts life; donating a kidney is seen as restorative, life giving, freeing. Some donors came to this realization early in their parent's, spouse's, or friend's kidney disease. Others watched the deleterious effects of dialysis on the patient for months or years and then realized they could donate and offered to do so—or then offered more insistently until the patient said yes.[41]

Clarity about the obligation to donate can emerge from and is intimately linked to a sense of family identity and solidarity, and adult children donors often voiced a connection between family solidarity, their sense of self, and their values. "We're full-blooded Greek [or Italian, Spanish, Dutch, or Japanese American]" are often followed by "so we stick by one another. Family is the most important thing, and this was a matter of the family unit." The ultimate importance of survival of the family unit was poignantly expressed in the unusual case of two sisters, each of whom donated a kidney, eight years apart, to their father: "When we came here from Denmark in the sixties, it was just the four of us. My sister and I were two and four years old. My dad had twenty-five dollars in his pocket and no job. That was the only time he was really scared. And he built his life, and we're a very close-knit family. . . . This journey is not about choice. It's just something that you do. We weren't forced to. . . . We were willing to sacrifice our lives to maintain the integrity of the family unit."

Family suffering and perseverance were additional themes when adult children told of their sense of obligation and solidarity as donors and prospective donors. Adult children understood their offer and gift in relation to what the family had been through already. Expressions of family solidarity, what you do for another family member, did not stop when a parent became older and sick with kidney disease. The gift of bodily substance allows family solidarity to be expressed. That is, the strength and compelling nature of a tie to a parent can be enacted in the transfer of a part of the body across generations, thus lending support and longevity to the entire family.

The timing of offers to give a kidney was variable, depending on when, during the patient's illness and medical workup, the donor realized he or she could or should make the offer. Physicians also play a role in this timing. Community internists, general practitioners, and other doctors outside the transplant world don't take a uniform approach to living donation. Recipients and donors I spoke with noted that some doctors suggested that the patient think in a general way about living donation. Others chose a time to mention a specific family member as an appropriate donor, for example, when end-stage kidney disease was diagnosed, when dialysis was imminent, or when dialysis had been under way for months. Other physicians outside the transplant world never mentioned living donors at all, or, if the patient raised the subject, suggested that he or she remain on dialysis indefinitely.

Speaking of how she timed making her own offer to donate, one daughter said, "We were watching him die. I could prevent his death. I wanted him around many more years. It was, in part, self-interest. I offered immediately, no doubts whatsoever in my mind about what to do. I volunteered before he, or anyone, raised the subject at all. I never was burdened or bothered by a sense of risk. There was no question in my mind." Another daughter explained how she chose when to make the offer: "When they told my mother she would have to start dialysis and go on the [cadaver] wait list I volunteered. They never mentioned [living donation] at the clinic when she went for her evaluation. I could save her life, and she wouldn't have to go on dialysis. My immediate reaction was to donate. 'You've got four kids'—and we all volunteered, but I always assumed it would be me. I'm the healthiest. My mother was, frankly, relieved." And another daughter donor said, "The moment he started dialysis, I offered. 'Dad, you need a kidney.' It was the obvious thing to do. You don't have something that your body needs to fully function, and it's quite possible that I might have something that you can use. I'm the youngest and I think it was, 'Nobody is cutting into my baby girl.' . . . But after nine months getting beaten up on dialysis, one day Dad said, 'This is getting old.' I said, 'Are you ready to get me tested?' And he said, 'Yes, I think I'm ready.' "

Another daughter recalled that the timing of her offer was based on her acknowledgment of her father's deteriorating health during his months on dialysis: "I could hear the desperation in my father's voice when he started dialysis. All of a sudden, his active life was gone . . . and to watch his deterioration was so hard. When I was being tested, he said, 'Let me know as soon as they say it's okay.' On the one hand, he didn't want to push. On the other hand, he wanted it so bad. The dialysis was driving him nuts."

After several years watching her husband undergo dialysis, a sixty-four-year-old woman was influenced to offer to donate to him when she recalled her mother's medical history:

My mother had one kidney. She had a kidney removed forty-two years ago, actually. And so I just got the idea one day that, well, if my mother can live with one kidney, well, I said, "I'll give you one kidney." And he said, "I don't know about that." But I said, "It's something we might think about." He was in dialysis for two and a half, three years before I really thought about it. I said, "It's getting ridiculous. I'll just give you a kidney, if that's what it takes." He wasn't receptive at first. He thought it was kind of risky. He was very worried about me. But I thought, people take risks every day. That's when we started testing. . . . If my family hadn't had this experience, I don't think it would ever have dawned on me. I probably never would have thought about it unless the doctor had said, "What about your wife?" Then I would have been willing. But I was the one who initiated it.

Future risks to their own health never weighed heavily (if considered at all) on these donors. Most of them expressed their unequivocal trust in the transplant team. They said they had no doubts about the outcome of surgery for themselves or the recipient. None worried about the issue of possible long-term effects.[42]

Few of the people I spoke with expressed any ambivalence about volunteering to donate. One instance, however, was in direct response to the age and frailty of the prospective recipient. A woman who had already donated a kidney to her sister talked about her brother's hesitancy to donate to their mother:

> My mom has a number of brothers and sisters. We wanted them to step up to the plate. But there's only so much—it's a strange dynamic, where you don't want to overtly pressure somebody. I think it's hard for the person needing the transplant to sometimes ask for it. I know my brother, when he went through this process with my mom, and he got matched—it was a very hard decision for him because in his mind, my mom had lots of complications. She's already quite frail, and the issues—is the kidney gonna do her any good—he was weighing that factor. And he's thinking we have a family history of high blood pressure. What if he develops kidney disease later on? And he was getting married, and so, all those factors kind of played into it. . . . It's interesting. My mom didn't want it from my brother. She felt like, if something happened to him, she would feel responsible. So she actually declined it from him. She's on the cadaver list.

In this case the son apparently weighed the urgency of donation against the long-term health risk to himself. His mother reasoned similarly, it seems, and she may have been affected also by the son's ambivalence and lack of enthusiasm about donation.

But some donors did indicate that they felt pressured to donate. The oldest of four daughters of a seventy-five-year-old woman felt pressure from two sources. First, the mother assumed her children would offer, and without prompting she told the doctors and nurses in the transplant evaluation clinic, "I'm thrilled that my daughters want to donate—that all the sacrifices I've made for them are worth it. I feel wonderful that they want to show their love to me in this way." Second, this daughter told me that her three younger sisters had expressed their extreme ambivalence about donation, so she felt the burden of responsibility weighed heavily on her shoulders: "I have grown kids. My three sisters all have little kids, though, in grade school and high school. So, God willing, and being the oldest, I will be the one who can donate. My sisters have concerns because of the younger kids. They are worried about it."

Like recipients, donors described how a hierarchy of donation within the family was established before medical testing for an adequate match began. An ethic of appropriateness had to be worked out: "All of us [siblings] wanted to give to Dad. We argued among ourselves about who should be tested first, who should get to donate. It was always a matter of which one of us gets to donate, not *if* we should donate." A daughter who donated to her father said, "We all have different roles in the family. My brother's married and has two young children. And I think if the chips had really come down, he might have stepped forward. My sister is married. I'm single. I had nobody else to consider. I didn't have to consult anyone. So that's just the way it was. And so many people said, 'Are your brother and sister getting tested?' And it was kind of like, well, I worked out. Why bother?" A seventy-five-year-old man who donated to his seventy-year-old wife said, "Naturally the kids said, 'Take me.' That was a given. They automatically offered. We didn't talk about it much. But we didn't want the kids. They're young, they have their own lives, and they may need their kidney later on. We both felt that if I was compatible, I would do it. And they were very happy with that. I was really worried, during the testing, that they would find something, or I would be too old, or I would have an abnormality in the other kidney and I wouldn't be able to give. And it didn't happen, and we were very pleased. And I'm sure the kids were relieved."

While donors mostly offer and give "without question," that giving is intimately tied, I found, to perceptions of how one will be judged within the family. Both donors and recipients exercise a moral calculus: the possibility of *receiving* another's body part leads patients to weigh the donor's potential risk and sacrifice of bodily integrity in relation to their own longer life and improved well-being. In contrast, the possibility of *giving away* a part of the body becomes implicated both in the demonstration of care and love and in the ability and responsibility to prolong another life.

Claims and the Ethic of Appropriateness across Generations

Thus to be confronted with end-stage kidney disease (one's own or another's) means to be aware that love and familial duty include the *potential* of the transfer of bodily substance, regardless of whether or not the acts of giving and receiving actually occur. How the ethics of appropriateness organize our claims on one another are perhaps most starkly revealed in the living donor example: having an "extra" kidney, the rationales for refusing and accepting an offer, the creation of hierarchies of potential donors, the zeal with which one pursues living donation.

Although the meanings inherent in "flesh of my flesh" arose long before the new biotechnologies, there is no question that emerging clinical techniques contribute to our changing sensibilities about what that phrase means.[43] Modern medical interventions simply provide one contemporary location for family relations and obligations to be expressed.[44] Living kidney donation is one way of demonstrating love and care. It extends the boundaries of what can be given and what can be received. It expands the logic (for recipients, donors, and health professionals) of the act of organ transfer to include assumptions about the routineness and naturalness of the generational direction of the gift, but the expanded logic also de-emphasizes the permanence of the gift and the finite character of this particular resource.

Everyone who engages the world of transplant medicine makes moves to include and exclude, to name and rank those who will be considered worthy of giving and receiving.[45] Love, obligation, altruism, family solidarity, bodily risk, and assumptions about the naturalness of both mortality and transplantation each play varying roles in individuals' moral reckonings. The nature of obligation—from generation to generation— was perhaps expressed most clearly by a fifty-four-year-old woman who donated a kidney to her employer and friend (the man who had solicited twenty-five potential donors), a person who, she noted, was *like* family. Though she thought about the impact her donation would have on her own daughter and her daughter's children, she did not think about it for very long:

He said that he had a kidney problem and that he was gonna look for a donor because he didn't want to be on dialysis. He gave me something to read, I think. But before then, I said yes. . . . I've known [him] for a long, long time. We're like family—it wasn't a question. It was an easy decision. It prolongs the average recipient's life by about sixteen years, I was told. . . . My daughter has one kidney. She had cancer when she was six years old, and they took a kidney out. That was thirty years ago. So I know a little bit about it. Knowing that no harm was going to come to me and knowing that, if down the line my daughter needed a kidney, she [would have] some sort of backup, I think that's what made it easy. I knew all of that. . . . I discussed it with my daughter and my son—what I was gonna do, how they felt about it. My daughter was totally for it, and she and I talked about it and I didn't even have to say anything. She was the one who said, "Well, I have two sons, you know, if I need a kidney. . . ." And that made me even more comfortable.[46]

This donor's decision was not troubled by the fact that her daughter had only one kidney. She was not unique among those I spoke with in assuming that the transfer of her own kidney to another could inspire a similar decision in those of a younger generation, to donate to older kin and like-kin in the future. That assumption, that others will give of their body, is now an ordinary part of the (global) cultural landscape.

The old question—What are our obligations across generations?—has not disappeared. As ever we must decide on and demonstrate the ways we care for older members of our families and our societies. But more than ever before, and because of available, routine procedures, we are now both being asked and are demanding to share in the extension of those lives in terms of bodily substance.

Living donor kidney transplant is one more technique linking how we understand the arc of human life to clinical opportunity and personal obligation. There is nothing inherently good or bad about living donation to an older generation, and I am not opposed to that direction of giving. After all, like nearly everyone else today I could become a donor or recipient, could welcome the opportunity to offer and give or to accept and receive a kidney. The important point is that, in this example, we are all the subjects of an experiment in ordinary medicine that is taking place on a broadening social scale. A price is paid for investing certain kinds of expectation in clinical technique. Those who have given or received a kidney (or piece of a liver), or have contemplated doing so, have likely already encountered elements of that price through the bodily enactment of love and commitment. The long-term impacts on generational relations cannot be foreseen in our aging society, which is only just beginning to pay attention to the effects of best evidence on patterns of health care delivery, on the problem of equity within scarcity, and on the quandary of social justice—all of which are churning in ordinary medicine's wake.

7

INFLUENCING THE CHARACTER OF THE FUTURE

Prognosis, Risk, and Time Left

———

By shaping the patients' understanding of their own
experience, physicians create the conditions under which their
advice seems appropriate.
—Paul Starr, *The Social Transformation of American Medicine*

To be normal is to be in a state of risk, a state that at some
inevitable future time will be fulfilled as a state of
disease or death.
—Kathleen Woodward, *Statistical Panic*

Simply by offering us prognoses and potentially life-extending treatments and then offering more treatments after that, medicine asks us to imagine different future scenarios for ourselves and our loved ones. Then it asks us to decide among them. Through those offers, medicine is reshaping the character of the future and our experience of it.

The timing of death has become a major cultural preoccupation in the United States, and although absolute control of the length of a life span mostly evades us, medicine today allows us, indeed incites us to consider as was never before possible *how much longer* we want to live. Medicine motivates us to function as if we could control our date of death. Then it asks that we act on that consideration, *do* something about it. Medicine permits us, implores us, invites us to negotiate with time. These are big demands, and they are another example of the profound way ordinary medicine influences, indeed shapes us.

The Paradox of Prognosis: Inescapable yet Nonpredictive

Prognosis (from the Greek; literally, foreknowing) plays a large part in shaping our expectations and actions, and it is inherent in how doctors make sense of evidence. People commonly associate prognosis with a prediction of mortality and the timing of death: "How much longer do you think I'll live, Doctor?" But the work of prognosis is more nuanced than that. Because doctors understand the usual and anticipated course of disease treatments, as well as what will happen if disease is left untreated, prognosis entails describing to patients what is likely to happen if they do or do not treat their condition and what can be expected from the different treatments available.[1] Prognostic details about the course of treated or untreated disease are the means by which physicians seek to persuade patients to move forward with treatments. They are also one reason patients and families come to expect (more) treatments to be offered in the future.

Prognosis is everywhere in our "society of statistics." It is part of "the omnipresent discourse of medical statistics" with which we're inundated:[2] one in nine women will develop breast cancer sometime during her life; one out of three people will face some form of cancer. It is embedded in one-year and five-year survival rates, in statistics about average life span and years remaining, in medical screening techniques and risk-reduction strategies of all kinds, and in the fact that today many of us live with the awareness that we know something about the probability of death in the context of specific diseases: "At your age, chemotherapy is only 40 percent effective"; "She has a 10 percent chance of survival." There are also life span predictor websites with provocative names like Death Clock and Living to 100. In this sense prognosis is an inescapable part of the fabric of contemporary life.

But prognosis is a notion that's too slippery to apply purposefully to any individual. Although risk awareness and future-thinking can be said to dominate contemporary thinking, specific, individualized prognoses about the timing of death are difficult if not impossible to pin down. Physicians can talk about the trajectory of disease and offer population statistics, but they cannot predict when death will occur (or disease will recur) for any one of us, and they have learned not to prognosticate in individual cases. The evidence of treatment benefit that emerges in clinical trials has repeatedly been shown to be nonpredictive in individual cases and for particular groups of patients, especially older patients.

How, then, does prognosis make itself felt in the clinic today? How does it influence us?

Prognosis is thoroughly embedded in doctor-patient dialogue, even though it may not be made explicit, even if doctors are unaware of that embeddedness, and, importantly, even though formal studies and plenty of doctors' informal accounts have shown that physicians are loath to prognosticate directly or candidly. Nevertheless prognosis "permits clinical work to take place. . . . It forms the basis for the clinician to treat and for the patient to respond."[3] Diagnostic technologies produce prognostic information, and because clinic conversations about life-threatening disease often focus on procedural options and what comes next, physicians are under greater pressure than ever before to say something to patients about the different kinds of future that are likely to emerge with different treatments or without treatment.

Diagnostic tests and discussion of their results instigate future-thinking. (If you have not yet heard your doctor say, "Let's do this test, *then* we'll decide," you likely will someday.) For persons over seventy the future already has a foreshortened horizon. And that future is brought into the present in the joined scenarios that medicine sets up for the seriously ill: the risk of death and the potential of avoiding death a bit longer. Medicine thus "materializes" and actualizes time,[4] causes it to be made real by the interventions that offer the possibility of a certain number of additional weeks, months, or years. The lure of more future must be grappled with in detail in the clinical sphere: doctors must think about what to offer patients and patients must decide what to do. Both the lure and the grappling with it are results and expressions of ordinary medicine.

The foreseeing of next treatments that are required by standard medical practice takes up considerable discussion time in clinics these days simply because there are very often next treatments to contemplate. The more screening and diagnostic tools that are available, the more often doctors make use of them to plan what should come next. Because diagnoses are more thorough and can be made earlier in a disease's trajectory than ever before, a fundamental task for doctors is to think about and anticipate what to do next after administering and then learning the results of tests, scores, and scans. In this sense prognosis is a form of anticipation—about disease, treatment, and the patient's future life span—and it is ever present in medical thinking. The more diagnostic information that is available, the more the physician needs to anticipate therapy (and the therapy that will follow that one) and to consider the patient's future condition with or without that therapy. Prognosis involves apprehending the effects of treatment on the disease, the body, and the life of the patient. It works in conjunction with diagnosis and extends the work of diagnosis.[5] For patients, who mostly want to keep living, the earlier the diagnosis, the more time there may be to think about future treatments and be engaged in treatment regimens.

The Demands of Time and of Unimaginable Futures

Clinical experience and scientific evidence together inform doctors that time is critical to therapy, and they always speak of next steps for patients in the context of the timeliness of treatments. When they lay out options, they are recommending courses of timely and time-limited action. For doctors future-thinking is considered best practice: "If you don't do the surgery within three months at the most, it is likely that the cancer will spread too far to allow us to operate"; "Let's do this now. I want to avoid a big surgery later."

But beyond settling on a course of therapy are the demands, always unspoken, that medicine makes on patients' imaginative powers to project themselves, their medical condition, and their feelings about that condition into multiple kinds of future so that they can "choose" one kind over another. This, of course, is impossible to do, as Mr. Jones discovered while grappling with his doctor's prognosis that unless he got an ICD immediately, he would die.

Cancer and heart disease are the two leading causes of death in the United States. They are also the arenas in which most of us will ponder and negotiate the timing of our own ends. The choices we make will be time sensitive. Time is active and prospective, and ordinary medicine hands us the responsibility of time.

The following four stories illustrate ways this responsibility plays out for patients, families, and doctors. They reveal the kinds of demand medicine sets up as it anticipates the course of a patient's disease and outlines the treatments available and as it asks patients to consider the control they have over the time that is left, even when that control may be an illusion. The previous examples of clinic dialogue have illustrated that from the physician's point of view discussion with the patient (and the family) often is about the need for them to know, in as much detail as they can absorb, what will or might or could happen if the patient chooses this treatment, that treatment, or no treatment at all. Each of the following stories highlights an aspect of the relationship of prognosis to evidence and provides an example of the way that relationship is enacted by the patient or family. Each illustrates also how prognosis settles on the patient and family as a question, often a burdensome one: "Should I try to go through three months of radiation therapy to stop the spread of cancer?" "Should I have the ICD to prevent sudden death?" In short, "What shall I do about the potentially open-ended future that medicine describes?"

Potential and possibility are what organize how we engage with medicine and the future. Not very long ago we died from heart attacks, cancer, and most every other disease without ever having to choose among potential futures, without having to consider managing the timing of our death. What ordinary medicine has done is complicate our approach to the inevitable. It has created a path that leads into a maze of complex decision points.

The First Demand: Knowing the Steps to Death

If you don't do something, it's disease progression all the way to death.
—Ninety-year-old cancer patient

Cancer specialists' knowledge about the course a disease takes without treatment and about the role of different interventions in potentially slowing or stopping its spread influences how they understand the windows of opportunity for certain interventions, the approximate time frame within which the disease will be manageable and responsive to specific procedures. This dual awareness—of the specific course of untreated disease progression and its somatic effects and of the importance of the timing of treatments—is a focus of their discussion with patients, and it opens up the possible future scenarios for patients to ponder. The physician is mapping a life-extending treatment pathway, and if a patient decides to forgo interventions at any point along the way, the physician's mandate is to ensure that that patient considers what will happen. One of ordinary medicine's demands is that we learn the details of the course of untreated disease "all the way to death." The doctor's ability to transmit that knowledge step by step is a recent development in medicine, and many physicians see doing so as a responsibility. Absorbing that information is part of what it means to be an informed patient in our age of so much precise yet paradoxically and ultimately indeterminate information about the future of our own body and life.

Mrs. Heath: The Path If You Forgo Treatment

Ninety-eight years old, petite, well-dressed, partially blind, and somewhat frail, Mrs. Hattie Heath had been diagnosed with bladder cancer and told that one possible treatment was to remove the cancer by surgically removing the bladder. Her son and daughter-in-law had seen the doctor a few weeks earlier, without the patient, to say they did not want their mother to have the surgery. The doctor replied that he could not make that decision without the patient present. She is competent to make that choice, he said, and the decision should be hers. Later they all came to the outpatient oncology clinic for a follow-up visit to discuss the surgical option so Mrs. Heath could come to some decision about a treatment plan. While I sat in the small exam room with the family, waiting for the doctor to arrive, I learned from Mrs. Heath that she lived in her own home with a daytime caregiver. She spoke intelligently and sat, stood, and walked unaided. Though somewhat forgetful, she was socially engaging and quite delightful.

The doctor arrived wanting to present a clear choice for the patient and settle on a plan. He began by asking Mrs. Heath, "Do you know what you've got?" She replied, "Cancer." He continued, "Yes, bladder cancer. We need to decide what we're going to do about it, if we are going to do anything about it, if we're going to do surgery to remove the bladder. I wouldn't advise surgery. If you were younger I'd say, 'Let's take out the bladder.'"

Mrs. Heath responded, "I don't want to be cut. I don't want surgery." The doctor continued, "So I want to discuss all the options. Chemotherapy? Radiation? These are no walk in the park for someone your age. Or cut it out? We're loath to go down the path of getting tissue, a biopsy, if we're not going to do anything afterward. If we don't do anything, there are two sets of consequences. First, the local. You will have more pain. You'll start to bleed more. If you bleed a lot and get weak, you'll have to come to the hospital for blood transfusions. Second, there are the systemic effects. Cancer could, actually it will spread beyond the bladder. It will eventually spread."

"And kill me," Mrs. Heath finished the thought. She was as calm throughout this conversation as if it were about the weather or plans for the week. The doctor emphasized, "If we're going to do nothing, we have to do it with the full understanding of what will happen." Mrs. Heath asked, "At my age, would you say, 'No surgery? Let things fall where they may?'"

The doctor gave what has become a standard reply in our era of patient-centered health care delivery in which patients have the right to choose: "I can't make that decision, and I can't decree which path to go down." He elaborated, "Quality of life is as important as quantity of life. Any treatment carries some risk. And some treatments you won't be able to tolerate because of your age. I would not advise surgery because of your age, though I have to say I just did surgery on a ninety-six-year-old lady. I went kicking and screaming, didn't want to do it, but she wanted it. I took out her bladder. I don't think anyone would give you chemo. It's too toxic. I think we should take a tissue sample, a biopsy, make sure it's cancer. Then give you radiation. I can tell you right now it is cancer, and I don't need the tissue sample. But they won't give you radiation without doing a biopsy for proof of the cancer. You'd have to have that proof. Radiation would be once a day for five or six weeks. There could be burning, pain, diarrhea. So the question is, is it worth it to do a biopsy? It's not worth it unless you are going to get radiation."

The patient's son and daughter-in-law insisted that she couldn't do radiation: "It would be too hard on her." But then they asked what the cure rate is. The doctor said that it is around 40 percent and added, "If she were younger, we would give it in combination with chemo, for better results." Mrs. Heath interjected, "I don't want surgery, really."

"The bigger issue," the doctor said, "is whether you are willing to do anything at all. Are you willing to have the side effects of radiation?" Mrs. Heath easily responded, "I don't have any pain now. I should just let nature take its course."

Being thorough, the doctor described what would occur without some kind of intervention. "If you do nothing, the course will be like this: We'll watch her blood level. If she loses too much blood, she'll get weak, then there is danger of falls, and she'll need a blood transfusion. She'll make less urine, a sign of kidney failure. The kidneys will get involved. They will eventually fail. She may get jaundiced if it goes to the liver. If the kidneys fail, that's not a bad way to go. The cancer may go to other places. She'll experience weight loss." He continued, "As I understand it now, you want to leave well enough alone. Very soon we can't change our minds and turn around on that path. I don't know when, but the path will get more rocky. It will get worse. It's a Hobson's choice. You need to know what's coming. It will get worse. You will get pain, blood loss. We will control the pain."

The conference concluded with Mrs. Heath confirming that she did not want surgery and the family declaring that radiation was out of the question. Mrs. Heath died five months later, following one hospitalization for a blood transfusion.

There is controversy within medicine and within families about how aggressively to treat cancers at older ages, and doctors, patients, and families are often uncertain about how to proceed.[6] The Cleveland Clinic website summarizes this impasse: "Even as the field of geriatric oncology grows, its goals are not uniformly stated. Some healthcare professionals assert that treatment of elderly cancer patients should aim to maintain or augment quality of life; others emphasize identifying effective treatments for the geriatric population as the goal, implying that any divergence from the approach taken with younger cancer patients reflects rationing or age-related bias."[7]

The political debate about age rationing sets up a dichotomy: on one side is the argument that rationing is necessary to ensure the solvency of Medicare, and on the other that any limitation of treatment to older persons is to be considered age discrimination and is against our principles of individual rights. Both sides often clash with the physiological realities of advanced age and the associated worries about the logic of undergoing additional technological intervention. Meanwhile there is no question that more and more older patients are in treatment and are growing older while in treatment.

If Mrs. Heath and her family had wanted surgery to remove the bladder, the doctor might not have tried to talk them out of it and might have complied. He raised the topic of surgery as an evidence-based option and felt obliged to mention it. As a number of physicians have noted, once options are on the table, patients consider them even when doctors do not specifically recommend them. At present there are no bureaucratic or other barriers that would prevent aggressive treatments for patients at any age, and physicians are loath to deny standard-of-care therapy to any patient.

The Second Demand: Confronting the Risk of Death

You can decide to do nothing, but that's a risk.
—Cancer specialist to eighty-year-old patient

Risk awareness and assessment and evidence-based medicine guide much of physicians' thinking, and as we have seen, conversations about risk structure a great deal of the doctor-patient encounter. Sometimes those conversations clarify for patients what to want. Often, though, they simply heighten patients' ambivalence regarding what to do.

The contemporary era, social scientists note, is a time of unprecedented risk awareness: we understand the world as full of risks of all kinds (environmental, financial, medical, etc.); a great deal of social, political, and economic life is devoted to defining, accounting for, and sometimes even mitigating those risks; and as individuals we encounter risks and experience the impact of risk awareness all the time. The notion of risk, perhaps more than anything else, has come to inform our thinking about health and disease.[8]

Medical technologies and techniques, including diagnostic procedures, enhance awareness of the risks of death and complicate our relationship to our own mortality. Over the past several decades the general turning toward risk assessment, risk reduction, risk management, and risk-prevention strategies has happened so seamlessly in the culture of medicine and, more broadly, in contemporary life that we do not think about it much. Most of us do not realize how much of the health care delivery enterprise and how much individual behavior in relation to medical intervention are devoted to risk management. Medications to lower cholesterol and blood pressure, screenings of all kinds (breast, colon, prostate, etc.), diagnostic workups, therapies to reduce future risk, tests for genetic probability, prophylactic treatments, and more are all about mitigating risk. Ultimately the biggest risk, the endpoint of all risks, is the risk of death, that is, the idea that death will come *too soon*.

The more tools medicine gives us with which to see risk—from genetic and imaging technologies to epidemiological studies, clinical trial results, and analyses of behavioral characteristics through surveys and questionnaires—the more risks to health emerge and the more of them we confront *personally* as individuals. In one sense health risks come into our awareness because medicine gives us the tools to find, measure, and define them. Diagnostic tests have enabled us to see disease states and to experience risk long before (sometimes decades before) any symptoms arise at all (if they ever do). After all, we do not feel the risks posed by high blood pressure, genetic markers, or small cancer tumors. It is medical testing that enables us to know we are at risk of disease or are in a high-risk group. And if that testing shows that we have a particular condition, or even a borderline condition or a predisposition to a condition, it confronts us with the risk of more serious disease in the future, whether sooner or later.

The predictions inherent in medical testing have enabled us also to become aware of the risks of death and then to consider how to act in light of that awareness. Ironically this ability to locate and calculate ever more risk has not led to a greater sense of well-being or to better health, as many observers have noted. On the contrary, reports describe a growing sense of dis-ease in general because as risks, diagnostic tests, and treatments proliferate, so too does our awareness of disease probabilities, disease recurrence statistics, and the unrelenting need to monitor and treat chronic and symptom-free conditions so that future risks, potential risks, are kept at bay.[9]

In another sense risks also exist because we suffer from chronic ailments, some of which can kill us if we do not pay attention to the risks they contain. Diabetes, degenerative kidney disease, heart disease, and many cancers have all become chronic illnesses that are sometimes responsive to life-prolonging treatments and may go on for decades. But the risks of exacerbation, metastases, recurrence, and often death are always present, and doctors and patients together must be vigilant about them. What has emerged in our risk-aware society in its medical environment full of tools to measure risks and to do something about them is our understanding that when a condition is made evident as a risk of death, it can almost always be treated and should be.

Our risk-aware society is also an aging society, so a great deal of the organization of health care delivery concerns avoiding, managing, and ameliorating the risks of death. This, of course, is what we want medicine to do. When patients are older and face serious and life-threatening illness, talk about reducing the risk of death—or, like Mrs. Heath, deciding not to—fills up much of the doctor-patient encounter. In recent years however, the goal of risk reduction has come face to face with late life, with more end-stage disease, with the problem of understanding the limits to interventions, and with the quandary of what constitutes too much treatment. The risk-reduction goal also has to take into account the fact that reducing one kind of risk leads not to freedom from disease, and not necessarily to longer life, but rather to other complex health problems and more risk later. The example of kidney dialysis for those in late life with multiple health problems offers a clear illustration of these hurdles.

Mr. Dunbar: Technology Organizes Risk Awareness

Patients who are guided by doctors and technology to confront the risk of imminent death must weigh that risk against the potentiality, but not certainty, of longer life. They are challenged to imagine worse health, better health, and death, and then to make a decision about what to do.

Mr. Lewis Dunbar, age eighty-six, was not feeling well following a bout with pneumonia. He asked his daughter to take him to the local hospital. He was then "shipped," I learned from hospital staff, to the hospital where we eventually met. Mr. Dunbar had congestive heart failure, had recently suffered a heart attack, and was about to undergo a diagnostic cardiac catheterization that would insert a catheter through the groin up through a blood vessel into his heart. At his bedside the cardiologist emphasized that Mr. Dunbar did "not have to make a decision today" regarding what to do after the procedure. The doctor did not want to rush him into making treatment decisions.

When catheterization laboratories came into being in the last quarter of the twentieth century, their single purpose was to perform diagnostic angiograms that could see and thus diagnose specific cardiac problems. At that time the only treatments for cardiac disease were medications and coronary bypass operations. Today cath lab procedures are curative and preventive as well as diagnostic; balloons and stents routinely open up clogged coronary arteries, enabling patients to breathe more easily and live longer. Cath labs perform four times as many procedures as they did twenty years ago, and the patients are older, often in their eighties and early nineties, and have multiple health problems in addition to cardiac disease. The cardiologist I was following did four to six procedures that day. The hospital she worked in did more than three thousand cardiac catheterization procedures in 2010. (Insurance reimburses doctors and hospitals by procedure.) Approximately 10 percent of the patients in this cath unit are ninety and older. These numbers and ages are typical across the United States. This is the socioeconomic-medical scene in which Mr. Dunbar had to strategically decide how or whether to attempt to manipulate the time he had left.

Mr. Dunbar was wheeled on a gurney into the cath lab, and I watched the procedure from behind a window in the lead-shielded control room, where technicians monitored him and the procedure. Lying on his back, he could turn his head to watch a big screen where still and moving pictures the doctor took throughout the procedure were displayed. Larger than life, the patient's beating heart and coronary arteries were clearly visible there in black and white, as was the placement and movement of the catheter. Mr. Dunbar and the rest of us could view his constricted arteries and muse, along with the doctor, about how to interpret the facts of his body and his disease. The medical truths of the body have never been more prominently displayed, more "in your face" than was evident there.[10]

Forty-five minutes after the procedure began, the doctor told Mr. Dunbar, "There is a tight narrowing in the left main coronary artery due to plaque. It is very dangerous. The right artery is also completely blocked—it is not supplying any blood to the heart. This is a dangerous matter. Typically bypass surgery is considered the safest. But technically we could use stents [placed by a catheter] to open the arteries. But if there is a problem it could be fatal. It is high risk for both procedures. You can think about it. If we're going to treat it, we should do something before you leave the hospital. Unless, philosophically, you want to let nature take its course. And then we can treat it with medications."

Like so many other patients who are faced with choices that are frightening, possibly life-threatening, and nearly impossible to make, Mr. Dunbar responded, "What would you advise?" The doctor said it was hard to know what to advise in this case. Theoretically bypass surgery would be the safest. But the stent procedure has a lower morbidity, lower risk of disease problems, than open heart surgery. During the stent procedure blood flow in one major artery would be clamped for a few seconds. Since the other major artery would be completely blocked, Mr. Dunbar could die in those few seconds without blood flow to and through the heart.

The doctor continued outlining the situation: the surgeons would not want to do bypass surgery; it is major surgery requiring general anesthesia. The patient had had pneumonia for two weeks, so he was not in great condition for major surgery. Mr. Dunbar could decide to opt out of having any procedure. In that case medications such as nitroglycerin would be palliative. They could help keep the arteries open a little bit, for a short time. "But if he goes home and has the big one, that's it."

Knowing such details creates the need to anticipate, think about, and decide certain matters, to consider life in corporeal terms and imagine how things might proceed, both to better health and to death. In a very short time Mr. Dunbar had progressed from simply not feeling well and asking to be taken to the hospital to having a procedure that produced the knowledge that he is between a rock and a hard place. Such knowledge is experiential for the patient but clinical and ordinary for the medical team. Decisions must be made.

The option of no decision was not allowed in this case because standard hospital procedure, indeed good medicine, creates a list of risks that must be acknowledged and provides an array of interventions that physicians and patients must choose from. The problem was that all the options seemed equally risky. Yet although no hierarchy of risk was apparent, paradoxically Mr. Dunbar could not go home without articulating a desire for one thing over another. The clinic sets up a risk-based deliberative process, and patients *must* engage it (or someone must do it in their stead). They must apprehend the likely or possible scenarios for their future. If Mr. Dunbar chose to go home without having anything else done in the hospital, it would be, could only be with the knowledge that he had made a conscious decision to take his chances in the face of the relative nearness of a fatal heart attack. It would also be with the knowledge that the other two options (bypass surgery or stents placed by catheter) could bring about immediate death or could instead relieve his condition and stave off death.

The dark side of patient autonomy is revealed here. The doctor wanted the patient to know which medical interventions were possible and available. That is, she guided Mr. Dunbar to consider the risks of death and the risks of life extension and then to voice an opinion. The following day Mr. Dunbar rejected the surgical bypass operation. Three days later he elected medical management only and was discharged from the hospital.

The tools of the clinic provide simultaneously bodily knowledge, risk awareness, and the imperative of autonomous choice. With Mr. Dunbar's potential cause of death visible on the operating room screen, his doctor asked him to do the impossible. Though she did not pose the question directly or prognosticate explicitly, she asked him to imagine death, and also—far easier—to imagine longer life. Many clinic and hospital discussions set up this choice, which, for patients and families, serves as a potential means for controlling the timing of death. At the same time, doctors acknowledge that they cannot know or control the exact timing of death. Yet paradoxically the clinic asks patients to attempt that control. Making this kind of impossible choice has become a common dilemma for those in late life.

The Third Demand: Bargaining with Time

In clinics today patients with life-threatening disease are presented, as a matter of course, with knowledge about the future path of their disease if it is left untreated, a path that is certain but with an unknown time line, inevitable yet impossible to comprehend existentially. In what has become an ordinary confrontation, that future path is discussed together with the demands and potential effects of treatment. Never before have we been able to learn, *must learn* in such exquisite detail the ways treatments might or will affect us, the ways our death could or will come about. As a result patients and their families learn to compare alternative time lines: How long can I live with treatment? Without treatment? How much longer do I want to try to live?

Mr. Trin: Linking the Value of Life to Age and "Time Left"

For some time, Mr. Thao Trin, age seventy-eight, and his physicians had been monitoring his liver cancer with vigilance through periodic blood tests and scans. When, a year earlier, the liver specialist he had been seeing for a decade began to talk about transplant as his "best option," Mr. Trin responded enthusiastically. At the time of this clinic visit, he had already had two rounds of chemotherapy infusion treatments directly into the liver in order to shrink the tumors while he waited for his name to rise to the top of the national waiting list for a liver transplant.

In the exam room Mr. Trin was accompanied as usual by his daughter, who would support any decision he made. His wife was also present. She did not want him to have a transplant because she feared for his life in such a complex surgery. The physician reviewed the most recent CT scans and noted that there was a new cancer tumor in a new location. "One of the tumors has grown a little in size. We're going to have to go in again and repeat the chemoembolization procedure. This is telling us that you have a liver that is prone to making tumors. And this tells us that a transplant is the best way to manage your cancer. These treatments can't control it."

The physician continued, "You could get an offer for a transplant in a couple of months. You should have the chemo procedure in the next couple of weeks." The daughter asked how the cancer would be treated if her father did not have a transplant. The doctor replied, "One of the risks is that the cancer can get ahead of us, and then the pace speeds up, and we can't control it and we can't predict how it will behave."

He then shifted the topic to speak about age and risk. "When we started with liver transplant, we didn't have any patients over fifty-five, then sixty. Now there is no age limit. But the older you are, the greater the risk. They have to clamp the largest vein in your body for forty-five minutes. And that puts a stress on your heart. So we want to do more tests, to see if you can withstand the surgery. If others on the team think he's a good candidate for a transplant, he should have one, and the sooner, the better. . . . The fact that they treated the tumor a couple of months ago and didn't knock it out, that hedges me over toward a transplant. In my experience you'd do well with a transplant."

Another doctor came in to discuss the different types of high-risk cadaveric donor livers that older patients especially may choose from. There was a high-risk donor form for Mr. Trin to fill out, and apparently there were choices he could make among livers that practitioners sometimes refer to as "in-between," that is, livers from donors with hepatitis B or C, from patients who died a cardiac rather than brain death, or from older donors with other conditions. "In order to use as many livers as possible, we use some of those in-between livers. They might not look good, but they might work well. We use our judgment. But the surgeon will give you the option. They will call you about these less than perfect livers, and you can decide if you want it." The doctor added, "When you get a call that a liver has been found, the surgeon does not bargain with you. You have fifteen minutes to decide."

Mr. Trin commented, "I've lived a good life to age seventy-eight. Now I leave it to the doctor." The doctor replied, "We won't offer you a liver that isn't good. You have to trust the surgeons. The science isn't perfect. The surgeon judges the context of the donor liver and your age and everything, and decides if the liver is good for you."

When the doctor left the exam room Mr. Trin reflected on the discussion. He pondered the next set of questions about control over "time left" and "additional" time that medicine opened up: "Maybe I should wait for a perfect, healthy liver. I want to wait. If I get a healthy liver, and it gives me five years, that's okay. If I live five years. My father died at seventy-seven.

If I live to eighty-two, that's good. If I had stayed in [another country], I wouldn't live this long. The medicines here have helped me live longer."

Mr. Trin's daughter said, "You have two things going against you if you wait for a 'healthy' liver. First, the cancer will grow, and second, you'll be older. If you turn down the first offer you get, and then need another infusion treatment before they offer you a 'healthy' liver, what would that be like? Healthy liver offers are more infrequent."

Mr. Trin mused, "To live past age eighty would be good." After a few seconds of reflection he changed his mind and said, "If I could get two added years with a nonperfect liver, living to age eighty, that would be okay."

How much potential additional time is worth the risks of transplant surgery? At first Mr. Trin thought five years, but then he quickly reconsidered and said that two years of life from a donor liver would be enough for him. Neither his range (two to five years) nor his recalibration (from five to two) is unusual for older persons who are considering major interventions. It seems that as they negotiate with themselves, older persons who seriously consider life-extending treatments confront several things simultaneously: the limits of medicine, yet the fact that life-extending interventions are normal and occur successfully every day; the feeling that even a relatively short future is worth the pain and the risk of death that may accompany major interventions; and the awareness that *time left* is a mandatory variable in calculations about risk, worth, and the best thing to do.

When the physician reentered the room, the daughter had questions: Can one have as long a life with a high-risk liver as with a "perfect" liver? The doctor replied that generally the longevity with a high-risk liver is as good as that from a perfect liver. Did her father get only one shot at a transplant because of his age? It depended. If he got a bad organ and there were immediate problems, he'd get another. If things went wrong later he'd probably not get another organ. What about cancer again, whether from his own or from a high-risk donor who had cancer? The doctor replied that one can have a recurrence of the cancer in the liver. "Even though this is the best treatment, we can't guarantee that he won't get a recurrence. But it's only a 10 percent or 20 percent chance of recurrence. If we don't do a transplant, we know his cancer will progress. The transplant is mostly curative, and we hope the cancer won't come back." What if the tumors got bigger? "We can't do a transplant if the tumors are bigger than five centimeters. Right now they are smaller and we can control it."

Two weeks after this clinic visit Mr. Trin had another chemotherapy infusion to reduce the size of the tumors. Four weeks later he had a successful liver transplant. He never filled out the high-risk donor form, so he did not learn what kind of liver he might have received if he had. Two years later he was enjoying life, without disease recurrence.

Mr. Trin confronted risk by negotiating with himself regarding how much remaining time was important to him, calculating desired "time left" in terms of age. He negotiated with himself about the value of life in relation to the amount of future he thought would be minimally acceptable in order to go ahead with transplant surgery, given his current age, his growing cancer, the risks of surgery, and the age of his father at death (a very common comparison point). He pondered and then decided quickly that the risks of transplant surgery would be worth it if he gained even two "additional" years of life. The structure of American health care delivery supports his calculations. Important too is the fact that his doctors were of the unanimous and strong opinion that transplantation would extend his life, and therefore it was the right thing to do.

The Fourth Demand: The Family's Dilemma

Ordinary medicine further complicates our approach to the inevitable with the demands that it places on how we interpret and express love. In addition to the bonds medicine forges among evidence, bodily commitment, and love that we saw in the example of living kidney transfer, medicine poses at least one additional demand on love when it forces the question: Does the expression of love mean supporting a patient's treatment choice, whatever that may entail? Family members often are caught in a tangled connection between love and treatment. In the U.S. context, which emphasizes the value of new technologies and the "more is better" ethos, the problem is that if a family member wants to encourage the patient to say no to treatment, it seems to imply a lack of love, or of enough love, for the patient. (Recall that in Mrs. Dang's case the family thought that if they said no to transplant surgery, they would be contributing to "killing" her.) Similarly if a patient rejects treatment, it seems to some families that he or she isn't trying hard enough to stay alive—for them.

In his poignant memoir *Swimming in a Sea of Death*, the journalist David Rieff candidly and with unresolved anguish portrays the contemporary sensibility of family surrounding the question of "doing the right thing." Like countless others, he was trapped and burdened by having to weigh the worth of more time, more life against the worth of more treatment and more suffering for a loved one. He was deeply perplexed about how to show "enough" love. His famous mother, Susan Sontag, refused to acknowledge that her final illness, myelodysplastic syndrome, was terminal, though she knew it was "a particularly lethal form of blood cancer," a "smoldering leukemia."[11] She chose to fight this disease as aggressively as she had fought breast cancer while in her early forties and uterine cancer six years before this final illness.

Rieff explicitly describes how, throughout Sontag's treatments and after her death, he pondered whether he had done the right thing, that is, whether he had remained too passive in his response to her desire for experimental and debilitating interventions that created immense suffering at her life's end. Should he have insistently presented her with the "truth," the fact that this time her disease was fatal? Should he have demanded that she acknowledge that truth? Should he have questioned the physicians' agreement to administer two kinds of aggressive treatments, first, a bone marrow transplant and then an experimental drug treatment, both with a very small, in fact infinitesimal chance of success? For at least two years after Sontag's death, he continued to dwell with the burden of those unresolved questions: "What I'm far less sure of is whether I did the right thing in going along with and in fact doing what I could to abet her in her refusal to contemplate the prospect that this third time around she would die of her cancer. . . . Did I do the right thing? Could I have done more? Or proposed an alternative? Or been more supportive? Or forced the issue of death to the fore? Or concealed it better? The unanswerable questions of a survivor."[12]

His memoir is a revelation of his own lingering doubt and guilt about his complicit role in his mother's final cancer treatments and final days. At the end of his story he states, "My failing was that my own ambivalence about the choice she had made often rendered me almost mute. . . . But I am anything but certain that I did the right thing, and, in my bleaker moments, wonder if in fact I might not have made things worse for her by endlessly refilling that poisoned chalice of hope."[13] He and his readers are left without a definitive answer regarding either his role or the role of family in general. The lack of resolution that he so strongly articulates highlights pressing medicoethical quandaries of our aging society: How long should we continue to fight death using medicine's growing armamentarium of interventions? Especially when evidence shows they will not provide benefit? When does one know that a treatment is "unnecessary" or "overused" or "futile," and who decides that? Where does the responsibility for more or less treatment reside? Sontag was not unusual in her quest for life-extending treatments. Research shows that thousands of patients overestimate their survival probabilities and thus seek treatment they hope will ensure life extension.[14] She was seventy-one at the time of her final treatments, and she had the resources to pay for the interventions she chose and received just before her death. Those treatments did not extend her life. They made her dying longer and more excruciating.

But is it the doctors' responsibility to do what the patient wants, to participate in a *folie à deux* in which physicians offer certain extreme interventions—because they exist—and hold out hope when there is none in order to go along with a patient's wishes?[15] Is moving on to the next therapy because a patient wants to keep going with high tech and aggressive treatments an expression of clinical (and emotional) commitment to the patient? According to Rieff's account, Sontag's doctors offered and did not discourage her from getting the bone marrow transplant and, several months later, the experimental drug.

Rieff quotes the physician Diane Meier, a leader in palliative medicine, confronting those questions directly in her explanation of what happens when doctors speak with critically ill patients:

> As a physician, you don't want to impose your quantitative, Cartesian view of probabilities on an individual person who says, "That's probabilities, that's not me. I'm a fighter. I want that thousand to one chance and who are you to say that it's not worth it? Whose life is it anyway?" The result is that, as doctors, we wind up through that kind of thinking becoming unwitting participants in a folie à deux with patients and family of caving to the desire to live because it is respectful of the patient and who she or he is and their perception of the right way to live, while realizing, in the other part of your brain that there's essentially no chance that this is going to help, that it's definitely going to cause harm and side effects, that it's hugely expensive out of the public trough, and it is a very wearing kind of cognitive dissonance.

Ordinary medicine has set up a particularly odd situation for physicians in the United States in that they sometimes feel that they are compelled to act against their better judgment. Meier goes on to speak of

> the denial, the kind of winking that goes on, where, yeah, we all know the patient's going to die, but we're all going to pretend like there's hope, so we're all going to go through these rituals because that's what we believe that the patient wants. In the meantime the patient is watching the doctor, who is offering this treatment, and clearly thinking to himself, if the doctor didn't think it would work he or she wouldn't offer it, but what the doctor's not saying is that the odds are minute and that he is trying to be responsive to the needs of the patient for hope. It's like a minuet. It's surreal.[16]

In the end, how often does this folie à deux, the inability of everyone to say no, trump the evidence and thus foster the question: Did we do the right thing? Oncologists (and other specialists) practice in the midst of a profound cultural tension that surrounds the relationship of medicine to longevity and mortality. The broad and always growing array of treatments complicates what physicians and patients alike consider appropriate, even for advanced disease, even while articles written by physicians and published in medical journals argue for the need to better integrate palliative care with oncology.[17] Studies show that patients do not understand that chemotherapy for incurable cancers, while perhaps providing weeks or months of palliation, is not curative. This lack of understanding prevents informed decision making and augments the "more is better" perspective that some patients and families embrace.[18] Other studies illustrate that large numbers of patients receive aggressive cancer treatments up until weeks and days before death. Physicians are pondering how to stop that practice, given the lure of more treatment, the lack of patient understanding about the capabilities of treatments, the belief that "more is better" despite the inevitability of death.[19]

The physician and ethicist Paul Helft draws attention to this problem and to the folie à deux between doctors and patients in his discussion of the benefits of "necessary collusion." This collusion is a form of prognosis by which physicians avoid or delay "discussing a definitive . . . estimate of life expectancy" so that painful information emerges over time and patients' hope is thus preserved.[20] This style of communication, while it preserves physician control of information, allows patients to accept the flow of prognostic information and thereby, it is hoped, avoid futile and painful treatments.

Yet Rieff offers a different view of who is in charge as he describes how the collusion worked in his mother's case. When Sontag asked her oncologist whether she would survive, "he, whether it was through force of personality, long experience, or psychological acuity, or some combination of all of these . . . managed to make the question 'unaskable' on some deep level."[21] He never addressed it directly but rather reframed it in ways that apparently relieved Sontag's mental anguish. Rieff was aware of how the doctors guided the discussions and determined their outcome in favor of more treatment.

Rieff's disquiet settles ultimately on two sets of questions. First, how relevant is the evidence to actual patient care in situations of life-threatening illness? How important is it for the "best practices" of medicine (and for the solvency of the U.S. health care delivery system) that Sontag (and many others in similar circumstances) refused to acknowledge the truth and *was refused* the truth? Rieff's story reveals that the value and use of scientific evidence, while a lynchpin of ordinary medicine, can be minimal, even nonexistent, when both life and hope are at stake. Patients' and families' sensibilities, their acknowledgments and judgments are certainly part of the equation. In the end evidence-based medicine simply does not, and perhaps cannot, guide all, or most, of medical practice.

Second, Rieff's lack of certainty about his own response to his mother's condition and his unease about the doctors' actions point to even more fundamental questions: "What does it mean to be a good doctor? To treat a patient? What is the sense of therapy?"[22] Aggressive cancer treatments, especially chemotherapy, offered and received near the end of life bring those latter questions poignantly into view.

Countless others share Rieff's inability to settle on a definitive response to the quandary of what to do and how to proceed when a loved one is given a prognosis *but is also given choices*. Not only must patients and their families consider the opposing offers of imminent death or treatments they are led to believe offer hope, but families must also consider their own role in decision making: either they facilitate another's longevity (and perhaps with added suffering), or they suggest a halt to treatment, thus acknowledging and abetting death. Often families are torn either way. Which action expresses love, or expresses it the best? Who is or should be responsible for such choices in the first place? With regard to such quandaries, Rieff's memoir stands as a cultural document of the contemporary era.

————

Ever more diagnostic tools produce ever more prognostic data and more pressure to imagine different futures and to choose among them. Yet prognostication has its limits, and uncertainty, always a staple of medicine, is shifted onto the patient and family through access to bodily details never before imaginable or visible. Perhaps more than ever before, patients and their families are plunged into debate about how much more time is wanted, how much is enough, and how the family must be involved. Contemplating "time left" is how, in the present, we confront the evidence presented to us about the future and about a sort of surplus of life in the context of life-threatening disease. Organizing both "more" time and the timing of death has become a contemporary imperative. In all this the future is characterized by certain kinds of investments and decisions,[23] but only *within the possibilities that medicine provides*. This is how we "make" longevity now, and this is the way the future does a great deal of its cultural work today.

8

FOR WHOSE BENEFIT?

Our Shared Quandary

————

To ask whether a society is just is to ask how it distributes
the things we prize. . . . The hard questions begin when
we ask what people are due, and why.
—Michael J. Sandel, *Justice*

To be a medical citizen is to concern oneself both with the realm
of politics and social justice and with clinical judgment. . . .
We are in this sense all medical citizens, each one of us capable
of using medicine as a way of thinking about society, and of
society and politics as ways of understanding
medical outcomes.
—Charles E. Rosenberg, *Our Present Complaint*

The story of our troubled health care enterprise does not end with the quandary for individual patients, families, and doctors about crossing the line of "too much" treatment. The chain of health care drivers and its ever present ethical field raise questions, as we have seen, about the goals of medicine itself in an aging society. When we widen our lens to look beyond the quandary facing individuals we see another one that asks: For whose benefit? What is deemed right for one patient is not necessarily considered right for society. The value accorded to the individual's right to treatment, expressed most clearly through Medicare reimbursement, collides with a different imperative: fairness. How can fairness, that is, equitable access for all, coexist with the normalcy, the ordinariness of so many expensive life-extending procedures? With what has become standard medical treatment for older persons? With what we have come to want and our growing need to have it?

Fairness has become a growing concern in debates about Medicare re-form and in debates about health care reform generally. In 2010 the Centers for Disease Control estimated that approximately one in five U.S. residents under sixty-five lacked health insurance (a percentage that had held steady for several preceding years).[1] Since people began enrolling in health coverage under the Affordable Care Act (July 2013 to June 2014) 9.5 million fewer adults (ages nineteen to sixty-four) were uninsured, reducing the adult uninsured rate from approximately 20 percent to 15 percent of the U.S. population.[2] Despite this overall decrease in the numbers of Americans who lack health insurance, such statistics make the challenges of achieving fairness in health care delivery for the un-insured and underinsured obvious. For those with Medicare insurance, our collective ethics are more complicated because, for them, *eligibility* for medical procedures has reorganized fairness in our aging society.

The implantable cardiac devices, aggressive cancer treatments, and organ transplants that are now in ordinary use for our older citizens are expensive and growing ever more so, but although reining in costs generates the most debate in the search for solutions to what ails health care delivery, costs actually represent only part of the problem. These treatments and devices also provoke questions about rationing—about how to achieve, or more accurately how to approach societal fairness in the form of equitable access to all kinds of therapeutics. In the world of transplantation there are ongoing debates about what is fair and just, and practices among donors, recipients, doctors, and institutions are always shifting. These activities show the concept of fairness in the actual process of being reinvented—in the kinds of bodily demands one citizen is making on another and in how the medical profession is fostering and facilitating those demands. Organ transplantation is perhaps the prime example today of biomedical advances creating more rather than fewer instances of lifeboat ethics, that is, allocation and rationing decisions made amid scarce resources.

Kidney Transplantation Redux: Modeling the Issues of Access and Scarcity

I return to the subject of kidney transplantation because developments in that realm so starkly illustrate how medical practice, individual expectation, and the public marketplace are responding right now to the quandary of access in an environment of increasing organ scarcity. Attempts to redefine fairness in organ allocation are emerging as our national institutions struggle to embody fairness in policies about access to organs. At the same time, individual recipients and donors are forging their own kinds of access as they proactively seek to give and receive organs, whether through their personal relationships or through the public marketplace of the Internet. Medical practitioners are responding to the problem of equity in allocation when increasing numbers of patients in need are beyond seventy but deceased organs are mostly from younger people; to the phenomenon of Internet solicitation; and to the broad challenge of the need for more organs generally.

The site of public concern about allocation decisions has moved far from its focus in the 1960s, which was on the need to ration maintenance dialysis due to a shortage of equipment. Today that concern is focused on the transplant arena, where the values question centers on age and the public good, in that the good of longevity making also contributes to shortages and death. This is the most recent iteration of the rationing and allocation problem, and it will grow rather than abate. In the United States persons over sixty-five are projected to be nearly 20 percent of the population by 2030, up from 12.4 percent in 2000.[3]

Throughout this book I have focused on events unfolding in the realm of transplantation precisely because developments there reveal so dramatically the quandary of deciding and then inventing and organizing what constitutes a *good enough ethics* regarding both access and limits to life-prolonging treatments. The various expressions of societal values in the world of kidney transplantation illustrate the benefits of the procedure and the quandary-provoking consequences of ordinary medicine at work today. Of particular note for any discussion of fairness and equitable access are the ways *evidence of benefit* is taken up in American life and the shifts in how certain kinds of therapeutic-cultural practices come to be considered morally and socially justifiable.

The success of medicine is clearly visible in the lives prolonged and made better by organ transplantation. There is no question about that. Yet in normalizing transplantation and other complex therapies for older adults, in moving in that direction, we have created new problems and unintended effects, new costs in terms of the quandary of fairness in an aging society. The politics of who benefits is intertwined with that quandary, as the following developments illustrate.

Age, Utility, Equity: Attempts to Organize Fairness

In February 2011 the Organ Procurement and Transplantation Network of the United Network for Organ Sharing (OPTN/UNOS) released "Concepts for Kidney Allocation" online to the public. This detailed proposal was designed to achieve greater fairness in the U.S. kidney donor allocation program, which was not making the best possible use of the country's supply of deceased donor kidneys in light of growing need, increasingly inadequate supply, and especially the growing numbers of older patients needing and receiving kidneys. The concepts, developed by the Kidney Transplantation Committee of UNOS, were based on nearly seven years of research, statistical modeling, and public debate and included careful consideration of demographic, disease, and current allocation trends among kidney donors and recipients in the United States. Since the national allocation and distribution system began in 1986, kidneys have been allocated primarily on a first-come, first-served basis. Simply stated, the longer one is on the waiting list, the closer one moves to the top of the list, and the person at the top is eligible to receive the first available, medically appropriate organ.[4] It was widely agreed among members of the UNOS Kidney Transplantation Committee that that method for allocation had become less efficient (in terms of individual patient survival) and less equitable (in terms of fair distribution) as the decades passed.[5]

For years fairness was made manifest in the amount of time spent waiting. The problem with this system, which UNOS began to reconsider in 2005–6, is that *age has become central to its waning fairness*. Demographics, evidence, medical practice, and our understandings of ordinary longevity have changed since 1986. The majority of kidney recipients today are over fifty. Persons sixty-five and older have been joining the waiting list in increasing numbers and have been receiving more kidneys each year from the pool, which has not grown fast enough to keep up with demand. They also receive an increasingly greater proportion of the total number of available deceased donor kidneys: 3 percent in 1988, 15 percent in 2011.[6]

Europe faces similarly shifting demographics. In Europe's version of UNOS, Eurotransplant, the percentage of the available kidneys going to recipients over sixty-five rose from 3.6 percent in 1991 to nearly 20 percent in 2007.[7]

The number of persons on the UNOS waiting list age fifty and below has remained constant since the turn of the millennium; the number sixty-five and above has tripled.[8] Other than assuring a good biological match, kidney allocation is keyed only to waiting time, and because of this, older persons receive more "younger" organs from the pool than ever before. Thus a seventy-five-year-old patient may receive a kidney from a twenty-five-year-old donor. That patient may gain ten or even fifteen years of life, but the organ could "live" decades longer in a younger body, according to the UNOS statistical analyses of the potential years of life of transplanted organs. Thus its potential for giving life is "wasted," as critics of the status quo phrase it, on an older person. In contrast, an organ from a sixty-year-old donor placed in a twenty-five-year-old patient may fail long before the recipient reaches old age, thereby creating the need for an additional organ at age fifty or so. In this scenario even more strain is put on the already untenable UNOS system, which, at the time of this writing, has a waiting list of over one hundred thousand names and a rotating supply of only about thirteen thousand available deceased donor kidneys.

The scheme OPTN/UNOS proposed in 2011—but rejected in 2012—had two parts. First, 20 percent of the kidneys with the longest potential life span would be offered to candidates projected to have the longest survival time with the organ. That part of the proposal favored younger patients. Second, the remaining 80 percent of kidneys in the pool would be "age-matched" to within fifteen years of the candidate's age. Thus a forty-year-old patient would be eligible for a kidney from a donor between twenty-five and fifty-five; a seventy-five-year-old patient would be eligible for a kidney from donors sixty or older. Age-matching would slightly shift donations to younger age groups by directing donor organs with the longest "useful" life to younger recipients. It would also reduce the number of unused, "wasted" kidneys, those from older donors declined by people at the top of the waiting list who prefer to wait for a younger and thus seemingly better one. That feature of individual patient choice was a major cause for the discarding of 2,644 deceased-donor kidneys in 2011.[9] (Because the window for a kidney to be accepted and transplanted is just a few hours, declined kidneys are discarded.)

In 1972, after twelve continuous years and in direct response to consumer advocacy, Medicare passed a law ending dialysis rationing.[10] The case of transplant scarcity can have no comparable resolution because there will never be enough organs and demand will continue to increase. The 2011 "Concepts for Kidney Allocation" attempted to make existing resources more effective and to make the system more equitable in terms of actual age distribution. It would have favored utility by maximizing the lifetime of an organ, and thus the UNOS distribution system potentially would have gained tens of thousands of future kidney life years. But it would also have de-emphasized all-around equity, that is, equal access to transplant for every person listed, regardless of the projected outcome.[11] The proposal did not claim to be ideal or to solve the problem of scarcity, and it generated considerable debate. When it was presented to community focus groups in 2007, it received mixed responses from groups of older persons around the country. One transplant surgeon noted at that time, "It would appear that the public has a strong sense of entitlement to receive the best care possible, and the concept of an organ allocation system driven primarily by utility is unacceptable."[12]

In August 2011 the U.S. Department of Health and Human Services, along with its Office of Civil Rights, expressed concern that the fifteen-year age-matching strategy "did not meet the requirements of the Age Discrimination Act of 1975." The problem, the government noted, was both that the fifteen-year algorithm seemed arbitrary and that this scheme did not take all-around equity into consideration. Equity is a particularly thorny issue here because, while the number of patients over fifty on the waiting list has grown and continues to grow rapidly, most organs from deceased donors come from younger persons. The scheme did not correct for the mismatch in age distribution of donors and potential recipients, and so it was considered discriminatory because it would disproportionately allocate deceased donor kidneys to young candidates.[13] Politically the evidence for enhanced utility could not overrule the specter of age discrimination. The individual right to young kidneys won that debate.

A new scheme, proposed in 2012 and accepted as UNOS policy in June 2013, tackles the problem of age discrimination less directly. Similar in part to the 2011 version, it will "enhance post-transplant survival benefit" and "increase utilization of donated kidneys" but without direct age-matching.[14] Like the previous plan, it strives to eliminate the worst mismatches by directing the highest quality 20 percent of organs to recipients thought to be likely to live the longest. But the other 80 percent will not be age-matched and will be distributed largely as they always have been.

Several new features aim to strengthen equity in the system; they address factors such as underserved groups and people with rare blood types and broaden the search criteria for patients willing to accept "lowest quality" kidneys. The new proposal is projected to add an additional 8,380 "life years achieved annually from the current pool of deceased donor kidneys" (considerably fewer than the 2011 projection) and will, it hopes, reduce the discard rate. Those who proposed it consider it to be a compromise that tweaks the status quo slightly in order to achieve greater utilization of organs but does not change it enough to get maximum utility at the expense of age equity.[15]

The example of kidney transplantation in the United States offers a microcosm of the broader health equity predicament. Those over sixty, seventy, and eighty constitute more and more of the public in aging societies and will continue to do so. How, then, are we to reconstitute health care delivery practices and the idea of the public good when the public purse is shrinking dramatically even as the successes of medicine, and with them our expectations about longevity and medical promise, continue to expand? As a cause of scarcity and of the quandary about allocation, age contributes both to new expressions of self-interest, obligation, and altruism and to the new societal mechanisms for allowing that expression. Perhaps, in our aging society, the idea of public health needs expanding as well.

The Tyranny of Potential: Does It Trump Organized Fairness?

As the example of kidney transplantation reveals, the unprecedented ability to extend older lives using medical technique is connected to the dilemma of the worthiness and value of those older lives in relation to younger lives. This dilemma has been brewing for decades but first gained wider public attention in 2006, when the Los Angeles Times reported the story of an eighty-five-year-old retired doctor who wanted a kidney and was at the top of the UNOS waiting list in his region.[16] Dr. Guthrie was active until the age of eighty, when he underwent cardiac bypass and valve replacement surgery. Following that intervention, his kidneys failed, and he had been on hemodialysis for five years, hoping for a transplant. His wife, son, and sister-in-law had offered him one of their kidneys, but he was reported to have told them, "I'm not selfish enough to consider that." However, his decision to wait on the national list illustrates what has become, because of growing scarcity, a different form of selfishness, mostly not acknowledged as such by those who are waiting. It is the selfishness of wanting and expecting to take a scarce resource from the anonymous commons rather than from within one's circle of friends and family. Persons needing transplants can be caught in an ethical tangle if and when they acknowledge that taking a kidney from either source can be considered a selfish act.

Two transplant centers in different states had refused to accept Guthrie on their waiting lists because of his age, but the hospital in Colorado that had performed his cardiac surgery offered him a place in line. Guthrie was at the top of the list on the morning a kidney from a thirty-year-old motorcycle accident victim became available, and a member of the transplant team phoned to offer him the organ. The team member justified the age discrepancy by pointing out that the patient had been on the list for three years, his overall health was good enough to survive the surgery, it was his turn, and, besides, no one knows how long a different potential recipient, of any age, might live. The goal of medicine and the physician's duty, this doctor opined (as do most others), was to provide the best medical care for the patient at hand at this moment. The conflicting goal—to ensure that each transplanted organ achieves the greatest life span possible—was a lesser imperative.

Another transplant physician at the same hospital decided to fight that logic. Guthrie was eighty-five; the kidney was thirty. What was the sense in offering a perfect organ to someone who would die soon, thus "wasting" the full life of the organ, probably decades, when hundreds of younger people waited for one? It was unreasonable and unethical. The two transplant surgeons were at an impasse until the doctor favoring the transplant backed down. With the support of the rest of the transplant team, Guthrie was denied the organ. Within a few months that hospital had revised its transplant access policy, which it had the legal authority to do: patients between seventy and seventy-nine would be offered only "expanded criteria" deceased organs, that is, organs from people sixty and above or that carried a history of some diseases. Patients eighty and above would be denied kidneys. Not all hospital policies are similar. The *Los Angeles Times* article reported that a Pennsylvania hospital transplanted a deceased donor kidney into a ninety-year-old that same year.

Guthrie lived two and a half more years, remaining on dialysis. When he died of a heart attack at age eighty-eight, the surgeon who had favored the transplant noted that prolonged dialysis puts a strain on the heart and perhaps Guthrie could have lived more years with a viable kidney.[17]

The dilemma of the best use of a younger organ plays out in transplant centers daily. One transplant surgeon I spoke with in 2011 expressed the anguish this problem of age and allocation caused him:

I had a patient who was listed at age sixty-seven. He waited eight years on the UNOS list and came to the top of the list at age seventy-five. The kidney offered was a thirty-year-old kidney. The second patient on the waiting list is at the hospital nearby, and he is twenty-nine years old. The kidney is definitely right for him. What am I supposed to do? That kidney is also the *right one for my patient*. It will work right away; he will spend less time in the hospital, thereby saving money; it will improve his health and his life. But what's right for my patient is not right for society. This happens all the time—seventy-year-olds are getting forty-year-old kidneys *a lot*. I wish someone would stop me from taking that kidney for my seventy-five-year-old patient. But I gave it to him.[18]

The conflict of imperatives is stark: whether to do "the best thing" for an individual patient or to contribute to greater equity in the transplantation system by age-matching. That conflict was not anticipated when the UNOS allocation and distribution program was established in the 1980s. This doctor's choice was in keeping with the dual aspect of the status quo: the older patient's right to a younger kidney and the doctor's traditional mandate "to do what is right" for the patient in front of him. The field of liver transplantation is facing the same conflict. One transplant surgeon noted in a discussion published in the *Archives of Surgery*, "One question is that a 70-year-old really doesn't need 30 years of liver function. Do you think we should, as transplant professionals, even be allowed to take a 20-year-old liver for a 73-year-old recipient when that liver might, more utilitarianly speaking, be useful in a 35-year-old recipient? Obviously, you are going to get better results with the 70-year-old if you take a nice young donor, but is that something that we ought to be doing?"[19]

The conundrum of individual versus societal benefit, which age exacerbates and these stories illustrate, may be resolved, in part and for a time, with a new UNOS policy. However, growing need amid increasing scarcity will continue to shape clinical decision making, patient activism, and how fairness continues to emerge and be contested.

The notion of medical potential drives biomedical science and clinical choice. It is also growing more powerful as a determinant of intervention because we are learning more and more about specific disease trajectories and treatment capabilities. In the case of organ transplantation, *potential* carries with it both the awareness of our human connection to others, known and unknown, and the question, with its variable answers, of whom to give to and accept from. Ordinary medicine in general creates a tyranny of choice for patients and doctors. The ordinariness of organ transplantation at older ages also organizes a tyranny of choice on the part of government and society because that ordinariness links the concepts of rights, scarcity, and interdependence with our notions of the public good. That link has not been discussed widely.

The Gift, the Market, and the Shifting Bases of Altruism: Newer Responses to Scarcity

In addition to the ordinary development of living kidney donation from younger to older persons, another now ordinary development has taken hold as well: living donation among unrelated strangers. In this instance new expressions of altruism and market forces are both in play. Both forms of donation illustrate how standards and norms regarding what is owed, what is available, and what is wanted and expected continue to emerge. Both demonstrate the fluid boundaries and intertwining of altruism and self-interest. Finally, both show that our notions of fairness about procurement and payment, worthiness and justice are mutable.

Ever since the first successful kidney transplant was performed in 1954, the medical profession and kidney transplantation's material supporters (UNOS, procurement organizations, other health workers, non-profit advocacy groups) have provided the moral logic, the language, and the organizing principle for the national system of voluntary donation that enables the extraordinary act of transferring organs from one body to another. From the beginning the goal of those groups was to encourage voluntary donation. Their rhetoric provided donors, recipients, families, transplant teams, and the public with a vocabulary—the "gift of life"—for the profound experience of giving and receiving a part of the body.[20] Procurement organizations specifically emphasize language that presents the organ donation as a means for survivors to achieve a positive experience following a loved one's death. For example, the website of the Association of Organ Procurement Organizations in the United States declares:

> There are over 115,000 listings across the country for people who are waiting for the call that will save their life. Some people wait days, many wait years, and thousands of people each year die while waiting

for an organ transplant. In these same communities, many families are answering a call no one wants to receive. Someone they love has died. *Hope lives where these two worlds come together, creating miracles out of tragedy.*

The generosity of donors and their families make the gifts of organ and tissue donation possible. Organ procurement organizations (OPOS) are the stewards of these precious gifts that are given with love and received with hope. Together, we put hope within reach to tens of thousands of people across the country.[21]

Yet the "gift of life" masks a broader spectrum of feelings about uses of a dead body and about the relationship of the family to the deceased. The language of altruism and "voluntary gifting" has performed extraordinary cultural work over the past half century: it has made the taking and exchange of body parts from the living and the recently dead socially acceptable and morally standard.[22]

The goal of UNOS is "to increase and ensure the effectiveness, efficiency and equity of organ sharing in the national system of organ allocation, and to increase the supply of donated organs available for transplantation."[23] The rhetoric of unsullied altruism dominates UNOS, which depends, for the time being, entirely on voluntary gifting. Its website states, for example, "Because transplantation depends on the generosity of the American public, UNOS promotes organ donation on an ongoing basis and pays tribute to our nation's organ donors and their families. . . . In 1992, UNOS founded Donate Life America, now an independent organization devoted solely to inspiring people to save and enhance lives through organ, eye and tissue donation."[24] Relatives of deceased donors receive no monetary compensation. In the 1990s proposals began to be floated to increase the organ supply by providing direct or indirect "incentives" and compensation to the donors' families, including funeral payments, reduced life insurance payments, tax credits, and early Medicare eligibility. All such proposals have been hotly debated and then abandoned.[25] Still, some patients who have sought and received organs are trying to shift institutional thinking so that the "gift of life" can receive some form of compensation in order to increase supply.[26]

Opposition to all such schemes remains strong, however, and comes from various quarters, illustrating the strong bond between the voluntary exchange of organs and its moral underpinnings. The tenacity with which volunteer giving is defended is perhaps especially surprising because in all other aspects of the organ transfer system—from the procurement organizations that distribute organs, to the doctors, teams, and institutions that transplant them—the participants are paid for their work.[27] Moreover "85 percent of the fifty-nine non-profit organ procurement agencies in the United States have established lucrative sources of income by selling body parts such as bone, skin, heart valves, veins, and tendons directly to for-profit biomedical firms or to tissue banks with corporate connections."[28] The phrase *gift of life* remains the moral lynchpin and organizational directive for the transplantation enterprise—a justification for an exceptional act performed in an otherwise complex, multibillion-dollar commercial industry of professionals, organizations, and health care delivery.

NEW KINDS OF *GOOD ENOUGH* DONORS EMERGE

As greater demand began to far outpace a nearly flat supply of deceased donor organs throughout the 1990s, hospitals and renal transplant groups gradually relaxed their formal requirements for what kind of "relatedness" was good enough for a prospective living donor. Immunosuppressant drugs had already changed the safety and survival equation, and now almost anyone could donate to anyone else. Genetic and familial relatedness no longer mattered medically. At first, the kinds of "non-biologically related" donors who dominated U.S. and other industrialized nations' transplant clinics included spouses, in-laws, adopted children, and close friends who were "just like" family. By 1999 or 2000, however, the demand for organs and the pressure to procure them overwhelmed the kin and kin-like boundaries that restricted the search for living donations to those with social or emotional connections to the recipient. So some people began to advertise in the media for donors. Transplant teams at medical centers were quite aware that sometimes a prospective donor-recipient pair were not cousins or childhood friends but represented a contractual arrangement between two people in need—one of money, the other of a kidney. A "don't ask, don't tell" practice took hold. One person who works in the transplant field put it this way: "Patients sometimes try to talk to me about that, and I say the federal government frowns on that. So if you have a private contract between yourself and someone else, then that's your business and you need to keep it private."

In collaboration with the American Society of Transplant Surgeons and other groups, UNOS held a conference of health professionals in 2006 to try to adjust to the shifting ethical field. Language emerged to cope with the realities on the ground as well as to keep *altruism* as the primary motivator for donation, and the "nontraditional" or "altruistic" living donor became part of the transplantation enterprise. At the same time, news of the illegal and often criminal global market in organ sales was appearing on the front pages of newspapers and gaining exposure in medical and academic journals, making more U.S. patients aware that they could "just go and buy a kidney" outside the United States.[29]

In 2003 a wealthy philanthropist, Zell Kravinsky, took philanthropy to a new extreme, and in doing so raised alarming questions about the limits to organ sharing. He persuaded the Albert Einstein Medical Center in New York to allow him to make a "non-directed" kidney donation to a poor stranger in need. When he first made his offer, the transplant center staff demanded extensive psychiatric testing and put him off for weeks while they deliberated his strange request. Motivated to give away as much as he could of what he owned, and specifically targeting a hospital in a poor neighborhood that served minority patients, Kravinsky was among the first wave of a still small group of proactive altruists, now termed "Good Samaritans," who approached hospitals.[30] His act tested notions of what constitutes "enough" altruism and raised questions about who can dictate limits to it. It also provides evidence of how a successful medical technique, transplantation, has expanded citizens' moral claims on one another. And it shows too that neediness dwells in donors as well as recipients.

WEBSITE SOLICITATION OF STRANGER DONORS

Then in 2004 the world of transplantation became even more complicated with the creation of MatchingDonors.com, the first U.S.-based website that enabled strangers to solicit, offer, and accept organs from one another. This was not like the Kravinsky example—a gift to someone, anyone, in need without knowing who the recipient would be. Rather the website joined gifting with the market. It provided a new kind of public marketplace for gifting by bringing those in need in contact with potential donors, and it allowed both commerce in and the commoditization of the body to flourish in the world of transplantation medicine. Suddenly not only could one choose to solicit a donor, but donors could also choose a specific recipient. Not only could one bestow the gift, but a pair could also exchange payment. Although direct cash payment for organs remains illegal in the United States, it did not take long before solicitation and contract making became normalized by the medical establishment as part of the scarcity-equity equation. A mere seven months after the website was launched, a Denver hospital performed a transplant involving a recipient (who had been searching for a kidney for five years) and a donor (who had failed to pay child support payments) who had made an agreement (reimbursement for donor expenses only, so they said). By agreeing to perform that transplant, the hospital opened the doors to stranger solicitation and contract making in the name of saving lives.[31] One transplant professional noted to me that private contracts are an asset to the UNOS list "because the people with private contracts are not staying on the deceased donor list. It may actually take some burden off the list. And poor people without family or resources would stay on the list, which would be shorter as a result."

By now many kidney and liver transplants are enabled by direct solicitation. Payment in those exchanges, when it occurs, remains below the radar. While most living donors are still related to recipients by blood, marriage, or a personal bond, the number of living donor transplants between strangers has increased. There were 12,284 potential donors and approximately 597 potential recipients registered on MatchingDonors .com on January 30, 2014. This was up from seven thousand potential donors registered in 2009. By 2011 MatchingDonors.com has facilitated 141 paired surgeries.[32] By May 2012 they had facilitated over two hundred matches for prospective surgery.[33] The UNOS system, though it still dominates allocation and distribution, is no longer the only game in town.[34]

Altruism is the moral value that is deemed essential and is touted as primary to the transplant enterprise; when "the gift" entered the marketplace and assumed the additional dimensions of solicitation, choosing among potential recipients, and negotiating payment, altruism became more difficult to interpret.

The broadening—from blood relative to stranger—of the medicoethical eligibility criteria for donation and the active solicitation of organs mark a dramatic change in the credit-debt dimension of the tyranny that accompanies the gift. As donation between strangers becomes normalized, new questions emerge as part of the cultural fabric: What do I owe to others from my own body, and to which others? What can I accept and demand from them? And from whom, specifically? What good can I do in the world? Such questions shape interpersonal relations and give rise to new forms of tyranny and to new parameters by which to measure fairness and examine the contours of social justice.

Taken together financial need, the normalcy of transplantation, and the venues that enable anyone to be a donor have strengthened the idea that we all—including older donors—have an "extra," "spare" kidney. That idea guides some people to conclude that donation to a stranger is obligatory for them, a necessary component of a fulfilled existence in which one is not "guilty" of neglecting those in need. Stories now abound of donors and prospective donors who want to do something significant with their lives, who want to perform an extraordinary act of generosity to save a life, and who are brought to the act through an evolving personal philosophy or a compelling desire to pay society back for previous misdeeds or a search for self-redemption.[35] There are also accounts of donors whose friends think they are mentally ill. Some donors have been accused of profound egotism or of "playing God" because rather than giving anonymously they picked their recipients from a website and chose who would live. Some donors report being shocked by the animosity they encounter; some say they experienced unexpected confusion or a feeling of devastation because of the kind of relationship (or nonrelationship) that develops afterward with the recipient.[36]

HOSPITAL SOLICITATION OF STRANGER DONORS

Hospitals have now joined in the task of active solicitation of individuals willing to donate a kidney to strangers—a huge cultural shift from the hospital staff's reaction to Kravinsky's offer in 2003. For example, the University of Minnesota Medical Center, which performs the largest number of living-donation transplants in the United States, encourages volunteers to come forward to donate through their website: "One of the programs we are proud of at our institution is our non-directed donor program in which donors can offer to give a kidney to anyone on the waiting list. We began this program over 10 years ago, and since then over 55 "heroes" have donated a kidney to someone they had never met and had no promise of meeting, and for no other reason than the joy of doing something that was of benefit to another person. Similar programs now exist throughout the world."[37]

In some regards such programs are using the normalcy that has come to accompany Internet solicitation (but without payment and without donor choice of recipient) to enhance their own transplant enterprises, and their active solicitation has come to be regarded by their peers as an ordinary part of that enterprise. The normalcy of website solicitation illustrates another dimension of how the fulfillment of need (both for oneself and another) and the expression of moral claims have come to be practiced.[38]

A few years after the emergence of MatchingDonors.com and solicitation on hospital websites, a group of surgeons and other health care professionals took the potential for the expansion of citizens' moral claims on one another in an entirely different direction. In a journal article they proposed inviting patients undergoing elective gall bladder surgery to donate a kidney at the same time, thus making a kidney available for transplantation.[39] This idea has been discussed in the medical literature but is too controversial at present to move beyond that arena for debate. Nevertheless it opens the possibility for a new source of altruism by identifying volunteer living donors among those who need elective surgery. The organ shortage motivated this proposal, and the authors note that if just 3 to 5 percent of gall bladder patients agreed to serve as living donors, the national supply would increase dramatically. They suggest that while this proposal is radical and ambitious, the history of medicine, and especially the history of transplantation, has been as well. Much of the medical community was against living organ transplantation during the 1950s, when the procedure was new and most patients died, and most continued to be against it in the following decade.[40] The proposal's authors note that from the beginning physicians have worried about subjecting healthy donors to risk, about flouting the most basic principle in medicine: to do no harm.

The authors also present a long list of medical and ethical challenges to the idea, with the goal of opening discussion. They note that combining two procedures ordinarily never performed together would entail innovative, experimental surgery, adding additional risks for the patient donor. They acknowledge that the invitation to donate an organ could easily be considered coercive because patients do not want to go against physicians' suggestions; thus informed consent would be difficult to achieve. They mention that general surgeons would be reluctant to let their patients undergo combined, experimental surgery with increased and unknown risks. They also provide suggestions for ways to circumvent all those problems. Critics of the proposal have articulated additional concerns: those who need elective surgery generally have other problems that can increase their surgical risks; most gall bladder patients are women, which raises questions about unequal burdens being placed on female patients; trust in medicine could plummet if patients fear that their doctors will simply take organs from them while they are anesthetized.[41]

The authors acknowledge that their suggestion "could founder because of a lack of patients willing to take an increased risk in order to donate to strangers."[42] They also note, however, that altruistic donation, in which individuals do take on risk, has become normative and point out that a number of hospitals now solicit "Good Samaritan" donors on their websites. They suggest that if "surgical altruism" proves feasible (for all the reasons they enumerate) and if enough volunteers come forward, this innovative source of organs not only could increase supply but would also have additional positive public effects: it could reduce the need for direct organ sales or for expanded criteria living donors (that is, older, sicker donors), thus reducing the risk to medically and socioeconomically vulnerable donors who seek compensation for their donation. If a sufficient number of volunteers came forward, the collective risk associated with kidney donation could decrease "because fewer healthy persons would undergo surgery solely for the purposes of kidney donation."[43] Thus "surgical altruism" could theoretically promote lower collective risk, although it would pose a greater risk to individual donor patients.

While it is a given that healthy persons are considered the best potential organ donors, our cultural knowledge about the ordinariness of kidney transplantation together with widespread living donation have made *everyone* a potential donor and recipient today. What this proposal has done is open the way for surgical patients to be seen as repositories of "spare" organs as well. The potential sources of organs appear to be boundless.

> One does not have to be governed or preoccupied by such ideas
> [as death-defying technologies] in order to be aware of their significance;
> it is sufficient that they have been conceived, expressed and thus made
> available as vehicles for further ideas. The issue, then, is not whether
> these technologies are good or bad, but with how we should think them
> and how they will think us. The issue is the forms of thought they present
> through which we shall look on other aspects of human affairs.
> —Marilyn Strathern, "Reproducing the Future"

The clinical success of living donation performs radical cultural work; it both holds and unleashes potential to see one's body as the vehicle for another's health and life and to understand that mortality can and should be pushed back by this act. Surgical altruism is merely the most recent emergent idea. It is thinkable because each preceding move did the cultural work necessary to pave the way for considering novel ways to expand the supply of organs.

The social changes that the transplantation enterprise has accomplished occurred in several moves. First, the institutions for organ procurement, disbursement, and regulation produced the opportunities for altruism to be expressed,[44] and they made altruism the driving force that enabled both cadaveric and living transplantation to take hold as an ordinary practice and response to the donor shortage. The increasing shortage and better immunosuppressive drugs then paved the way for the next move, in which living donation came to be seen as "the normal, natural thing to do, no question about it," as many donors claim. An increase in the number of older people seeking organs and the direction of giving from younger to older followed seamlessly. No one noticed. Donations by unrelated but known donors became normalized at about the same time, pushing the cultural work of organ transfer to yet another new, "natural" form of understanding and acceptance about whose body and which kinds of social relatedness "counted" and could be used. Each new category of person that came to be considered appropriate as a donor opened up societal thinking about *what categories of persons* are appropriate for this task, while still accommodating the emotion and value of altruism.

But each move also complicated our understanding of altruism and its relationship to self-interest. Each move made medicine more deeply complicit in shaping the future of human relations and human affairs in society. If neighbors, church and business associates, and others not connected by blood or family were donating "naturally," if families were contacting everyone they knew, related or not, by email and other social media to ask for potential donors, it was only a small step to advertise need and actively solicit an organ from a stranger. The transplant enterprise both went along with and stimulated all this because of the growing shortage, increasing need, and ever-present clinical evidence of good outcomes. Anonymous stranger donation ("I just wanted to do something for someone") and hospital solicitation of "Good Samaritan" donors quite easily followed.

The now accepted, ordinary knowledge that everyone has a "spare" kidney has made the active search for additional sources of healthy organs thinkable, and the thousands of individuals undertaking gall bladder surgery are simply the newest site where this intervention into ideas has settled. While elective surgical patients are not (yet) actively solicited, the idea travels—between doctors, among medical institutions and journals, and ultimately to discussions with patients—and no doubt will eventually become part of a moral calculus for some surgical patients.

These are the steps, in the realm of kidney transplantation at least, by which we have learned to take more longevity for granted. These are also the steps by which our basic notions of health, the right to health, and the public good have been and are being subtly, or not so subtly, changed. Overall there has been an insidious elision from one morally acceptable position to the next.

As the anthropologist Marilyn Strathern notes, it is sufficient that an idea be conceived and expressed to make it available as a vehicle for further ideas. There is no question that intervention in this sociomedical arena has produced fantasies and doomsday scenarios about extreme uses of the body. The politics of potential amid scarcity, desire, and the logic of allowable policy all inspire doctors, patients, and medical institutions to organize the "good" of transplantation practices in new ways, thus generating additional expressions of individual rights, public benefits, and the work of the marketplace.

We may ask whether these steps take us incrementally closer to the dystopia that Kazuo Ishiguro describes in his novel *Never Let Me Go*, in which society easily thinks about, indeed creates a cloned population from which to harvest useful body parts. Or perhaps what is happening now is closer to what the science fiction author Bruce Sterling depicts in *Holy Fire*, in which the elderly rule the world, and even at age ninety-five and beyond full-body rejuvenation is a choice, a right, and entirely doable.

In their separate ways the UNOS concepts of 2011 and 2012 (evidence-based, statistically oriented attempts to address equity issues) and the surgical altruism idea (to access healthy organs from a small percentage of elective surgery patients) are attempts to provide more transplants to more people and thus to impact the health of the public. Each scheme describes a way to organize the "good" of more transplants, of more lives saved. Whether either one succeeds will be a matter of politics and how quickly and to what degree the social changes they entail come to be accepted, as well as whether citizens and institutions will permit the cultural work of transplantation medicine to move in those directions.

Beyond Kidneys: Ordinary Medicine's Ongoing Invisible Metamorphosis

The cultural moves that rationalize the "good" and "just" aspects of living donation echo other moves in medicine that I have described. Each of those moves shows how what becomes thinkable builds on what is considered appropriate and normal, on what activities are already embedded in and expressed through the chain of health care drivers. For instance, consider the moves from pacemaker to implantable cardiac defibrillator, to cardiac resynchronizing therapy device, to the recent left ventricular assist device. Each of those devices further prolonged the lives of patients with ever more severe heart failure, and the development of those successively more complex, expensive, and invasive devices was enabled by the growing role of the medical device industry, the production of evidence, and Medicare reimbursement criteria. Another example is the use of maintenance dialysis for ever older and sicker patients because it is available and paid for by Medicare but also because the ethos of medicine surrounding dialysis, established a half century ago to treat younger persons, is only now beginning to change in response to the aging population. For a different kind of example showing how the thinkable emerges from the ethical field and then is strengthened by ordinary medicine's logic, consider the ways that logic organizes and rationalizes families' thinking as they face the quandaries posed by their felt complicity in extending or shortening a life, their contribution to suicide or murder, to death or longer life, and their ruminations over what acts show enough duty and love.

The complex drivers that have created today's ordinary medicine and will propel it into the future do their work beneath almost everyone's radar. I hope to have made clear that the judgments and commitments inherent in medicine's organizational linkages—among evidence-based medicine, Medicare payment criteria, standards, and necessity—are built on values, on political and economic decisions regarding who should benefit, and on the pressures of the public marketplace and the potential for donation from surgical patients. If this is understood, perhaps more of us will be able to see how those judgments underlie actual, everyday health care delivery. Then perhaps more of us will be able to see how those judgments are shaping the quality of our aging experience and our relationships with intimates and strangers and at the same time are contributing to the debates about medicine's relationship to fairness, social justice, and the public good. The content of those judgments and how they are driving health care delivery need to become the preeminent topics of our national conversation about health care reform.

CONCLUSION

Toward a New Social Contract?

———

Hope and reality have fused. Medical miracles are expected by
those who will be patients, predicted by those seeking research
funds, and profitably marketed by those who manufacture
them. . . . What the biologist Rene Dubos some decades [ago]
spoke of as "the mirage of health"—a perfection that never
comes—is no longer taken to be a mirage, but solidly out
there on the horizon.
—Daniel Callahan, *What Price Better Health?*

Our practices in medicine define the kind of society we have. Ordinary
medicine is emblematic of other trends in American society, and how
we shape the values and directions of the health care delivery enterprise will determine—and reveal—the kind of society we create in the
coming years. Because the trends that have brought us to this point are
ongoing—especially the dominance of private industry in health care
services, the priority given technology use regardless of cost, and the lack
of equity in the distribution of medical care—they continue to derail the
practice of medicine, indeed the entire health care delivery enterprise
as a social good. So our current state of affairs raises a critical question:
What values do we want to govern that enterprise?[1]

Observers of medical practice and health care delivery—from health
economists, policy analysts, and ethicists to journalists, doctors, patients,
and families—note that the necessity of cost control sits in tension with
the value we place on open-ended choice, individual rights, and always
escalating need.[2] To date the need for cost control and the tension between cost control and rationing have dominated the political debates;
some, however, have begun to argue that those debates should not be
centered on cost control at all. They point out that the cost issue deflects

us from considering the problem of health care services run amok, from focusing on dignity, suffering, and the role of medicine in society now.[3] Ultimately the focus on costs deflects us from linking health policy to social equity. While not regularly emphasized in political discourse, that linkage is essential if one of the values we wish to foster and preserve is that of medicine as a social good.[4] To that end, addressing the challenges of building fairness, equity, and sustainability into the entire enterprise remains an essential goal.

I have focused throughout this book on describing how the norms, the criteria for our business-as-usual health care delivery system become standard, entrenched, and thus unremarkable and largely invisible. My goal has been to make the fundamental features of ordinary medicine—the chain of health care drivers and the ethical field in which they operate—visible because ordinary medicine has an ever tightening grip on the practice of medicine and the lives of patients. Both the chain and its attendant judgments have pushed U.S. health care toward the condition I have been calling "postprogress," have caused a sea change in medical practice, patient care, and family concerns, and have done so below the radar. Together the chain and the ethical field wield enormous power over our lives: they shape what we want and how we act in the realm of health, illness, and life and have altered the very experience of growing old in the United States. I argue that ordinary medicine has altered and continues to shape vital components of what it is to be human—our relationship between body and self, our understanding of time and our future, and our most intimate family commitments. What values should govern an enterprise that can so profoundly influence how we relate to those we love?

Few would deny that ordinary medicine needs to be fixed. But it is difficult to repair what cannot be seen either clearly or in its entirety. By describing ordinary medicine and the diffuse ethical field that supports it, I am offering an opening for the goals of medicine to be further clarified and for drawing attention to the values we want to govern the enterprise.

Ordinary Medicine and Its Critics

Criticism of American health care is at an all-time high and is coming from every imaginable source: doctors, patients, families, economists, ethicists, policy analysts, and politicians. In the United States we rescue the desperately ill from death's door and stave off the end of life more often than in any other nation, and our diagnostic and treatment capabilities are magnificent, yet most observers agree that our system spends too much, relies on too much technology, and wastes an enormous amount of money on unneeded and inappropriate services. In addition many doctors, patients, and families are deeply unsettled by the pathways of care delivery they find themselves on. In general, although individual health care professionals work hard and often struggle to practice the kind of medicine they believe supports the public good, the *system itself* has lost any sense it may once have had of what medical goals are appropriate and what priorities are realistic for the delivery of services.

Consider the oncologist Siddhartha Mukherjee's illustration in *The Emperor of All Maladies* of how ordinary medicine's "more" perspective is seen as entirely reasonable:

> *"More is more,"* a patient's daughter told me curtly. (I had suggested to her delicately that for some patients with cancer, "Less might be more.") The patient was an elderly Italian woman with liver cancer that had metastasized widely throughout her abdomen. She had come to the Massachusetts General Hospital seeking chemotherapy, surgery, or radiation—if possible, all three. . . .
>
> The daughter was a physician . . . [who] wanted the best possible care for her mother—the best doctors, the best room with the best view of Beacon Hill, and the best, strongest, and toughest medicine that privilege and money could buy.
>
> The elderly woman, meanwhile, would hardly tolerate even the mildest drug. Her liver had not failed yet but was on the verge of doing so, and subtle signs suggested her kidneys were barely functioning. I suggested that we try a palliative drug, perhaps a single chemotherapeutic agent that might just ameliorate her symptoms rather than pushing for a tougher regimen to try to cure an incurable disease.
>
> The daughter looked at me as if I were mad. "I came here to get treatment, not consolations about hospice," she finally said, glowering with fury.[5]

The forces that make such demands appear reasonable are precisely those that make our health care system the entrenched, dysfunctional, "more is more" enterprise that it is today.

Like the furious daughter, the American public has never before expected—perhaps demanded—so much from the medical treatments that are at its disposal. Many of those treatments have changed how we understand terminal illness and chronic disease. Many, in recent years, have changed how we experience old age and the dying process. From the simple feeding tube to the high-tech heart pump, from cardiac bypass surgery to aggressive chemotherapy, we seek out, acquiesce to, and use today's therapies for a number of interlocking reasons: because they have become routine and ordinary; because often they quell the desperation that those who want to live often feel when faced with critical illness; and, because they often do prolong life, they have come to be considered medically necessary.

That sense of necessity has led not only to too much treatment but also to the quandary about crossing the line and taking a path that leads out of or away from too much treatment. It seems that for every person who gains wanted time from cardiac, cancer, and other aggressive interventions, there is someone who is wary about wanting "more." It is not apparent if one of those groups is larger and, if so, which one. The sociologist and author Lillian Rubin, age eighty-eight, echoed the thoughts of many in that second group in her contribution to the widespread conversation about whether or when to cross the line: "At 88-going-on-89 and not in great health, what's courageous about spending our children's inheritance just so we can live one more month, one more year? . . . Why at this advanced stage of old age do I have to add to my anxieties? . . . How can it be an affirmation of life when someone is in constant pain, when the mind is no longer fully functional, when the body can't do for itself the basic things necessary to sustain life?"[6]

Further complicating the quandary is the fact that no one has a crystal ball, and transplants, cardiac devices, cancer therapies, and many other interventions *do, often,* prolong lives. Thus looming questions about the values that govern the health care enterprise are raised by postprogress ordinary medicine: How is "successful treatment" to be defined, especially in an aging society? What is to be measured and against what standard?[7] And from whose perspective?

Ordinary medicine does not have a grounding philosophy; it was not created out of whole cloth in a premeditated way. It has evolved piecemeal over the past four decades or so in response to the perfect storm swirling through American cultural life: new technologies for diagnosis and treatment, the blossoming of the biotech industry and the clinical research engine, the expanding power and reach of industry, and, fueled by medicine's successes, the public's escalating expectations of its capabilities. It has evolved as well in response to our culturally ingrained idea that more is better, and thus its growth cannot be fully controlled by government, taxpayers, practicing doctors, or others. Is it any wonder that what the medical sociologist Arthur Frank characterizes as an "unthinkably broad array of knowledge and skills, professions, coalitions, and interest groups, fears and promises, fantasies and soon-to-be-realities, concrete and virtual institutions, folklores and sciences"[7] and the medical historian Charles Rosenberg calls an "infrastructure of ideas, practices, thresholds, and protocols" is so seemingly impossible to manage in terms of priorities, scope, and limits?[8]

None of the situations we find ourselves in was inevitable or the only way our health care system could have developed or the only logic possible. Other nations have developed different systems of payment and different priorities about the delivery of treatments, and many of them have higher life expectancies than does the United States.

Cost Controls and Appropriate Services: Reform Efforts to Date

Since the 1970s attempts have been made to craft health care policy that would contain costs and deliver more appropriate services, such as, for example, through HMOs, managed care, preferred provider organizations, diagnostic related groups, and, more recently, accountable care organizations, medical homes, comparative effectiveness research, and health information technology systems. (These are only examples; the list is far longer.) Recent reviews of these efforts demonstrate many of their positive and ongoing accomplishments in cost cutting, systems management, and improved quality of care. Thus in many respects reform is already under way. (President Obama's Affordable Care Act contributes to some of those efforts, especially in the area of access to health care services for those previously uninsured and with preexisting conditions.)[9]

The winds of change can also be seen in the attention paid to eliminating waste throughout the care delivery enterprise; the moves to reward doctors, hospitals, and provider groups for quality of care rather than quantity of procedures delivered; the greater priority given to evidence-based treatment recommendations; and the medical education efforts that link principles of cost awareness to evidence-based treatments.[10]

Yet there has not been, and cannot be, a single kind of solution that fully, or even significantly, alters the values that undergird the health care drivers I have described. However much we Americans continue to look for the "big fix" and the "holy grail," as two eminent health policy experts note in their reviews, "American health care is radically American: in-dividualistic, scientifically ambitious, market intoxicated, suspicious of government, and profit-driven," as Daniel Callahan, a longtime observer of our health care conundrums, has characterized it.[11]

Many have noted (often with alarm) the skyrocketing costs of drugs, devices, hospitalization, and hospital equipment and have proposed so-lutions based on evaluating their worth and reining in those ever rising costs.[12] However, the technological imperative, hospitals' competition for new technologies, the mechanisms of fee-for-service payment, and variations in physicians' patterns of practice all exert a powerful hold that mitigates any widespread and significant change. When those entrenched factors are added to the pattern of aggressive treatments near the end of life, the production of more medical specialists at the expense of primary care physicians and escalating patient demand and desire,[13] it is no wonder that no specifically targeted policy solution is equipped to bring about any significant change in the system.

For many of those seeking a corrective, "Less is more" is the new ral-lying cry. In other words, we should refrain from automatically employ-ing every available test and treatment; we should somehow rein in the patient's furious daughter. Yet resistance to such a corrective has been loud and relentless, and although increasing numbers of physician and insurance groups and medical centers have instituted some exemplary reforms in cost control and the delivery of care, their methods have not been broadly generalizable (at least not yet) to other institutions.[14]

The potency of the health care drivers and the values that shape and strengthen them not only stymie cost-control reform; they also explain why the field of bioethics has been unable to craft a solution to ordinary medicine's more intangible quandaries, for example, determining what counts as necessary treatment, wanted treatment, and successful treat-ment. Traditionally based on the principles of autonomy and individual-ism, bioethics has concentrated much of its work on the essential dyad—the doctor and the patient—in its efforts to examine and propose ways that medical decision making between those parties can be made more rational and thus more effective.[15] Yet in the 1970s critics began noting that what happens within the doctor-patient dyad has its source in the broader social and structural determinants of health and decision mak-ing: poverty, educational opportunity, access to medical services, racism, and more.[16] The critics demonstrated that solutions to decision-making quagmires can occur upstream from the dyad only by addressing the sociocultural and structural environment in which doctors and patients exist.

Valiant efforts have been made to try to learn what patients want in terms of aggressive interventions and comfort measures. Attempts to track, understand, and foster better communication between doctors and patients began in 1995 with the SUPPORT study, designed to examine the extent and content of doctor-patient dialogue about treatment preferences in the hospital setting.[17] The institutionalization of patient self-determination, advance directives, and living wills (beginning with the 1990 federal Patient Self-Determination Act) ensured patients' right to make their own treatment decisions. The bioethics-based perspective of the SUPPORT study (and countless others) assumed, or hoped, that improved doctor-patient communication could effect system change and that patients and their families always, or even sometimes, knew what they wanted in terms of intensive, life-sustaining therapies.[18] But in retrospect those two assumptions proved to be unfounded.[19]

Five years after the SUPPORT study was completed, the researchers realized that the course of hospitalized patients' care is guided not by individual "preferences" or shared decision making but by institutional patterns and routines; thus doctor-patient dialogue is not the key to more appropriate (and more welcome) forms of treatment. And when faced with the risk of death, many patients (and their families) would not or could not articulate preferences about what they wanted in the way of specific treatments; that is, patients mostly do not know what they want in terms of *whether and when to cross the line or say stop*.

Broadening the Focus

My own findings about what happens to patients as they seek or find themselves receiving life-prolonging procedures reveal similar patterns. As I hope has been clear in the patient stories I've presented, though many patients demand aggressive treatments, they are in fact asking for both care and hope through those demands. The treatments that doctors mention, offer, or feel they must perform or that patients and families read about and ask for are for them symbols of that hope. Because medical paternalism is no longer valued and because patient responsibility and shared decision making are encouraged,[20] patients and, perhaps more strikingly, their families feel a profound burden in saying no to life-extending treatments. And because there are more procedures and treatments available to choose from than ever before, patients and families are being asked to shoulder more decisions, more responsibility, despite the fact that they have the least knowledge of disease patterns, treatment outcomes, and the implications of crossing the line toward more treatment.

In a profound way ordinary medicine has off-loaded the traditional sphere and burden of bioethics onto patients and families, and the choices doctors now offer them seem to be about choosing *life* or *death*. They are expected to weigh the implications of one (potential) sort of death over another—sudden and without warning or drawn out and accompanied by distressing symptoms—and then decide. So one major effect of ordinary medicine plays out in our collective anxieties about crossing the line. This burden is not one that patients and families used to have to carry. Do we want it to remain a dominant feature of the health care enterprise?

Where amid the policy proposals and decision-making dilemmas do we find doctors? On the one hand, they direct the flow of therapies through the health care enterprise and are the gatekeepers (however unevenly) to the use of treatments. They have a great deal of authority in influencing the decisions of individual patients, and patients want their guidance. We want to continue to trust them, and we want them to show that they care, regardless of our prognosis. Yet, on the other hand, physicians act well downstream from the transformations that frame treatment decision making in the first place, and they must function within the pressures, values, and politics that undergird the health care enterprise. As we have seen, they may sometimes go against their better judgment in acceding to patient demands; they do but also do not follow evidence-based guidelines; they serve on national committees to ensure that treatments (even some that show equivocal benefit) are reimbursed by insurance. Their recommendations are channeled by the pressures of ordinary medicine and by the chain of transformations I have described. And so they act as delivery vehicles within the larger apparatus that is ordinary medicine.

Patients' anxieties and misgivings about crossing the line and doctors' downstream actions (perhaps especially those in which they contradict their own better judgment) are but two aspects of a much larger question, one that is missing from most societal debate: How, ultimately, do we want to live in relation to medicine's tools?

The Stakes of the Matter: Broadening the Basis of Reform

The work of ordinary medicine, the burden of responsibility that patients and families shoulder about crossing the line (to potentially more life or death), and the existential and societal question about how to live in relation to medicine's tools all urgently demand that we give deep consideration to our health care enterprise's reigning logic, its organizational drivers, and the values that support it. Then, having done so, we must consider what we want the role of medicine to be in relation to longevity making in an aging society. What kinds of claims on medicine and the health care delivery system can we continue to make? What kinds of claims on our own old age do we *want* to make?

The transformations that constitute ordinary medicine and the quandaries that result are reflected in our ongoing and seemingly recalcitrant political disputes over the right to life, the right to die, and the right to treatment, each of which has occupied large swaths of American civic life. Those still active disputes illustrate the shifting, conflicted battleground on which ideas about what constitutes successful therapy, evidence of therapeutic benefit, progress in medicine, human rights, and medicine's role in society form and change over time. Like many other cultural "truths" they do not settle or sit still, which leads me to think that change in the emphases of ordinary medicine is possible.

In order to craft a sustainable solution to the problem of rising costs, at least two points bear scrutiny. The first is the logic of the entire chain, a logic that (I must stress this again) *appears* to be based on scientific rationality but operates in the realm of ethical judgments. The second is that in the world of ordinary medicine *need* arises from the successes of clinical interventions, from escalating societal expectations about medical potential and health in later life, and from the transformations inherent in the medical-industrial system.

A successful approach to broad reform—not only cost control—would also have to consider the existence and powerful role of the ethical field in determining how medicine operates (including its waste and overuse), how need is governed, and how these factors shape our national impasse. For the judgments inherent in medicine's organizational linkages—among evidence-based medicine, Medicare payment criteria, standards, and necessity—are built on values, on political and economic decisions regarding who should benefit, on the pressures of the public marketplace, and on societal expectations about medicine and the aging experience. If and when these connections are understood, perhaps more of us (doctors, patients, and policymakers alike) will be able to see what is now largely hidden: how those inherent judgments underlie actual, everyday health care delivery. The ethical field needs to be acknowledged and become part of our societal conversation about health care reform.

If ordinary medicine continues on its current path, if we continue to allow the enterprise to be dominated by market priorities, if the cultural rhetoric continues to dwell on the primacy of individual rights (but only for those who have gained access to the system), then the stakes for our society are high indeed. At stake in ordinary medicine—that is, practice as usual—and at stake, ultimately, with regard to citizens' trust in the entire enterprise is the way our democratic values are (or are not) put into practice. Do we continue to allow the enterprise to be organized and driven by profit and market share? Is there a way to turn the cultural rhetoric away from the primacy of individual rights and toward the public good?

The task at hand is to further reinvent ordinary medicine in and for our aging society, a society in which we have such high expectations about the promise and potential of medicine and show such low regard for putting the brakes on costs. Ideas travel and change, and means and ends evolve. If we can refine our understanding of what drives ordinary medicine and take stock of the cultural pressures and organizational transformations that, for example, make chronic kidney dialysis, the LVAD, organ transplantation, and aggressive cancer treatments acceptable as normal or standard therapies even in very late life, or make surgical altruism a plausible idea, then perhaps we can discern the ways ordinary medicine no longer best serves the practice of medicine or the health of our society.

Any insights we gain may make it easier for us to see how those judgments and drivers are shaping the quality of our aging experience and our relationships with loved ones and strangers and at the same time are contributing to the debates about medicine's relationship to fairness, social justice, and the public good. The ethical field in which ordinary medicine operates needs first to become visible and then to take its place as the preeminent topic of our national conversation about health care reform.

NOTES ON THE RESEARCH

I began to think about the quandary of drawing the line while I was conducting my study of American hospitals and how death happens there
(published as . . . *And a Time to Die*). After that study was completed I
thought about ways I could understand and document both the sources
and effects of that quandary. I started paying close attention to those
sources that are located well beyond hospital walls, in the social and political arena of debates about health care access, Medicare solvency, and
who controls the end of life, in the ascendance of the value of evidence-
based medicine and the surge in clinical trials, and in the contradictory
fact that we desire advanced medical interventions without limit or end
yet protest the overuse or inappropriate use of those tools and the suffering they sometimes cause.

I wanted to construct the project so that the perfect storm of our aging
society, the escalating pace of clinical innovation, the technological imperative, and the changing relationship of medicine to old age would be
data I could scrutinize in the actual deliberations of doctors, patients,
and families and the conversations among them. My initial goal was
to examine how certain medical interventions, all of them on the rise
among older persons, were affecting patients and families and how those
treatments were shaping the practice of medicine. How did doctors and
their older patients decide to go forward with cardiac interventions, kidney transplants, and renal dialysis? What were doctors telling patients,
and how were patients responding? And then more broadly, what factors
in the clinical world and in American life were contributing to the fact
that increasing numbers of elderly patients were receiving high-tech,
life-sustaining treatments and at ever older ages? In short, what specific
factors were giving shape to the quandary of the line, and how were patients and families living in its midst?

The anthropological research on which this book is based was funded
in two phases, both supported by the National Institute on Aging. The

research received Institutional Review Board (Human Subjects) approval at the University of California, San Francisco, as well as at the institutions in which I gathered data.

In the first phase, from 2002 to 2006, two associates and I conducted the field research. I observed the conversations among health professionals, patients, and their families in kidney transplantation clinics at urban medical centers when patients came for initial evaluations and follow-up exams. I spoke with patients and families in waiting rooms, exam rooms, and following their appointments, sometimes briefly, sometimes for an hour or more. And I spoke with doctors, nurses, and health care professional staff on transplantation teams. In the clinics I was interested in learning what doctors and transplant team members told patients about their need and eligibility for the procedure and the different types of donation to consider. I focused on how patients and families processed the information they were hearing about need, quality of life, and where a kidney might come from. I began to learn the routine, standard pathways of care by which patients, especially older patients, receive organs. Outside the clinics I interviewed patients who had received transplants, patients who were prospective recipients, their family members, and kidney donors and prospective donors.[1]

One research associate, Ann Russ, conducted lengthy observations and interviews with patients, nurses, and doctors in two dialysis units in different cities, paying particular attention to the experience of older patients who came regularly for outpatient hemodialysis. My other research associate, Janet Shim, conducted in-depth interviews with academic, hospital-based, and community-based physicians in internal medicine and geriatrics and with cardiac specialists about the use of cardiac bypass, the ICD, and other cardiac procedures among older patients. She interviewed patients who had undergone bypass surgery, angioplasty, or a stent procedure or who had received a cardiac device, and some of their family members as well. During this first phase we observed, spoke with, and interviewed approximately 105 patients, forty-five family members, and thirty-five doctors and other health care professionals.

This first part of the project identified how physicians learn to evaluate patients for life-extending procedures and how those evaluations, and thus treatments, have changed in recent decades. It began to describe how medical choice is organized by structural features of the health care delivery system and how so many patients come to desire, but also acquiesce to, medical interventions when they are over seventy, eighty, and ninety years of age. As the research progressed, I sought to document the ways societal notions of old age and the normal life span were being expressed in the clinic by patients and families as they spoke with doctors and medical teams. And I wanted to learn how the medical care older patients were receiving was informing patient and family knowledge about health in later life and the possibilities and promises of medical intervention at ever older ages.

In the second phase, from 2007 to 2011, I examined the impacts on doctors, patients, families, and American society of additional procedures whose use among the elderly was an emerging and rapidly growing phenomenon. I continued to observe and interview doctors and patients in kidney transplantation clinics, this time concentrating specifically on the direction of living donation from younger to older persons. I also observed patients, families, and health care professionals in liver transplantation clinics because the age among liver transplant recipients has also been rising. I interviewed liver donors and recipients and their family members. I also focused extensively on the cardiac implantable devices, the ICD, CRT, and LVAD, because their use had expanded tremendously among the elderly in the early years of the new millennium. I interviewed doctors and medical teams who evaluate patients for these devices and who implant them, other health care professionals who care for patients with these devices, and forty-six patients who either have devices, are considering whether to receive a first device or a subsequent, more complex one, or have decided not to receive one. I interviewed a few people who decided to have an ICD deactivated. And I interviewed some of their family members. During this second phase I conducted research in several locations outside California.

My associate for this phase of the project, Lakshmi Fjord, observed doctors, nurses, and patients in several oncology clinics, paying close attention to the ways doctors talked about diagnosis, prognosis, and treatment options and what they recommended and how older patients and their families made decisions surrounding chemotherapy, surgery, and radiation in the short and long term. In this second phase we observed, spoke with, and interviewed more than two hundred patients, 150 family members, and sixty physicians and other health care professionals.

Throughout the project I attended lectures about trends in clinical medicine, biomedical research, aging, ethics, and health policy at my own university. During the second phase especially, and throughout the writing of this book, I read widely in the medical literature and news media on topics related to the research that have generated a great deal of societal angst and debate and have sparked so much discussion in medicine, bioethics, and health policy, including the skyrocketing costs of cancer drugs (some without much life-prolonging benefit), the safety of cardiac devices, the future of Medicare, the conundrum of knowing when to stop pursuing aggressive treatments, the expanding and tenacious use of expensive diagnostic (and sometimes disease-causing) technologies, and the powerful role of the pharmaceutical and device industries in doctors' practices and patients' lives.

As the book took shape I focused my analysis on how the ever mutable understandings of what constitutes standard-of-care treatments are formed through the mix of clinical innovation, Medicare reimbursement policies, and physician, patient, and family practices, including their ambivalence about moving forward with invasive therapies. I sought to emphasize the hidden ways standards in health care delivery become standard. To accomplish this I needed to portray what happens on the ground, in the work of medicine and the lives of patients. I also needed to step back and out, to describe how the structures of research, Medicare finance, and health care delivery influence so much.

Confidentiality

I have made every effort to maintain the anonymity of the medical centers, health care professionals, patients, and families involved in this project. To that end I do not specify the names or locations of the medical centers or physicians' practices in which this research was conducted. Most of the research was conducted in northern California in a variety of clinical settings and in patients' homes. Some of the project was carried out during several visits to midwestern and East Coast locations. All names are pseudonyms. I have omitted or slightly changed potentially identifying features of individuals. All quotations are based on taped and transcribed conversations or on verbatim note taking.

The fieldwork for this project could have been carried out in many places. The developments, debates, and quandaries I describe are located throughout the United States, and the conversations and events I portray at the specific sites I visited are similar to those that occur throughout the country every day. Many health care professionals, patients, and families will recognize them as similar to their own experiences of the quandary of the line.

Note

1 Additional information on the numbers of patients and doctors who participated in this project and other research details can be found in the following
notes: chapter 2, nn7,47; chapter 6, n3.

NOTES

Introduction: Diagnosing Twenty-First-Century Health Care

1 I collected most of the data reported here. Lakshmi Fjord, Ann Russ, and Janet Shim, research associates for different phases of this project, collected additional data included here. I am indebted to them for their astute observations and probing interviews, which extended the scope of this project.

2 This way of thinking about ethics, although it moves away from well-known conceptions and uses of bioethics, emerges from that older kind of ethics, including the debates in the 1960s about rationing kidney dialysis to "deserving" citizens and the concern, beginning in the 1970s with Karen Quinlan, about who has the authority to withdraw life-sustaining treatment from whom and when. See chapter 1 for additional details about the ethical field.

3 Both the quandary for patients and families about enough or too much treatment and when to stop and the forces of the health care system that perpetuate and strengthen the impasse that hinders reform have been developing for a long time. I examined one feature of this quandary in *. . . And a Time to Die: How American Hospitals Shape the End of Life*, my study of hospital death and the social and structural forces that shape the ways many of us die in the United States. In that volume I explain how, unless and until someone says stop, the bureaucracy of the American hospital itself "moves things along," channels both doctors and patients toward the most intensive, aggressive treatments— even for the very frail and elderly, even when people claim they do not want those treatments, even when death (which is rarely mentioned or expected) is imminent. But what happens in the hospital when a patient is near death provides only one piece of the answer to why the default setting of medicine is *more* treatment, and it is only one example of how that setting affects so many of us.

   Ordinary Medicine provides a companion volume and a prequel, so to speak, to *. . . And a Time to Die* in that it examines those upstream connections that shape the organization of medical treatments to which patients respond. While here too I portray interchanges among doctors, patients, and families, it is in encounters that happen well before the very end of life. Nevertheless, because my focus is on life-threatening conditions and their treatments, death is always a player on the stage.

Asked if they want their death to be preceded by a prolonged stay in a hospital intensive care unit, few would say yes; that is a situation in which more life would be unwanted. What I chart here, in contrast, is an infinitely more complicated situation because medicine's successes in extending *wanted* life, well before the very end, are all around us. Yet at the same time, the quandary of the line affects increasing numbers of us.

Chapter 1: Ordinary Medicine in Our Aging Society

1 See Fox and Swazey, *The Courage to Fail*; Rothman, *Beginnings Count*.
2 A normal rhythm then can resume, through either the pacing function of the device, which corrects the rhythm, or the heart's own return to a normal beating pattern. It has been commonly referred to as an "emergency room in the chest" and functions like the defibrillator paddles used for resuscitation in emergency rooms. Thanks to Paul Mueller for discussions about this. See Jeffrey, "Machines in Our Hearts"; Kamphuis et al., "ICD: A Qualitative Study of Patient Experience the First Year after Implantation."
3 See Butler, *Knocking on Heaven's Door* for a detailed memoir about the ramifications of a pacemaker.
4 Vice President Dick Cheney had one for twenty months before he received a heart transplant at age seventy-one, in 2012.
5 Administration on Aging, "Projected Future Growth of Older Population."
6 Centers for Medicare and Medicaid Services. "Medicare Enrollment Reports."
7 These developments occurred as well in a social environment in which preventive maintenance—of our cars, our computers, the roof over our heads, *and* our health—has become such a normal way of life for a broad middle class.
8 On the topic of objectivity in medical science and practice, see, for example, Lock and Gordon, *Biomedicine Examined*; Lock and Nguyen, *An Anthropology of Biomedicine*.
9 Butler and Puri, "Deathbed Shock."
10 Jeffrey, "Machines in Our Hearts," 258; Lefkowitz and Willerson, "Prospects for Cardiovascular Research."
11 Goldenberg et al., "Causes and Consequences of Heart Failure after Prophylactic Implantation of a Defibrillator in the Multicenter Automatic Defibrillator Implantation Trial II," 2810.
12 A national survey of hospices found that approximately half of patients near the end of life will be shocked by their ICD. See Goldstein et al., "Brief Communication."
13 Goldstein et al., "Management of Implantable Cardioverter Defibrillators in End-of-Life Care"; Goldstein et al., "'That's Like an Act of Suicide'"; Goldstein et al., "'It's Like Crossing a Bridge.'"
14 Gordon, "Tenacious Assumptions in Western Medicine."
15 Butler, "Do Health and Longevity Create Wealth?"
16 Crawford, "Health as a Meaningful Social Practice."

17 Beck, "Risk Society"; Beck, "Living in the World Risk Society"; Giddens, *The Consequences of Modernity*; Giddens, *Modernity and Self-Identity*.
18 Dumit, "The Depsychiatrisation of Mental Illness"; Dumit, "Normal Insecurities, Healthy Insecurities"; Rose, "The Politics of Life Itself."
19 Gifford, "The Meaning of Lumps"; Dumit, *Drugs for Life*.
20 Crawford, "Risk Ritual and the Management of Control and Anxiety in Medical Culture."
21 Armstrong, "The Rise of Surveillance Medicine"; Dumit, *Drugs for Life*.
22 Creatinine is a chemical waste product that is produced by muscle metabolism and to a lesser extent by eating meat. If kidneys are not functioning properly, an increased level of creatinine may accumulate in the blood. A serum creatinine test measures the level of creatinine and gives an estimate of how well the kidneys are filtering waste (glomerular filtration rate). Mayo Clinic Staff, "Tests and Procedures."
23 Denise Grady, "Deadly Inheritance, Desperate Trade-Off," *New York Times*, August 7, 2007; Shim, Russ, and Kaufman, "Risk, Life Extension and the Pursuit of Medical Possibility."
24 Lowy, *Preventive Strikes*.
25 Rose, "The Politics of Life Itself"; Dumit, "Normal Insecurities, Healthy Insecurities."
26 Dumit, *Drugs for Life*; Timmermans and Buchbinder, "Patients-in-Waiting."
27 Rothman, *Strangers at the Bedside*; Rosenberg, *Our Present Complaint*, 6.
28 Rothman, *Strangers at the Bedside*.
29 Beecher, "Ethics and Clinical Research."
30 Rothman, *Strangers at the Bedside*.
31 In my previous book, . . . *And a Time to Die*, I illustrate how those feelings and qualms are often evident at the hospital bedside, even when death is very near.
32 That limited idea of ethics set the stage in 2009 for the notion, still circulating widely, of "death panels." That epithet reflects the perception that life-and-death decisions about health care would be made by bureaucrats rather than by doctors if more health care services were organized and reimbursed by a government insurance system.
33 Bill Keller, "How to Die," *New York Times*, October 8, 2012.
34 There are no data for Medicare recipients about whether, and the extent to which, cost figures in their thinking about ethical dilemmas.
35 Interferon is a cytokine, a specific protein that the human body is constantly making. Interferon therapy is currently the gold standard in treatment for certain types of hepatitis B and C. Interferon helps the body distinguish between cells infected by the virus and noninfected cells, targeting infected cells for destruction. Cutler, "Understanding Hepatitis C Interferon Therapy."
36 In electrical current treatment, also called radiofrequency ablation, high-frequency electrical currents create heat that destroys the abnormal cells. It is commonly used to treat cancers that originate in the liver. Chemoembolization is a procedure done by an interventional radiologist. A catheter inserted through

the groin with contrast dye and chemotherapy goes to the liver, where the medication is injected. It poisons and starves the tumor of its blood supply. In radiotherapy ablation a probe through the skin is inserted into the lesion, and heated tongs in the probe burn the tumor.

Chapter 2: The Medical-Industrial Complex I

1 Until his death in 2014 he continued to crusade against commercial influences in medicine. See especially Arnold S. Relman, "How Doctors Could Rescue Health Care," *New York Review of Books*, October 27, 2011; Arnold S. Relman and M. Angell, "America's Other Drug Problem: How the Drug Industry Distorts Medicine and Politics," *New Republic*, December 16, 2002, 27–41.

2 Relman, "The New Medical-Industrial Complex."

3 de Lissovoy, "The Implantable Cardiac Defibrillator."

4 See, for example, Bardy et al., "Amiodarone or an Implantable Cardioverter-Defibrillator for Congestive Heart Failure"; Moss et al., "Prophylactic Implantation of a Defibrillator in Patients with Myocardial Infarction and Reduced Ejection Fraction"; Phurrough et al., "Decision Memorandum."

5 See especially comments by Mark Hlatky and Joanne Lynn in Phurrough et al., "Decision Memorandum," 15.

6 Janet Shim conducted the physician interviews excerpted in this chapter between 2002 and 2004. I selected excerpts from sixteen in-depth interviews with internists, general and interventional cardiologists, and cardiac surgeons who worked in a variety of practice settings, including academic medical centers, community hospitals, and private practice offices. See also Shim et al., "Risk, Life Extension and the Pursuit of Medical Possibility."

7 Starr, *The Social Transformation of American Medicine*, especially 338–47.

8 Kaufman, *The Healer's Tale*, 173.

9 Starr, *The Social Transformation of American Medicine*, 347.

10 Rothman, *Strangers at the Bedside*, 59.

11 Dorsey et al., "Funding of U.S. Biomedical Research, 2003–2008," 137. Other federal funders include the Department of Defense, of Agriculture, of Energy, and the National Science Foundation. Moses et al., "Financial Anatomy of Biomedical Research," 1335.

12 Lowy, "Trustworthy Knowledge and Desperate Patients," 54–55; Mukherjee, *The Emporer of All Maladies*.

13 Marks, *The Progress of Experiment*; Timmermans and Berg, *The Gold Standard*.

14 Randomization, the random assignment of each patient or healthy study participant to the experimental or the standard therapy group, decreases the chance of investigator bias. In most of these studies the patients or both the investigators and the patients do not know which group they are in while being treated. The greater the number of patients in a study, when coupled with their randomization into equal groups, the more solid the assurance that the idiosyncratic features of individual study participants—age, gender, ethnicity, medical condi-

tion, and so on—are equally distributed and will not unduly bias the researchers or the research findings. Epstein, *Inclusion*, 48–49.

15 Donald Mainland quoted in Marks, *The Progress of Experiment*, 157.

16 Marks, *The Progress of Experiment*, 132–33, 58–59.

17 Epstein, *Inclusion*; Lambert, "Accounting for EBM"; Lowy, "Trustworthy Knowledge and Desperate Patients," 50–51.

18 Rothman, *Strangers at the Bedside*, 63–64.

19 *Efficacy* refers to establishing a statistically significant finding through experimental procedures. *Effectiveness* refers to demonstrating the worth of a medical intervention (for a large population) outside the experiment. Epstein, *Inclusion*, 49.

20 Timmermans and Berg, *The Gold Standard*, 90, 166–67. And see Lowy, "Trustworthy Knowledge and Desperate Patients" for a history of this development.

21 Hurst quoted in Berg, "Turning a Practice into a Science," 450. To be sure, worry about the lack of a scientific basis for medicine motivated researchers for hundreds of years before the contemporary era.

22 Feinstein quoted in Berg, "Turning a Practice into a Science," 449.

23 Berg, "Turning a Practice into a Science"; Lambert et al., "Introduction." For a discussion of these shifts in medicine, see Arney and Bergen, *Medicine and the Management of Living*. Much earlier, however, in his landmark report on medical education of 1910, Flexner stated that the practice of science and the practice of medicine should use the same techniques. See Berg, "Turning a Practice into a Science."

24 Kaufman, *The Healer's Tale*, 241.

25 Kaufman, *The Healer's Tale*, 306–7.

26 Kaufman, *The Healer's Tale*, 304–37.

27 Kaufman, *The Healer's Tale*, 106.

28 Konner, *Becoming a Doctor*, 15–16.

29 Konner, *Becoming a Doctor*, 16.

30 Sackett et al., *Clinical Epidemiology*.

31 Lambert, "Accounting for EBM," 2638.

32 Evidence-Based Medicine Working Group, "Evidence-Based Medicine. A New Approach to Teaching the Practice of Medicine," in Lambert, "Accounting for EBM." The authors state, "Medical practice is changing and the change, which involves using the medical literature more effectively in guiding medical practice, is profound enough that it can appropriately be called a paradigm shift."

33 Timmermans and Berg, *The Gold Standard*, 86.

34 Sackett et al., "Evidence Based Medicine."

35 Timmermans and Mauck, "The Promises and Pitfalls of Evidence-Based Medicine."

36 Lambert, "Accounting for EBM," 2639.

37 Timmermans and Berg, *The Gold Standard*, 142.

38 Lambert et al., "Introduction."

39 Joseph and Dohan, "Diversity of Participants in Clinical Trials in an Academic Medical Center."

40 Epstein, *Inclusion*.

41 Mendelson and Carino, "Evidence-Based Medicine in the United States," 133–36; Field and Lohr, *Clinical Practice Guidelines*.

42 I am indebted to Alan Venook for conversations about cancer guidelines, the goals of academic clinical research, insurance reimbursement, and the weighing of research evidence.

43 Sackett et al., "Evidence Based Medicine"; Timmermans and Berg, *The Gold Standard*.

44 Data for this vignette and others throughout the book about cancer treatment options for patients seventy and older were collected by Lakshmi Fjord between 2007 and 2010. I selected these vignettes from field notes on 150 patient-doctor interactions at oncology clinics serving ethnically and economically diverse populations in an urban metropolitan area.

45 "A pathologist assigns a Gleason grade ranging from 1 through 5 based on how much the cancer cells under the microscope look like normal prostate cells. Those that look a lot like normal cells are graded as 1, while those that look the least like normal cells are graded as 5." American Cancer Society, Cancer Glossary.

46 The PSA test is used primarily to screen for prostate cancer. It measures the amount of prostate-specific antigen (PSA) in the blood. PSA is a protein produced in the prostate, a small gland that sits below a man's bladder. PSA is mostly found in semen, which also is produced in the prostate. Small amounts of PSA ordinarily circulate in the blood. The test can detect high levels of PSA that may indicate the presence of prostate cancer. http://www.mayoclinic.org/tests-proce dures/psa-test/basics/definition/prc-20013324. Accessed July 30, 2014.

47 Brachytherapy is "internal radiation treatment given by putting radioactive seeds or pellets right into the tumor or close to it. Also called interstitial radiation therapy or seed implantation. May be used along with external beam radiation therapy." American Cancer Society, Cancer Glossary.

48 Lin et al., "Why Physicians Favor Use of Percutaneous Coronary Intervention to Medical Therapy"; Moscucci, "Behavioral Factors, Bias, and Practice Guidelines in the Decision to Use Percutaneous Coronary Interventions for Stable Coronary Artery Disease"; Bates et al., "Ten Commandments for Effective Clinical Decision Support"; Broom et al., "Evidence-Based Healthcare in Practice"; Dopson et al., "Evidence-Based Medicine and the Implementation Gap." For specific examples of regional variation, see, for example, O'Hare et al., "Regional Variation in Health Care Intensity and Treatment Practices for End-Stage Renal Disease in Older Adults"; Matlock et al., "Regional Variation in the Use of Implantable Cardioverter-Defibrillators for Primary Prevention."

49 Mendelson and Carino, "Evidence-Based Medicine in the United States."

50 Skinner and Fisher, "Reflections on Geographic Variations in U.S. Health Care." See also Gottlieb et al., "Prices Don't Drive Regional Medicare Spending Variations." In a striking example of this development, the surgeon and author Atul Gawande has shown that some practitioners in one Texas town, viewing medical practice as a business and revenue stream, employed all kinds of pro-

cedures more often than their colleagues in nearby locations, thereby ensuring greater profits in the procedure-driven U.S. reimbursement environment. The high costs of health care services in that community represented an extreme case, but it serves as an example of the way profit growth has become a "legitimate ethic in the practice of medicine" through the overuse of procedures. Gawande also documented other communities, clinics, and physician groups that worked proactively to keep costs down. A. Gawande, "The Cost Conundrum," *New Yorker* 1 (2009): 42, 36.

51 See, for example, Adams, "Against Global Health?"

Chapter 3: The Medical-Industrial Complex II

1 See Holmes et al., "Anthropologies of Clinical Training in the 21st Century." See especially Pine, "From Healing to Witchcraft."

2 Moses and Martin, "Biomedical Research and Health Advances."

3 Petryna, *When Experiments Travel*, 3; Moses et al., "Financial Anatomy of Biomedical Research"; Moses and Martin, "Biomedical Research and Health Advances," 567 68. Major research universities, perhaps especially my own, UCSF, do not reflect this trend; at UCSF the NIH contributes the major share of research dollars. Between 2007 and 2012 industry funding for human research at UCSF was approximately 25 percent of federal funding. Yet industry funding grew at my university campus over 300 percent between 2002 and 2012.

4 De Vries and Lemmens, "The Social and Cultural Shaping of Medical Evidence."

5 Lemmens, "Piercing the Veil of Corporate Secrecy about Clinical Trials."

6 See, for example, Lemmens, "Piercing the Veil of Corporate Secrecy about Clinical Trials"; De Vries and Lemmens, "The Social and Cultural Shaping of Medical Evidence"; Elliott, *White Coat, Black Hat*; Angell, *The Truth about the Drug Companies*; Bodenheimer, "Uneasy Alliance"; Krimsky, *Science in the Private Interest*; Daniel Carlat, "Dr. Drug Rep," *New York Times Magazine*, November 25, 2007, 64–69; Healy, "The New Medical Oikumene"; Fisher, *Medical Research for Hire*; Arnold S. Relman and M. Angell, "America's Other Drug Problem: How the Drug Industry Distorts Medicine and Politics," *New Republic*, December 16, 2002, 27–41. For research on the impact of private industry on international research see, for example, Petryna et al., *Global Pharmaceuticals*; Petryna, *When Experiments Travel*; Adams, "Randomized Controlled Crime."

7 Dorsey et al., "Funding of U.S. Biomedical Research, 2003–2008," 140.

8 Moses and Martin, "Biomedical Research and Health Advances."

9 De Vries and Lemmens, "The Social and Cultural Shaping of Medical Evidence."

10 De Vries and Lemmens, "The Social and Cultural Shaping of Medical Evidence," 2695.

11 Angell, *The Truth about the Drug Companies*; Elliott, *White Coat, Black Hat*.

12 Epstein, *Impure Science*.

13 Established by the Food and Drug Administration Modernization Act, passed by U.S. Congress in 1997.

14 U.S. Department of Health and Human Services et al., "Guidance for Industry: Information Program on Clinical Trials for Serious or Life-Threatening Diseases and Conditions," 9.

15 "The term life-threatening is defined as (1) diseases or conditions where the likelihood of death is high unless the course of the disease is interrupted and (2) diseases or conditions with potentially fatal outcomes, where the endpoint of clinical trial analysis is survival." U.S. Department of Health and Human Services et al., "Guidance for Industry: Information Program on Clinical Trials for Serious or Life-Threatening Diseases and Conditions," 9.

16 McCray and Ide, "Design and Implementation of a National Clinical Trials Registry."

17 Butler and Nyberg, "Issue Brief"; Petryna, *When Experiments Travel*, 3; U.S. National Institutes of Health.

18 For anthropological studies of this trend, see Rajan, "Experimental Values"; Petryna, *When Experiments Travel*.

19 "Off-label" refers to physicians' prescription of drugs for conditions other than those approved by the U.S. Food and Drug Administration. Children, in addition to the elderly, are perhaps the prime targets of this trend. For example, the use of human growth hormone has spread to children who are short but are considered to be within the normal growth range, and psychiatric drugs not tested on children are in widespread use for controlling their behaviors.

20 Wilson Duff, "Patent Woes Threatening Drug Firms," *New York Times*, March 7, 2011.

21 Kaufman, "The World War II Plutonium Experiments"; Jonas, "Philosophical Reflections on Experimenting with Human Subjects"; Appelbaum et al., "False Hopes and Best Data."

22 See J. Groopman, "The Right to a Trial: Should Dying Patients Have Access to Experimental Drugs?," *New Yorker*, December 18, 2006, 40.

23 Keating and Cambrosio, "Cancer Clinical Trials," 100.

24 Gina Kolata, "Add Patience to a Leap of Faith to Discover Cancer Signatures," *New York Times*, July 19, 2011.

25 On February 3, 2014, ClinicalTrials.gov listed 13,175 cancer studies that were open for recruitment and a total of 38,710 studies that were open, active, recently completed, or withdrawn (U.S. National Institutes of Health).

26 "The Costly War on Cancer." Pharmaceutical and biotechnology companies are testing nearly nine hundred new cancer drugs, more than in any other disease category. Gardiner Harris, "Where Progress Is Rare, the Man Who Says No," *New York Times*, September 16, 2009.

27 "The Costly War on Cancer." *Big Pharma* is a term widely used today, and there is no question that it resonates with "Big Brother" as used in *1984* by George Orwell to characterize the power of government over intimate life and the absence of individual autonomy in all endeavors.

28 Keating and Cambrosio, "Cancer Clinical Trials," 216.

29 From their website, www.nccn.org, accessed March 21, 2012: "The National Comprehensive Cancer Network® (NCCN®), a not-for-profit alliance of 21 of

the world's leading cancer centers, is dedicated to improving the quality and effectiveness of care provided to patients with cancer. Through the leadership and expertise of clinical professionals at NCCN Member Institutions, NCCN develops resources that present valuable information to the numerous stakeholders in the health care delivery system. As the arbiter of high-quality cancer care, NCCN promotes the importance of continuous quality improvement and recognizes the significance of creating clinical practice guidelines appropriate for use by patients, clinicians, and other health care decision-makers. The primary goal of all NCCN initiatives is to improve the quality, effectiveness, and efficiency of oncology practice so patients can live better lives."

30 Histories have been written about the emergence of chemotherapy. See, for example, Keating and Cambrosio, "From Screening to Clinical Research"; Keating and Cambrosio, "Cancer Clinical Trials"; Mukherjee, *The Emporer of All Maladies*; Lowy, " 'Nothing More to Be Done.' " For a social history of changing conceptions of innovation and limits to treatment in cancer care, see Baszanger, "One More Chemo or One Too Many?"

31 Lowy, " 'Nothing More to Be Done,' " 231.

32 Mukherjee, *The Emporer of All Maladies*, 173.

33 Keating and Cambrosio, "Cancer Clinical Trials."

34 Thanks to Robert Martensen for emphasizing this point.

35 "Medical oncology was organized as a trial oriented professional segment." Lowy, " 'Nothing More to Be Done,' " 219.

36 Mukherjee, *The Emporer of All Maladies*, 173.

37 A recent development for a few kinds of cancer (lung, ovarian, multiple myeloma, and non-Hodgkin's lymphoma) is maintenance therapy, a treatment strategy encouraged by the pharmaceutical industry yet widely debated regarding its effectiveness. Chemotherapy agents are given continuously, not only until a cancer goes into remission or stops growing. Proponents of this strategy note that it can help turn cancers into chronic illnesses, keeping them under control even when not curing them. Others suggest that lack of strong evidence for benefit, as well as side effects, drug resistance, and cost, are reasons to be wary. Andrew Pollack, "Considering Longer Chemotherapy," *New York Times*, July 21, 2009.

38 Bailar and Smith, "Progress against Cancer?"; Mukherjee, *The Emporer of All Maladies*, 505.

39 Gina Kolata, "In Long Drive to Cure Cancer, Advances Have Been Elusive," *New York Times*, April 24, 2009.

40 Mukherjee, *The Emporer of All Maladies*, 401–2.

41 Kolata, "In Long Drive to Cure Cancer, Advances Have Been Elusive."

42 Peter B. Bach, Leonard B. Saltz, and Robert E. Wittes, "In Cancer Care, Cost Matters," *New York Times*, October 15, 2012. The authors, physicians at Memorial Sloan-Kettering Cancer Center, became so outraged at the price of the drug Zaltrap (jointly marketed by Sanofi and Regeneron) for advanced colorectal cancer—$11,063 for one month of treatment, with no demonstrated benefit over other therapies—that they refused to prescribe it for their patients.

43 Gapstur and Thun, "Progress in the War on Cancer." Lung cancer is the leading cause of cancer death in the United States today, followed by breast, prostate, and colon cancer. Kolata, "In Long Drive to Cure Cancer, Advances Have Been Elusive."

44 According to the SEER statistics from 2008, there were 13,397,159 persons with invasive cancer (prevalence—not incidence). Of those, 11,732,690 were over fifty, 9,532,820 were over sixty, and 6,116,039 were over seventy. See National Cancer Institute, Table: http://seer.cancer.gov/csr/1975_2011/results_single /sect_01_table.23_2pgs.pdf. Accessed July 30, 2014.

45 Gapstur and Thun, "Progress in the War on Cancer," 1084.

46 "The Costly War on Cancer," 67.

47 Chambers and Neumann, "Listening to Provenge."

48 "Extremely Expensive Cancer Drugs: Treatments with Limited Medical Benefits for Some Patients Could Be a Drain on Medicare," *New York Times*, July 7, 2011; Frederick Tucker, "Drugs and Profits," *New York Times*, May 25, 2011.

49 Naomi Kresge, "Billions Riding on Results of Breast Cancer Treatment," *San Francisco Chronicle*, September 25, 2012.

50 Hawthorne, *Inside the FDA*; Elliott, *White Coat, Black Hat*.

51 Epstein, *Impure Science*, 269. The quotation within this quotation is Epstein citing John James's analysis of the role of the FDA. See James, "DDC: AZT Combination Approval Recommended."

52 Many note that the FDA does not have sufficient funding to adequately evaluate emerging therapies and cite the problems inherent in the fact that industry pays the FDA to review its studies.

53 Epstein, *Impure Science*, 277.

54 Epstein, *Impure Science*, 274.

55 CD4 cells are a type of white blood cell that is specifically targeted and destroyed by HIV. A healthy person's CD4 count can vary from 500 to more than 1,000. Even if a person has no symptoms, HIV infection progresses to AIDS when his or her CD4 count becomes less than 200. Mayo Clinic Staff, "Test and Diagnosis."

56 Epstein, *Impure Science*, 275, quoting Martin Delaney.

57 Epstein, *Impure Science*, 277.

58 Mukherjee, *The Emperor of All Maladies*, 424.

59 Epstein, *Impure Science*, 278.

60 Until 2002 most of those drugs were granted accelerated approval on the basis of the "response duration" of the drug, usually is measured from the time of initial response until tumor progression is documented. See U.S. Department of Health and Human Services et al., "Guidance for Industry: Clinical Trial Endpoints for the Approval of Cancer Drugs and Biologics," 19.

61 According to Johnson et al., "Accelerated Approval of Oncology Products."

62 "If there is no available therapy that improves survival, an improvement in progression-free survival or time to progression of sufficient magnitude to assure a better quality of life and that possibly predicts improved survival may be the basis of regular approval." Johnson et al., "Accelerated Approval of Oncol-

ogy Products," 637. Yet this is a murky issue because PFS does not necessarily indicate improved quality of life, though it might.

63 Cited in Groopman, "The Right to a Trial." Also see Johnson et al., "Accelerated Approval of Oncology Products": "Progression-free survival and time to progression are frequent primary endpoints in clinical trials in advanced cancer and are the most difficult endpoints for the Food and Drug Administration (FDA) to interpret when considering a drug for either regular or accelerated approval. Progression-free survival and time to progression are potential surrogates for improved survival or a better quality of life. For some indications, progression-free survival or time to progression is accepted by the FDA as an established surrogate and is the basis for regular approval of a drug. For example, the FDA used progression-free survival as an established surrogate to grant regular approval for gemcitabine for the treatment of advanced ovarian cancer after failure of platinum-based chemotherapy" (637). Accelerated approval, rather than regular approval, was given at the time for Gleevec because the drug looked promising; that is, the degree of improvement for patients in the trials was "sufficient to be reasonably likely to predict a survival benefit superior to that with the available therapy" (637). Additional clinical studies did support that particular use of the drug.

64 Keating and Cambrosio, *Cancer on Trial*, 364–68.

65 Lowy, " 'Nothing More to Be Done.' "

66 Baszanger, "One More Chemo or One Too Many?," 868.

67 Baszanger, "One More Chemo or One Too Many?," 868–69.

68 Overall survival is the gold standard, but it does require a larger study sample and more time. PFS studies take less time.

69 Tucker, "Drugs and Profits."

70 Tucker, "Drugs and Profits"; Carpenter et al., "Reputation and Precedent in the Bevacizumab Decision"; D'Agostino, "Changing End Points in Breast-Cancer Drug Approval."

71 Tucker, "Drugs and Profits."

72 That is, as the primary endpoint in clinical trials for the approval of first-line chemotherapy for metastatic breast cancer. See Carpenter et al., "Reputation and Precedent in the Bevacizumab Decision"; D'Agostino, "Changing End Points in Breast-Cancer Drug Approval."

73 Joe Nocera, "Why Doesn't No Mean No," *New York Times*, November 22, 2011. Nocera mentions that nine of the thirty-two members on the NCCN breast cancer panel have financial ties to Genentech. Meanwhile more recent clinical trials keep unresolved the controversy about the benefit of Avastin (bevacizumab) therapy. See Montero and Vogel, "Fighting Fire with Fire."

74 Baszanger, "One More Chemo or One Too Many?," 868.

75 In Jacoby, *Never Say Die*, the author asks why the generation (baby boomers and older) that saw the demise of smallpox, polio, and other diseases shouldn't have high expectations.

76 Butler and Nyberg, "Issue Brief"; Schmucker and Vesell, "Are the Elderly Underrepresented in Clinical Drug Trials?"

77 American Geriatrics Society, "Issue Brief."

78 Epstein, *Inclusion*, 123.

79 Landers, "Trials of Treating the Elderly."

80 Schmucker and Vesell, "Are the Elderly Underrepresented in Clinical Drug Trials?"

81 Arnold and Vastag, "Medicare to Cover Routine Care Costs in Clinical Trials."

82 Butler and Nyberg, "Issue Brief."

83 Hubbard and Jatoi, "Adjuvant Chemotherapy in Colon Cancer"; Zalman et al., "Examining the Evidence." See also Taylor et al., "The Disappearing Subject."

84 De Vries and Lemmens, "The Social and Cultural Shaping of Medical Evidence," 2696.

Chapter 4: "Reimbursement Is Critical for Everything"

1 Callahan, *Taming the Beloved Beast*; Fuchs, "The Growing Demand for Medical Care"; Gillick, "The Technological Imperative and the Battle for the Hearts of America"; Rothman, *Beginnings Count*.

2 Rothman, *Beginnings Count*, 71.

3 The effects of that core value are seen in Medicare spending. According to the Congressional Budget Office, "Medicare," spending in 2012 was $555 billion. Medicare spending in 2012 represented 3.7 percent of GDP (Potetz et al., "Medicare Spending and Financing"), while overall "national health expenditure" was 18 percent (Centers for Medicare and Medicaid Services, "NHE Fact Sheet"). Together Medicare, Medicaid, and the Children's Health Insurance Program (CHIP) made up 21 percent of the U.S. budget in 2012. In comparison 19 percent was spent on defense, 22 percent on social security, and 2 percent on education (Center on Budget and Policy Priorities, "Policy Basics").

4 This is not to imply that life spans or life expectancy have been statistically increased, merely that older patients have gained *time* that they very much wanted.

5 That doctor later informed me that 25 percent of transplant patients who have hepatitis C get cirrhosis five to seven years after the transplant. In 5 percent of those patients, the hepatitis C comes back very severely, killing the patient in the first year following transplantation.

6 UNOS is the private, nonprofit organization that manages the nation's organ transplant system under contract with the federal government. Its mission is to regulate and oversee the effectiveness and equity of organ allocation and distribution in the United States (UNOS.org).

7 I never learned whether Mrs. Ames received a transplant.

8 Here I follow the work of Becker, "The Uninsured and the Politics of Containment in U.S. Health Care" and Shore and Wright, *Anthropology of Policy*, 11, in their conceptualizations of policy as a "political technology" that shapes action and subjectivity. I suggest that Medicare reimbursement policies act as a tool, a means of both ethical and rational power that affects doctors and patients.

9 Gillick, "The Technological Imperative and the Battle for the Hearts of America," 283.

10 While the FDA thus enables many new technologies to move through the health care delivery system, it does not serve as an agent of transformation—it does not act as a mechanism that converts research findings into evidence, or evidence into standards of care, and so on. Therefore it is not an element in the chain of transformations I describe here.

11 In addition medical specialties and subspecialties have proliferated over the years, and Medicare also funds clinical training and then pays for the often lucrative procedures that specialists perform.

12 Gillick, "The Technological Imperative and the Battle for the Hearts of America"; Tunis, "Why Medicare Has Not Established Criteria for Coverage Decisions."

13 Mendelson and Carino, "Evidence-Based Medicine in the United States."

14 Gillick, "The Technological Imperative and the Battle for the Hearts of America"; Tunis, "Why Medicare Has Not Established Criteria for Coverage Decisions"; Centers for Medicare and Medicaid Services, "Medicare Evidence Development and Coverage Advisory Committee."

15 Mendelson and Carino, "Evidence-Based Medicine in the United States."

16 Hlatky, "Evidence-Based Use of Cardiac Procedures and Devices."

17 "No payment may be made . . . for any expenses incurred for items or services, which . . . are not reasonable and necessary for the diagnosis or treatment of illness or injury or to improve the functioning of a malformed body member." Sec. 1862(a) of the Social Security Act, cited in Neumann and Chambers, "Medicare's Enduring Struggle to Define 'Reasonable and Necessary' Care," 1775. See also Gillick, "The Technological Imperative and the Battle for the Hearts of America."

18 Gillick, "The Technological Imperative and the Battle for the Hearts of America"; Tunis, "Why Medicare Has Not Established Criteria for Coverage Decisions"; Foote, "Why Medicare Cannot Promulgate a National Coverage Rule."

19 Tunis, "Why Medicare Has Not Established Criteria for Coverage Decisions."

20 I discuss patient autonomy in greater detail in . . . And a time to Die, especially 71–75.

21 Bach, "Limits on Medicare's Ability to Control Rising Spending on Cancer Drugs"; Hlatky, "Evidence-Based Use of Cardiac Procedures and Devices"; Neumann et al., "Medicare and Cost-Effectiveness Analysis."

22 The history of stent use is one of rapid growth: from 85,000 procedures among those sixty-five and older in 1996 to 233,000 in 2010 (Kozak et al., National Hospital Discharge Survey; Centers for Disease Control and Prevention, "Rate of all-listed procedures for discharges from short-stay hospitals, by procedure category and age: United States, 2010." Accessed August 12, 2014. http://www.cdc.gov/nchs/data/nhds/4procedures/2010pro4_numberprocedureage.pdf.

23 Angioplasty.org, "Drug-Eluting Stent Overview."

24 Mayo Clinic Staff, "Drug-Eluting Stents"; Fogoros, "Controversy on Drug Eluting Stents Widens."

25 Redberg, "Editor's Note."

26 Rita F. Redberg, "Squandering Medicare's Money," *New York Times*, May 26, 2011.

27 See Prasad et al., "Reversals of Established Medical Practices"; Ioannidis, "Why Most Published Research Findings Are False."

28 Redberg, "Squandering Medicare's Money."

29 Gordon, "Tenacious Assumptions in Western Medicine."

30 Cassell, "The Nature of Suffering and the Goals of Medicine"; Rosenberg, *Our Present Complaint*; Callahan, *Taming the Beloved Beast*.

31 Callahan, *Taming the Beloved Beast*; Gillick, "Medicare Coverage for Technological Innovations"; Gillick, "The Technological Imperative and the Battle for the Hearts of America."

32 Koenig, "The Technological Imperative in Medical Practice," 467, 86.

33 Callahan, *Taming the Beloved Beast*; Gillick, "The Technological Imperative and the Battle for the Hearts of America." For a recent discussion of the medical pros and cons of device replacement in elderly patients, see Kramer et al., "Time for a Change."

34 Kaufman et al., "Ironic Technology."

35 Lefkowitz and Willerson, "Prospects for Cardiovascular Research."

36 Goldstein and Lynn, "Trajectory of End-Stage Heart Failure."

37 Goldman et al., "Consequences of Health Trends and Medical Innovation for the Future Elderly."

38 Most medical centers had declared a moratorium on those transplants by 1970. Gillick, "The Technological Imperative and the Battle for the Hearts of America"; Fox and Swazey, *Spare Parts*.

39 Gillick, "The Technological Imperative and the Battle for the Hearts of America," 281.

40 Gillick, "The Technological Imperative and the Battle for the Hearts of America," 280.

41 Fox and Swazey, *The Courage to Fail*.

42 Gillick, "The Technological Imperative and the Battle for the Hearts of America," 282.

43 Only certain facilities are eligible for Medicare reimbursement for the costs of implanting the LVAD.

44 Hunt et al., "ACC/AHA 2005 Guideline Update for the Diagnosis and Management of Chronic Heart Failure in the Adult."

45 Heart Failure Society of America, "HFSA 2006 Comprehensive Heart Failure Practice Guideline." According to the device manufacturer's website, in 2006 two hundred patients received LVADS (Thoratec Corporation, "Heartmate II Clinical Outcomes"). Eight hundred forty-seven patients who received the device as destination therapy have been registered on intermacs.org (accessed May 31, 2012). The Interagency Registry for Mechanically Assisted Circulatory Support (Intermacs) was created with support from the National Heart, Lung and Blood Institute, FDA, CMS, the device industry, and health care providers. In June 2006 this registry began to collect information about patients, devices, and outcomes, including adverse events. The registry is focused on use of

FDA-approved ventricular assist devices, including destination therapy. The registry meets the CMS mandate that all hospitals in the United States that provide mechanical circulatory support as destination therapy enter their cases into a national audited registry. During the six-month period from January to June 2010 (shortly after FDA approval of the new continuous-flow device, HeartMate II), there was a nearly tenfold increase in the number of registered uses for destination therapy. All registered cases during this period received the newer FDA-approved HeartMate II ventricular assist device. As of June 30, 2011, 126 medical centers had registered patients, 101 of which centers were approved by CMS to provide destination therapy. A total of 847 patients treated with destination therapy had been registered, and all recent cases employed the FDA-approved continuous-flow ventricular assist device, presumably HeartMate II. No VA medical centers were listed by the registry as of November 28, 2012 (University of Alabama at Birmingham School of Medicine, Intermacs). Patients receiving a continuous device as destination therapy had significantly worse survival rates than those receiving a continuous device as a bridge to transplant (Rector et al., "Use of Left Ventricular Assist Devices as Destination Therapy in End-Stage Congestive Heart Failure").

46 Hospitalization costs for implanting the LVAD in a person sixty-five or older were reported in 2011 to be approximately $195,000. Slaughter et al., "Temporal Changes in Hospital Costs for Left Ventricular Assist Device Implantation."

47 One end is attached to the left ventricle, the chamber of the heart that pumps blood out of the lungs and into the body. The other end is attached to the aorta, the body's main artery. Blood flows from the heart's ventricles into the pump, which passively fills up. When the sensors indicate it is full, the blood is ejected out of the device to the aorta. MedicineNet, "Left Ventricular Assist Device (LVAD) for Heart Failure."

48 The equipment today is much lighter.

49 Hernandez et al., "Long-Term Outcomes and Costs of Ventricular Assist Devices among Medicare Beneficiaries."

50 Kaufman et al., "Old Age, Life Extension, and the Character of Medical Choice"; Shim et al., "Clinical Life."

Chapter 5: Standard and Necessary Treatments

1 Kaufman, *The Healer's Tale.*

2 Latour and Venn, "Morality and Technology."

3 The anthropologist Marilyn Strathern expresses this idea well in "Reproducing the Future," 5: "For the intervention is also into ideas, including ideas about the future itself—what it is that we are laying or seeding for generations to come."

4 The creation of the category of knowledge "brain dead" by a Harvard committee of surgeons, ethicists, and others seeking to make organ transplantation an ethical practice is a story in its own right. See Lock, *Twice Dead.*

5 Lock, *Twice Dead*; Kaufman, "In the Shadow of 'Death with Dignity'"; Kaufman, . . . *And a Time to Die.*

6 Rothman, *Beginnings Count*, 112.
7 Latour and Venn, "Morality and Technology," 252.
8 Data for this clinic vignette were collected by Lakshmi Fjord.
9 Rosenberg, *Our Present Complaint*, 198.
10 Buchhalter et al., "Features and Outcomes of Patients Who Underwent Cardiac Device Deactivation"; Butler and Puri, "Deathbed Shock"; Goldstein et al., "Brief Communication."
11 See Kaufman, . . . *And a Time to Die* for examples of these kinds of patients.
12 Weber et al., "Who Should Be Treated with Implantable Cardioverter-Defibrillators?"
13 Dickerson, "Redefining Life While Forestalling Death," 365.
14 Katz and Marshall, "New Sex for Old."
15 Shim et al., "Clinical Life."
16 Pollock, "The Internal Cardiac Defibrillator."
17 Kaufman et al., "Ironic Technology"; Goldstein et al., "Brief Communication"; Goldstein et al., "Management of Implantable Cardioverter Defibrillators in End-of-Life Care."

    Patients tend to choose deactivation under certain circumstances when that option is discussed with them by their physician. See Dodson et al., "Patient Preferences for Deactivation of Implantable Cardioverter-Defibrillators." See also, Buchhalter et al., "Features and Outcomes of Patients Who Underwent Cardiac Device Deactivation"; Butler and Puri, "Deathbed Shock."
18 Caverly et al., "Patient Preference in the Decision to Place Implantable Cardioverter-Defibrillators"; Goldberger and Fagerlin, "ICDs—Increasingly Complex Decisions."
19 Jeffrey, "Machines in Our Hearts," 4.
20 Katy Butler, "My Father's Broken Heart," *New York Times*, June 20, 2010.
21 In 2008, 339,076 Americans received the device (Hlatky, "Evidence-Based Use of Cardiac Procedures and Devices"). This was up from seventy-five thousand in 2001 (Grant, "Ethical and Attitudinal Considerations for Critical Care Nurses Regarding Deactivation of Implantable Cardioverter-Defibrillators"). Seventy-eight percent of those who received the device in 2011 had it implanted because they were considered at high risk for a potentially lethal arrhythmia (Hammill et al., "Review of the Registry's Fourth Year, Incorporating Lead Data and Pediatric ICD Procedures, and Use as a National Performance Measure"). See also Grant, "Ethical and Attitudinal Considerations for Critical Care Nurses Regarding Deactivation of Implantable Cardioverter-Defibrillators"; Swindle et al., "Implantable Cardiac Device Procedures in Older Patients"; Hammill et al., "National ICD Registry Annual Report 2009."
22 Swindle et al., "Implantable Cardiac Device Procedures in Older Patients."
23 Goldstein and Lynn, "Trajectory of End-Stage Heart Failure."
24 Bristow et al., "Cardiac-Resynchronization Therapy with or without an Implantable Defibrillator in Advanced Chronic Heart Failure."
25 Buxton, "Implantable Cardioverter-Defibrillators Should Be Used Routinely in the Elderly"; Sohail et al., "Mortality and Cost Associated with Cardiovascular Im-

plantable Electronic Device Infections"; Yarnoz and Curtis, "Why Cardioverter-Defibrillator Implantation Might Not Be the Best Idea for Your Elderly Patient."

26 Chan et al., "Impact of Age and Medical Comorbidity on the Effectiveness of Implantable Cardioverter-Defibrillators for Primary Prevention."

27 Krahn et al., "Diminishing Proportional Risk of Sudden Death with Advancing Age." The authors note that for those persons over eighty in their study population, only 26 percent of deaths could be classified as "sudden." Patients under fifty were twice as likely to die due to arrhythmia (that is, sudden death) and thus were more likely to benefit from the device. The study suggests that benefit of the device decreases with advancing age.

28 Heidenreich and Tsai, "Is Anyone Too Old for an Implantable Cardioverter-Defibrillator?"

29 Harvard Health Newsletters, "Who Needs an Implantable Cardioverter-Defibrillator?"

30 Deactivation entails reprogramming the device so that it does not deliver a shock to abort a potentially lethal rhythm. Goldstein et al., " 'It's Like Crossing a Bridge' "; Barry Meier, "Lifesaving Devices Can Cause Havoc at Life's End," *New York Times*, May 14, 2010; Withell, "Patient Consent and Implantable Cardioverter Defibrillators."

31 Goldstein et al., " 'That's Like an Act of Suicide' "; Mueller et al., "Deactivating Implanted Cardiac Devices in Terminally Ill Patients"; Meier, "Lifesaving Devices Can Cause Havoc at Life's End."

32 Eckert and Jones, "How Does an Implantable Cardioverter Defibrillator (ICD) Affect the Lives of Patients and Their Families?" Although the bioethics literature notes that the deactivation of the device can be classified as the forgoing of extraordinary means of care, and thus is acceptable ethically and is a patient's right and choice. Mueller et al., "Deactivating Implanted Cardiac Devices in Terminally Ill Patients"; Sulmasy, "Within You/Without You." The bioethicist D. P. Sulmasy writes, "Both physicians and patients view the deactivation of the device as something *different* from the withdrawing of other life support technologies, and therefore, as problematic," 70. The fact that the device is inside the body and is programmed to abort a lethal rhythm makes deactivation confusing and morally troubling for some when considering deactivation near life's end. See also Goldstein et al., " 'That's Like an Act of Suicide' "; Goldstein et al., " 'It's Like Crossing a Bridge' "; Meier, "Lifesaving Devices Can Cause Havoc at Life's End"; Withell, "Patient Consent and Implantable Cardioverter Defibrillators."

33 Swindle et al., "Implantable Cardiac Device Procedures in Older Patients."

34 Timmermans, *Sudden Death and the Myth of CPR*. Sociologist Stefan Timmermans traces the history of the origin of that assumption, both in Europe and the United States, to the 1960s, with the normalization of emergency cardiopulmonary resuscitation. He shows how the technology of emergency CPR moved into the hospital and quickly became the default practice there, enabling sudden death to be framed as "one more road block waiting to be cleared by modern medicine" (53), regardless of the patient's age, frailty, or otherwise terminal condition, and regardless of mounting evidence showing that the vast majority of

patients who receive emergency resuscitation in the hospital never leave the hospital alive.

35 Goldenberg et al., "Causes and Consequences of Heart Failure after Prophylactic Implantation of a Defibrillator in the Multicenter Automatic Defibrillator Implantation Trial II," 2810; Goldstein and Lynn, "Trajectory of End-Stage Heart Failure"; Kirkpatrick and Kim, "Ethical Issues in Heart Failure"; Withell, "Patient Consent and Implantable Cardioverter Defibrillators."

36 See Butler, "My Father's Broken Heart" for a poignant tale of the effect of a pacemaker on the ethics of caregiving.

37 Much of this section on dialysis is adapted, updated and reworked from Russ et al., " 'Is There Life on Dialysis?' " Ann Russ drafted that article in 2005 with participation from Janet Shim and me. She collected all the data reported here on dialysis patients and their providers. Her analysis and interpretation form the basis of this section, and I am indebted to her and Janet Shim for allowing me to rework and augment the article in a different form here.

38 Germain et al., "When Enough Is Enough."

39 The forty-three patients interviewed ranged in age from seventy to ninety-three. There were twenty-six women and seventeen men; twenty-four were Caucasian, thirteen African American, five Asian, and one Latino. All interviews took place within the dialysis units while patients dialyzed.

40 U.S. Renal Data System, "USRDS 2012 Annual Data Report."

41 Patel and Schulman, "Invited Commentary."

42 Germain et al., "When Enough Is Enough"; Germain and Cohen, "Maintaining Quality of Life at the End of Life in the End-Stage Renal Disease Population."

43 Rothman, *Beginnings Count*.

44 Rothman, *Beginnings Count*; Gordon, "The Political Contexts of Evidence-Based Medicine."

45 Rothman, *Beginnings Count*, 90.

46 Germain and Cohen, "Maintaining Quality of Life at the End of Life in the End-Stage Renal Disease Population."

47 Fox and Swazey, *The Courage to Fail*, 217.

48 Fox and Swazey, *The Courage to Fail*, 203. It preceded the left ventricular assist device, another "halfway technology."

49 Through government-mandated cost control and age rationing in the government-funded health care system.

50 "In 1973 the program served 10,000 patients at a cost of $229 million. By 1990, it was serving 150,000 patients at a cost of $3 billion" (Rothman, *Beginnings Count*, 107). Today that cost is $32.9 billion (U.S. Renal Data System, "USRDS 2012 Annual Data Report").

51 For example, Germain et al., "When Enough Is Enough"; Schell et al., "An Integrative Approach to Advanced Kidney Disease in the Elderly"; Germain and Cohen, "Maintaining Quality of Life at the End of Life in the End-Stage Renal Disease Population." Exceptions are Cohen et al., "Practical Considerations in Dialysis Withdrawal"; Davison, "Quality End-of-Life Care in Dialysis Units."

52 Rothman, *Strangers at the Bedside*, 150.

53 See Jonsen, *The Birth of Bioethics*.

54 A notable exception is the groundbreaking work of the Renal Palliative Care Initiative. See Cohen et al., "Practical Considerations in Dialysis Withdrawal"; Poppel et al., "The Renal Palliative Care Initiative"; Cohen and Germain, "Measuring Quality of Dying in End-Stage Renal Disease."

55 Russ et al., "'Is There Life on Dialysis?'" The ability to delay the onset of dying—sometimes, it seems, indefinitely—opens new arenas of responsibility for patients and families who increasingly must authorize and "choose" death and the time for it. Ironically even while the time of dying is, in those units, made indistinct—as living and dying increasingly shade into one another—the time of death in life is expanded for older patients.

56 Kaufman, . . . *And a Time to Die*.

57 Official literature distributed by the National Kidney Foundation indicates that it is unknown how long people can live on dialysis and that it may be possible for some dialysis patients to live as long as people without kidney failure. Survival rates on dialysis depend on a variety of factors, including age, method and duration of access, and other medical conditions. At one clinic clinicians reported that one older man had been on dialysis nearly twenty years. Yet "in people over 75 years old starting dialysis, the mortality rate in the initial 6 months on dialysis has increased dramatically over the past 10 years" (Germain and Cohen, "Maintaining Quality of Life at the End of Life in the End-Stage Renal Disease Population," 133).

58 Fox and Swazey, *The Courage to Fail*, 277–79.

59 Kutner and Jassal, "Quality of Life and Rehabilitation of Elderly Dialysis Patients," 108; Kurella et al., "Octogenarians and Nonagenarians Starting Dialysis in the United States"; Germain and Cohen, "Maintaining Quality of Life at the End of Life in the End-Stage Renal Disease Population"; Germain et al., "When Enough Is Enough."

60 Levy, *Living or Dying*, 4.

61 Between 1977 and 1995 in the United States the numbers of new patients with end-stage renal disease ballooned from sixteen thousand to seventy-two thousand. By 2002 nearly half the U.S. dialysis population was over sixty-five, and patients over seventy-five were the fastest growing group of recipients in the United States and in Europe and Australia (Oreopoulos and Dimkovic, "Geriatric Nephrology Is Coming of Age"; Sims et al., "The Increasing Number of Older Patients with Renal Disease"). The number of persons with end-stage renal disease will continue to increase as the U.S. population ages. The rate of disease among those sixty-five to seventy-four has increased 28 percent since 2000, while the rate among those seventy-five and older has increased by 37 percent. Among those twenty to forty-four and forty-five to sixty-four, in contrast, growth has been 13 and 20 percent, respectively (U.S. Renal Data System, "USRDS 2011 Annual Data Report"). In 2011 prevalence of ESRD in the United States for ages sixty-five to seventy-four was 130,583; for ages seventy-five and older it was 98,248 (U.S. Renal Data System, "ESRD Quarterly Update."

62 Kurella et al., "Octogenarians and Nonagenarians Starting Dialysis in the United States."

63 Knauf and Aronson, "ESRD as a Window into America's Cost Crisis in Health Care."

64 Gina Kolata, "Asking Kidney Patients to Forgo a Free Lifeline," *New York Times*, July 19, 2011. Yet Mr. Tolleson (chapter 1) refused to start dialysis, much to the consternation of his children.

65 Davison et al., "Nephrologists' Reported Preparedness for End-of-Life Decision-Making."

66 Kolata, "Asking Kidney Patients to Forgo a Free Lifeline."

67 O'Hare et al., "Trends in Timing of Initiation of Chronic Dialysis in the United States."

68 Rosansky et al., "Early Start of Hemodialysis May Be Harmful."

69 O'Hare et al., "Trends in Timing of Initiation of Chronic Dialysis in the United States."

70 Samstein and Emond, "Liver Transplants from Living Related Donors."

71 Incidence rates of liver and intrahepatic bile duct cancers are rising, with annual changes greater than 2 percent (as is kidney cancer). "Cancer Trends Progress Report."

72 Dienstag and Cosimi, "Liver Transplantation." See also "Liver Transplantation NIH Consensus Statement Online 1983 Jun 20–23."

73 Starzl et al., "Liver Transplantation."

74 Coyne et al., "Decision Memorandum."

75 Organ Procurement and Transplantation Network, "Concepts for Kidney Allocation."

76 According to analysis by the Centers for Medicare and Medicaid Services. See Organ Procurement and Transplantation Network, "Concepts for Kidney Allocation."

77 Organ Procurement and Transplantation Network, "Concepts for Kidney Allocation." Also in 2000–2001 the first adult living donor liver transplants were performed, thereby creating a way to ease the problem of deceased donor organ scarcity and the increasing waiting time for an organ from the national UNOS waiting list.

78 Organ Procurement and Transplantation Network, "Concepts for Kidney Allocation."

79 Ly et al., "The Increasing Burden of Mortality from Viral Hepatitis in the United States between 1999 and 2007." See also Centers for Disease Control and Prevention, "Hepatitis B Information for Health Professionals." Accessed August 12, 2014. http://www.cdc.gov/hepatitis/HBV/HBVfaq.htm#overview.

80 Centers for Disease Control and Prevention, "Viral Hepatitis." See also Centers for Disease Control and Prevention, "Surveillance for Acute Viral Hepatitis, United States, 2007."

81 Keswani et al., "Older Age and Liver Transplantation"; Lipshutz et al., "Outcome of Liver Transplantation in Septuagenarians."

82 MedicineNet, "Liver Cancer." See also Centers for Disease Control and Prevention, "Surveillance for Acute Viral Hepatitis, United States, 2007"; Mukherjee, *The Emporer of All Maladies*, 340. Thanks to Scott Biggins and Michael Thaler for discussions about the causes of liver cancer.

83 Biggins, "Pretransplant Evaluation and Care." Those pretransplant interventions enabled Mr. Carter (chapter 1) and Mrs. Ames (chapter 4), both with liver cancer resulting from hepatitis C, to remain eligible for and ultimately to receive liver transplants.

84 Chemoembolization is a procedure done by an interventional radiologist. A catheter inserted through the groin with contrast dye and chemotherapy goes to the liver, where the medication is injected. It poisons and starves the tumor of its blood supply. In radiotherapy ablation, a probe through the skin is inserted into the lesion. Heated tongs in the probe burn the tumor.

85 Cardenas and Gines, "Predicting Mortality in Cirrhosis"; Biggins, "Pretransplant Evaluation and Care."

86 Nensi and Chandok, "Liver Transplantation in Older Adults." See also Lipshutz et al., "Outcome of Liver Transplantation in Septuagenarians." The authors conclude that age alone should not be used to limit liver transplantation. Yet they note as well that advancing age is a risk factor for cardiovascular disease and cancers.

Chapter 6: Family Matters

1 Fox and Swazey, *The Courage to Fail*; Rothman, *Beginnings Count*.

2 Tan and Chertow, "Cautious Optimism Concerning Long-Term Safety of Kidney Donation."

3 Segev et al., "Kidney Paired Donation and Optimizing the Use of Live Donor Organs."

4 Organ Procurement and Transplantation Network, "Data."

5 The situation is similar in Europe: in 1999, 12.5 percent of all transplantations reported to the Eurotransplant registry were for persons over sixty-five. Schratzberger and Mayer, "Age and Renal Transplantation."

6 Compare with 1988, when the ratio of living to deceased donors, for all age groups, was 32 to 68 percent. By 2000 the ratio of living to deceased donors was approximately 50–50.

7 The actual number of older kidney recipients (of both deceased and living donor organs) in the United States (sixty-five and over) has grown in the past two decades (from 213 in 1988 to 2,950 in 2011). For all age groups the interpersonal sources of living donation have shifted in the past decade. For example, spouse donations have increased over time from 4 percent in 1993 to 12 percent in 2011. Adult child donors constituted 13 percent of donors to recipients both under and over sixty-five in 1993 and 15.3 percent in 2011. Unrelated living donors have increased from 2.4 percent in 1993 to 34.6 percent in 2011 and are the group that has shown the greatest increase. Organ Procurement and Transplantation Network, "Data."

8 Mandal et al., "Does Cadaveric Donor Renal Transplantation Ever Provide Better Outcomes Than Live-Donor Renal Transplantation?"

9 For reports on donations to strangers, see Ian Parker, "The Gift," *New Yorker*, August 2, 2004, 54–63; Strom, "An Organ Donor's Generosity Raises the Question of How Much Is Too Much." See also "Transplant Arranged via the Internet Is Completed," *New York Times*, October 21, 2004. The gift relationship is shaped with increasing regularity by poverty, coercion, and the global market between "bioavailable" kidney sellers and needy and ready buyers (Cohen, "Operability, Bioavailability, and Exception"). In the context of the illegal market, the kidney is not a gift on the part of the seller but represents a temporary reprieve from debt or economic ruin or the promise of economic gain. Relinquishing the "gift" under those circumstances is often fraught with shame, chronic debility, and severe ostracism. Often the relinquishing is coerced. Cohen, "Where It Hurts"; Scheper-Hughes, "The Last Commodity."

The literature on the worldwide traffic in illegal organs in general, and on the causes and consequences of that organ trade, has grown enormously since the early 2000s. See, for example, Larry Rohter, "Tracking the Sale of a Kidney on a Path of Poverty and Hope," *New York Times*, May 23, 2004; Cohen, "Where It Hurts"; Cohen, "Operability, Bioavailability, and Exception"; Scheper-Hughes, "The Global Traffic in Human Organs"; Scheper-Hughes, "Keeping an Eye on the Global Traffic in Human Organs"; Scheper-Hughes, "Parts Unknown"; Danovitch, "Who Cares?"; Moniruzzaman, "'Living Cadavers' in Bangladesh"; Lock, "The Quest for Human Organs and the Violence of Zeal"; Shimazono, "The State of the International Organ Trade." There is also a feature film about the globalization of the illegal kidney market, *Dirty Pretty Things*.

10 Maureen Dowd, "Our Own Warrior Princess," *New York Times*, June 1, 2003; Denise Grady, "Transplant Frontiers: A Special Report. Healthy Give Organs to Dying, Raising Issue of Risk and Ethics," *New York Times*, June 24, 2001.

11 According to the NIH, a kidney transplant is an operation that places a healthy kidney in the body. The transplanted kidney takes over the work of the two kidneys that failed ("Kidney Failure"). During a transplant the surgeon places the new kidney in the lower abdomen and connects the artery and vein of the new kidney to the recipient's artery and vein. Often the new kidney will start making urine as soon as blood starts flowing through it, but sometimes it takes a few weeks to start working ("Kidney Transplantation").

12 Nathan et al., "Organ Donation in the United States"; Prottas, *The Most Useful Gift*, 12.

13 Most kidney transplant candidates (92.5 percent), regardless of age, are eligible for Medicare, which generally covers 80 percent of the cost of transplant surgery and 80 percent of the cost of antirejection medications for three years. In some cases the costs of antirejection medications are covered for as long as needed. In some cases Medicaid covers the costs of treatments for those ineligible for Medicare. And in some cases Medicaid covers the 20 percent of the costs of surgery and medications that Medicare does not cover. Medicaid and veterans' benefits vary considerably from state to state.

See National Kidney Foundation, "A to Z Health Guide"; Medicare Rights website; Medicare.gov.

14 Chapter 8 explores the issue of the broadening scope of social obligation and altruism beyond family.

15 This is, not only to get well but to stay that way. As the sociologist Talcott Parsons so famously noted, "To be sick . . . is to be in a state which is socially defined as undesirable, to be gotten out of as expeditiously as possible. No one is given the privileges of being sick any longer than necessary but only so long as he 'can't help it.' . . . The sick person makes the transition to the additional role of patient. He thereby, as in all social roles, incurs certain obligations, especially that of 'co-operating' with his physician—or other therapist—in the process of trying to get well" ("Illness and the Role of the Physician," 456). Writing in the early 1950s, Parsons could not have envisioned the kinds of life-sustaining technologies now available and the quandaries they produce for elderly patients, especially, today.

16 Laqueur, "From Generation to Generation."

17 Fox and Swazey, *Spare Parts*; Fox and Swazey, *The Courage to Fail*.

18 Mauss, *The Gift*.

19 Fox, "Afterthoughts," 254; Sharp, *Strange Harvest*.

20 Siminoff and Chillag, "The Fallacy of the 'Gift of Life.'"

21 Chkhotua et al., "Kidney Transplantation from Living-Unrelated Donors"; Mandal et al., "Does Cadaveric Donor Renal Transplantation Ever Provide Better Outcomes Than Live-Donor Renal Transplantation?"; Wolfe et al., "Comparison of Mortality in All Patients on Dialysis, Patients on Dialysis Awaiting Transplantation, and Recipients of a First Cadaveric Transplant."

22 Mandal et al., "Does Cadaveric Donor Renal Transplantation Ever Provide Better Outcomes Than Live-Donor Renal Transplantation?"

23 Arns et al., "'Old-for-Old'"; Morrissey and Yango, "Renal Transplantation"; Saxena et al., "Renal Transplantation in the Elderly."

24 Davis, "Evaluation of the Living Kidney Donor"; Davis and Delmonico, "Living-Donor Kidney Transplantation."

25 According to UNOS policy, however, donors who eventually need a kidney themselves go to the top of the recipients' list.

26 Tan and Chertow, "Cautious Optimism Concerning Long-Term Safety of Kidney Donation"; Wolfe et al., "Comparison of Mortality in All Patients on Dialysis, Patients on Dialysis Awaiting Transplantation, and Recipients of a First Cadaveric Transplant."

27 I discuss the utility question in detail in chapter 8.

28 In 2011, of 8,029 deceased donors, 22.8 percent were expanded criteria donors, according to Organ Procurement and Transplantation Network and Scientific Registry of Transplant Recipients, "OPTN/SRTR 2011 Annual Data Report." See also Metzger et al., "Expanded Criteria Donors for Kidney Transplantation"; Ojo, "Expanded Criteria Donors."

29 Fox and Swazey, *The Courage to Fail*; Summers et al., "Analysis of Factors That Affect Outcome after Transplantation of Kidneys Donated after Cardiac Death in the UK."

30 Wolfe et al., "Comparison of Mortality in All Patients on Dialysis, Patients on Dialysis Awaiting Transplantation, and Recipients of a First Cadaveric Transplant."

31 Segev et al., "Kidney Paired Donation and Optimizing the Use of Live Donor Organs"; Wolfe et al., "Comparison of Mortality in All Patients on Dialysis, Patients on Dialysis Awaiting Transplantation, and Recipients of a First Cadaveric Transplant."

32 I collected most of the data reported here between 2002 and 2008. The small, opportunistic interview sample consisted of recipients, prospective recipients, donors and potential donors. The thirty-five kidney recipients between the ages of seventy and eighty-one (twenty-four men, ten women; one had two transplants from two live donors) mirrors the U.S. national profile in terms of the ratio of living to deceased donor organs transplanted: 20 to 15. Fifty-eight persons (seventy to eighty) were in the process of medical evaluation for a kidney transplant. I spoke with twenty-six of their family members or nonkin who had already offered to donate a kidney. Ethnically our entire sample of recipients, donors, prospective recipients, and their potential donors reflects the broad diversity found in metropolitan California: African American, Euro-American, Chinese American, Japanese American, Hispanic, Filipino, Samoan, and immigrants from Afghanistan, China, Europe, and Vietnam.

33 Thanks to Ann Russ for helping to clarify these points.

34 Nolan et al., "Living Kidney Donor Decision Making."

35 Yet gender is implicated in the donor and prospective donor response to the need for a kidney simply because more men than women have kidney disease, leading them to need kidneys and preventing them from becoming donors. This biomedical fact needs to be considered in an analysis of gender and the tyranny of the gift. UNOS statistics show that men receive about one-third more kidneys (both cadaveric and living) than do women because of greater disease incidence. In 2011, 10,240 men and 6,573 women, of all ages, received kidney transplants. Of living donors in 2011, there were 2,218 men and 3,551 women, all adult ages. Organ Procurement and Transplantation Network website.

36 A fistula, or graft, is usually placed in the arm. It involves the surgical creation of a permanent connection between an artery and a vein under the skin, which enables adequate blood flow for dialysis. Fistulas are the preferred vascular access for long-term dialysis patients because they last longer than other forms of access and are less prone to infection and clotting. Russ et al., " 'Is There Life on Dialysis?' "

37 Creatinine is a chemical waste product that is produced by muscle metabolism and to a lesser extent by eating meat. If kidneys are not functioning properly, an increased level of creatinine may accumulate in the blood. A serum creatinine test measures the level of creatinine and gives an estimate of how well the kidneys are filtering waste (glomerular filtration rate). Mayo Clinic Staff, "Tests and Procedures."

38 Data collected by Janet Shim.

39 Katz and Marshall, "New Sex for Old"; President's Council on Bioethics (U.S.), "Beyond Therapy."

40 Biehl, "Life of the Mind."

41 The three comments from donors are all from women. Within my sample wives offered and donated more often to husbands than husbands offered and donated to wives. Among siblings, women offered to donate to their parents before their brothers did, and they did so more easily, enthusiastically, and insistently. They were also more adamant than their brothers that a parent accept their gift, and they expressed no reservations about giving. Their brothers, we were told, did not offer as quickly and were more reticent about giving at all.

42 See Gretchen Cuda-Kroen, "Organ Donation Has Consequences Some Donors Aren't Prepared For," NPR, July 2, 2012 (accessed January 14, 2013). http://www.npr .org/blogs/health/2012/07/02/155979681/organ-donation-has-consequences -some-donors-arent-prepared-for.

43 Brodwin, *Biotechnology and Culture*, 10.

44 Laqueur, "From Generation to Generation."

45 Carsten, *After Kinship*, 180.

46 Data collected by Janet Shim.

Chapter 7: Influencing the Character of the Future

1 Previous scenarios provide extended examples.

2 Woodward, "Statistical Panic," 197.

3 Christakis, *Death Foretold*.

4 Wilk, "It's about Time."

5 Christakis, "The Ellipsis of Prognosis in Modern Medical Thought"; Christakis, *Death Foretold*; Adams et al., "Anticipation."

6 See, for example, Nordin et al., "Do Elderly Cancer Patients Care about Cure?."

7 Cleveland Clinic, "Bioethics Reflections."

8 Yet even in our era of widespread risk awareness and assessment, some observers note that the concept of medical risk does not inform our actual judgments and choices a great deal.

9 See also Dumit, *Drugs for Life*; Rosenberg, *Our Present Complaint*; Shorter, *Bedside Manners*; Jain, "Living in Prognosis."

10 For analyses of the different kinds of effects of body-imaging technologies on patients and health professionals, see Cartwright, *Screening the Body*; Joyce, *Magnetic Appeal*; Dijck, *The Transparent Body*.

11 Rieff, *Swimming in a Sea of Death*, 47.

12 Rieff, *Swimming in a Sea of Death*, 21.

13 Rieff, *Swimming in a Sea of Death*, 110, 69.

14 Weeks et al., "Relationship between Cancer Patients' Predictions of Prognosis and Their Treatment Preferences."

15 The French phrase refers to "a madness shared by two," used here not to refer to a psychiatric symptom but rather to behavior that seems delusional.

16 Quoted in Rieff, *Swimming in a Sea of Death*, 113–14.

17 Ferris et al., "Palliative Cancer Care a Decade Later." For a history of the relationship between palliative care and chemotherapy in particular, see Baszanger, "One More Chemo or One Too Many?"

18 Weeks et al., "Patients' Expectations about Effects of Chemotherapy for Advanced Cancer."

19 Corn, "Ending End-of-Life Phobia"; Earle et al., "Trends in the Aggressiveness of Cancer Care near the End of Life"; Harrington and Smith, "The Role of Chemotherapy at the End of Life"; Matsuyama et al., "Why Do Patients Choose Chemotherapy Near the End of Life?"

20 Helft, "Necessary Collusion," 3147.

21 Rieff, *Swimming in a Sea of Death*, 112.

22 Baszanger, "One More Chemo or One Too Many?," 869.

23 Brown, "Shifting Tenses."

Chapter 8: For Whose Benefit?

1 Centers for Disease Control and Prevention, "Vital Signs."

2 The number of uninsured young adults dropped the most, from 28 percent to 18 percent. S. R. Collins, P. W. Rasmussen, and M. M. Doty, "Gaining Ground: Americans' Health Insurance Coverage and Access to Care After the Affordable Care Act's First Open Enrollment Period," The Commonwealth Fund, July 2014. http://www.commonwealthfund.org/publications/issue-briefs/2014/jul/health-coverage-access-aca. Accessed August 15, 2014.

3 Administration on Aging, "Projected Future Growth of Older Population."

4 Medical criteria are also part of the equation.

5 Kevin Sack, "Kidney Transplant Committee Proposes Changes Aimed at Better Use of Donated Organs," *New York Times*, September 22, 2012.

6 Organ Procurement and Transplantation Network website.

7 In 1999 Eurotransplant instituted a set of policies called the Eurotransplant Senior Program, in which organs from donors sixty-five and older were allocated to candidates of the same age. Since this program was instituted, there has been a substantial increase in the number of organs from older donors (de Fijter, "An Old Virtue to Improve Senior Programs"). The number of older kidney donors has tripled since the policies were introduced, and discard rates are far lower than they are in the United States (Sack, "Kidney Transplant Committee Proposes Changes Aimed at Better Use of Donated Organs"). The proportion of older deceased donors (over age sixty-four) increased significantly during those years as well—in Europe, from just over 2 percent in 1991 to 18 percent in 2007 (de Fijter, "An Old Virtue to Improve Senior Programs"); in the United States, from 0.8 percent (thirty-three of 3,876) in 1988, to 5.6 percent (421 of 7,433) in 2011 (Organ Procurement and Transplantation Network, "Concepts for Kidney Allocation").

8 Saxena et al., "Renal Transplantation in the Elderly."

9 Sack, "Kidney Transplant Committee Proposes Changes Aimed at Better Use of Donated Organs."

10 Rothman, *Beginnings Count.*

11 Stegall, "The Right Kidney for the Right Recipient."

12 Freise, "Commentary on 'Outcome of Liver Transplantation in Septuagenarians,'" 782.

13 Ross et al., "Equal Opportunity Supplemented by Fair Innings."

14 Organ Procurement and Transplantation Network, "OPTN/UNOS Board Approves Significant Revisions to Deceased Donor Kidney Allocation Policy."

15 Organ Procurement and Transplantation Network, "OPTN/UNOS Board Approves Significant Revisions to Deceased Donor Kidney Allocation Policy"; Organ Procurement and Transplantation Network, "Proposal to Substantially Revise the National Kidney Allocation System"; Sack, "Kidney Transplant Committee Proposes Changes Aimed at Better Use of Donated Organs."

16 Alan Zarembo, "How Old Is Too Old for a Transplant? Kidneys Are Scarce. Elderly Patients May Get Fewer If Rules Change," *Los Angeles Times*, November 5, 2006.

17 I never met a patient who received a kidney at or beyond the age of eighty-five. I did meet scores of patients between 2003 and 2010 at several clinics in the United States who were in their mid- to late seventies, and I met three persons who had received kidneys at eighty to eighty-one. I also met two patients who had received deceased donor livers at age seventy-eight.

18 I do not know if this surgeon asked the older patient if he would prefer that the young organ go to the younger patient. Certainly physicians do not pose that question routinely.

19 Hirose, "Commentary on 'Outcome of Liver Transplantation in Septuagenarians,'" 782.

20 Fox and Swazey, *The Courage to Fail*, ix.

21 Association of Organ Procurement Organizations, "Hope within Reach."

22 Healy, *Last Best Gifts*; Sharp, *Strange Harvest*. And it has allowed for the individual expression of this kind of extraordinary generosity. See Bramstedt and Down, "The Organ Donor Experience."

23 United Network of Organ Sharing, "OPTN."

24 United Network of Organ Sharing, "Awareness and Promotion."

25 Healy, *Last Best Gifts*, 36–37.

26 Satel, "Supply, Demand and Kidney Transplants"; Sally Satel, "A 'Gift of Life' with Money Attached," *New York Times*, December 22, 2009.

27 Healy, *Last Best Gifts*; Sharp, *Strange Harvest*, 50.

28 Fox and Swazey, *The Courage to Fail*, xvii. "While it is illegal to buy and sell human tissue, fees to recover, sterilize, process, store and transport the tissue can add up. The industry estimates it's worth more than $1 billion a year, and industry experts estimate one body can generate revenues of more than $80,000." For example, heart valves sell for $12,000 each, and "bone grafts are priced according to size and use, from $300 to $5,000." National Public Radio, "Interactive: The Anatomy of Human Tissue Profits," July 17, 2012, accessed March 18, 2013, http://www.npr.org/2012/07/17/156837673/interactive-the-anatomy-of-human -tissue-profits.

29 Cohen, "Where It Hurts"; Cohen, "Operability, Bioavailability, and Exception"; Delmonico et al., "Ethical Incentives—Not Payment—for Organ Donation"; Larry Rohter, "Tracking the Sale of a Kidney on a Path of Poverty and Hope," *New York Times*, May 23, 2004; Scheper-Hughes, "Parts Unknown." The possibility of buying an organ outside the United States is viewed as "another option," especially when circumstances limit access to other kinds of donors. A seventy-one-year-old man on dialysis following cardiac bypass surgery and subsequent kidney failure was told in the clinic that he had options: an expanded donor kidney from an older person or a living donor. His wife and his three children, in their twenties, all offered to donate a kidney to him. But his wife did not have health insurance. The patient's polycystic kidney disease made him wary that his children would also have the disease, and the transplant team would not consider them potential donors if they carried the gene for it. By 2006, when this man appeared at the clinic, kidney sales appeared normal to many. "I'm impatient," he said. "I already have an offer for a kidney from China, Pakistan, and India. The Internet makes this easy." Since he made that remark in 2006 the global, illegal market in kidneys (and other organs) has grown tremendously. See Kevin Sack, "Kidneys for Sale," *New York Times*, August 17, 2014.

30 His story was reported widely in the media. See Ian Parker, "The Gift," *New Yorker*, August 2, 2004, 54–63; Stephanie Strom, "An Organ Donor's Generosity Raises the Question of How Much Is Too Much," *New York Times*, August 17, 2003.

31 Steinbrook, "Public Solicitation of Organ Donors."

32 Katie Worth, "Altruistic Kidney Donations Are on the Rise, but Some Voice Ethical Concerns," *San Francisco Examiner*, February 6, 2011. According to CBS, they had matched "more than 150" (Jennifer Ashton, "More Organ Seekers Turning to Web to Find Them," CBS News, September 7, 2011, accessed May 30, 2012, http://www.cbsnews.com/stories/2011/09/07/earlyshow/health/main20102520.shtml?tag=contentBody;cbsCarousel). MatchingDonors.com now has the world's largest database of available altruistic donors (2,482 registered potential donors as of May 30, 2012) willing to take part in a paired kidney exchange. Due to incompatible blood types or antibodies, those potential donors cannot donate to a loved one, so they agree to be part of a larger exchange in which they donate to a compatible recipient, and their loved one also receives a medically suitable organ. See also Kevin Sack, "60 Lives, 30 Kidneys, All Linked," *New York Times*, February 19, 2012.

33 MatchingDonors.com.

34 More stranger kidney donations are occurring in the United Kingdom as well, as the result of a 2006 rule change at the Human Tissue Authority allowing unrelated individuals to become living donors. BBC, "Stranger Kidney Donations Rising," June 23, 2009, accessed March 10, 2011, http://news.bbc.co.uk/2/hi/health/8114688.stm.

35 Bramstedt and Down, "The Organ Donor Experience." There is no doubt that an ethics of generosity is fostered by transplant medicine, perhaps especially in the United States and other industrialized countries. The global traffic in illegal

organs, however, attests to other forces influencing donors and recipients, especially poverty, coercion, and the quick ethical acceptance of "bioavailable" kidney sellers and as the solution to the needs of buyers. Cohen, "Operability, Bioavailability, and Exception." See also Scheper-Hughes, "The Last Commodity."

36 Larissa MacFarquhar, "The Kindest Cut," *New Yorker*, July 27, 2009.

37 The website also states, "When our program was set up, we felt it was best if donor and recipient did not meet for at least 6 months. However, if the recipient wanted to send a letter of thanks to the donor, it would be sent via our transplant center. The donor might then respond, again via the transplant center. If both want to meet, we facilitate the meeting a minimum of 6 months after the transplant. To date, nearly half of the donor-recipient pairs have met." University of Minnesota Medical Center, "Transplant, Solid Organ."

38 While not actively soliciting, many hospitals now extol the virtues of living donations on their websites. See, for example, Johns Hopkins Medicine, Comprehensive Transplant Center, "Benefits of Living Donation," http://www. hopkinsmedicine.org/transplant/living_donors/benefits.html; Mayo Clinic, Liver Transplant, "Living-Donor Liver Transplant," http://www.mayoclinic.org /liver-transplant/living-donor-liver-transplant.html; Columbia University Medical Center, Department of Surgery, "Renal and Pancreatic Transplant: Kidney Donation," http://www.columbiasurgery.org/pat/kidneypancreastx/donation .html; Hartford Hospital, "Good Samaritan Donation," http://www.harthosp .org/transplant/TransplantationResources/GoodSamaritanDonation/default .aspx; UCSF Medical Center, "Living Liver Donor Transplant," http://www.ucs fhealth.org/treatments/living_liver_donor_transplant/index.html (all accessed March 18, 2013).

39 Testa et al., "Elective Surgical Patients as Living Organ Donors."

40 Atul Gawande, "Letting Go," *New Yorker*, August 2, 2010, 36–49.

41 Gordon et al., "In Response to Testa et al."; Mortier and Rogiers, "Living Donation, Are There Limits?"

42 Testa et al., "Elective Surgical Patients as Living Organ Donors," 2402.

43 Mortier and Rogiers, "Living Donation, Are There Limits?"

44 Saxena et al., "Renal Transplantation in the Elderly."

Conclusion: Toward a New Social Contract?

1 See also Sandel, *What Money Can't Buy*, 9.

2 As we have seen in the cases throughout this book, costs of extraordinary treatments are not part of the ethical tangle among choice and need for Medicare recipients.

3 See, for example, Bill Keller, "How to Die," *New York Times*, October 8, 2012.

4 Callahan, *What Price Better Health?*

5 Mukherjee, *The Emporer of All Maladies*, 223–24.

6 Rubin, "Let's Talk about Dying."

7 Frank, *The Renewal of Generosity*, 10; Rosenberg, *Our Present Complaint*, 6.

8 Rosenberg, *Our Present Complaint*, 198.

9 The Affordable Care Act has brought the topic of health care reform into the public discourse.

10 See, for example, Moriates et al., "The Value in the Evidence"; Berwick and Hackbarth, "Eliminating Waste in U.S. Health Care"; Redberg, "Getting to Best Care at Lower Cost."

11 Marmor and Oberlander, "From HMOS to ACOS"; Schroeder, "Personal Reflections on the High Cost of American Medical Care"; Callahan, *Taming the Beloved Beast*, 7.

12 See, for example, Ezekiel J. Emanuel and Steven D. Pearson, "It Costs More, but Is It Worth More?," *New York Times*, January 3, 2012; Samuel D. Waksal, "Pay Only for Drugs That Help You," *New York Times*, March 7, 2012.

13 Schroeder, "Personal Reflections on the High Cost of American Medical Care"; Daniel Callahan and Sherwin Nuland, "The Quagmire: How American Medicine Is Destroying Itself," *New Republic*, May 19, 2011.

14 T. Marmor and J. Oberlander, "Treating You Better for Less," *New York Times*, June 3, 2012.

15 Jonsen, *The Birth of Bioethics*; Fox, "The Evolution of American Bioethics."

16 Fox, "Advanced Medical Technology"; Fox and Swazey, "Medical Morality Is Not Bioethics"; Hoffmaster, *Bioethics in Social Context*; Hoffmaster, "Can Ethnography Save the Life of Medical-Ethics?"

17 SUPPORT Principal Investigators, "A Controlled Trial to Improve Care for Seriously Ill Hospitalized Patients."

18 Kaufman, . . . *And a Time to Die.*

19 Lynn et al., "Rethinking Fundamental Assumptions."

20 Recently some have noted the difficulty or impossibility of patients being proactive about health care choices. See, for example, Nease et al., "Choice Architecture Is a Better Strategy Than Engaging Patients to Spur Behavior Change."

BIBLIOGRAPHY

Adams, Vincanne. "Against Global Health? Arbitrating Science, Non-Science, and Nonsense through Health." In *Against Health: How Health Became the New Morality*, edited by Jonathan Metzl and Anna Rutherford Kirkland, 40–58. New York: New York University Press, 2010.

Adams, Vincanne. "Randomized Controlled Crime." *Social Studies of Science* 32, no. 5–6 (2002): 659–90.

Adams, Vincanne, Michelle Murphy, and Adele E. Clarke. "Anticipation: Technoscience, Life, Affect, Temporality." *Subjectivity* 28, no. 1 (2009): 246–65.

Administration on Aging. "Projected Future Growth of Older Population." Department of Health and Human Services. Accessed May 30, 2012. http://www.aoa .gov/aoaroot/aging_statistics/future_growth/future_growth.aspx#age.

American Cancer Society. Cancer Glossary. Accessed May 5, 2012. http://www.cancer .org/Cancer/CancerGlossary/index.

American Geriatrics Society. "Issue Brief: The Underrepresentation of Older Adults in Clinical Trials." Accessed January 24, 2012. http://www.americangeriatrics .org/advocacy_public_policy/research/.

Angell, Marcia. *The Truth about the Drug Companies: How They Deceive Us and What to Do about It.* New York: Random House, 2004.

Angioplasty.org. "Drug-Eluting Stent Overview." February 2013. Accessed June 8, 2013 http://www.ptca.org/des.html.

Appelbaum, P. S., L. H. Roth, C. W. Lidz, P. Benson, and W. Winslade. "False Hopes and Best Data—Consent to Research and the Therapeutic Misconception." *Hastings Center Report* 17, no. 2 (1987): 20–24.

Armstrong, David. "The Rise of Surveillance Medicine." *Sociology of Health and Illness* 17, no. 3 (1995): 393–404.

Arney, William Ray, and Bernard J. Bergen. *Medicine and the Management of Living: Taming the Last Great Beast.* Chicago: University of Chicago Press, 1984.

Arnold, K., and B. Vastag. "Medicare to Cover Routine Care Costs in Clinical Trials." *Journal of the National Cancer Institute* 92, no. 13 (2000): 1032.

Arns, Wolfgang, Franco Citterio, and Josep M. Campistol. "'Old-for-Old'—New Strategies for Renal Transplantation." *Nephrology, Dialysis, Transplantation* 22, no. 2 (2007): 336–41.

Association of Organ Procurement Organizations. "Hope within Reach." Accessed November 8, 2012. http://www.aopo.org/.

Bach, Peter B. "Limits on Medicare's Ability to Control Rising Spending on Cancer Drugs." *New England Journal of Medicine* 360, no. 6 (2009): 626–33.

Bailar, J. C., 3rd, and E. M. Smith. "Progress against Cancer?" *New England Journal of Medicine* 314, no. 19 (1986): 1226–32.

Bardy, G. H., K. L. Lee, D. B. Mark, J. E. Poole, D. L. Packer, R. Boineau, M. Domanski et al. "Amiodarone or an Implantable Cardioverter-Defibrillator for Congestive Heart Failure." *New England Journal of Medicine* 352, no. 3 (2005): 225–37.

Baszanger, I. "One More Chemo or One Too Many? Defining the Limits of Treatment and Innovation in Medical Oncology." *Social Science and Medicine* 75, no. 5 (2012): 864–72.

Bates, D. W., G. J. Kuperman, S. Wang, T. Gandhi, A. Kittler, L. Volk, C. Spurr, et al. "Ten Commandments for Effective Clinical Decision Support: Making the Practice of Evidence-Based Medicine a Reality." *Journal of the American Medical Informatics Association: JAMIA* 10, no. 6 (2003): 523–30.

Beck, Ulrich. "Living in the World Risk Society." Paper presented at the Hobhouse Memorial Public Lecture, London School of Economics, February 15, 2006.

Beck, Ulrich. "Risk Society: Towards a New Modernity." *Theory, Culture and Society* 9 (1992): 260.

Becker, G. "The Uninsured and the Politics of Containment in U.S. Health Care." *Medical Anthropology* 26, no. 4 (2007): 299–321.

Beecher, H. K. "Ethics and Clinical Research." *New England Journal of Medicine* 274, no. 24 (1966): 1354–60.

Berg, M. "Turning a Practice into a Science: Reconceptualizing Postwar Medical Practice." *Social Studies of Science* 25, no. 3 (1995): 437–76.

Berwick, D. M., and A. D. Hackbarth. "Eliminating Waste in U.S. Health Care." *JAMA Internal Medicine* 307, no. 14 (2012): 1513–16.

Biehl, João. "Life of the Mind: The Interface of Psychopharmaceuticals, Domestic Economies, and Social Abandonment." *American Ethnologist* 31, no. 4 (2004): 475–96.

Biggins, Scott W. "Pretransplant Evaluation and Care." In *Zakim and Boyer's Hepatology: A Textbook of Liver Disease*, edited by Thomas D. Boyer, Michael P. Manns and Arun J. Sanyal, 1314. Philadelphia: Saunders/Elsevier, 2011.

Bodenheimer, T. "Uneasy Alliance—Clinical Investigators and the Pharmaceutical Industry." *New England Journal of Medicine* 342, no. 20 (2000): 1539–44.

Bramstedt, Katrina A., and Rena Down. *The Organ Donor Experience: Good Samaritans and the Meaning of Altruism*. Lanham, MD: Rowman and Littlefield, 2011.

Bristow, M. R., L. A. Saxon, J. Boehmer, S. Krueger, D. A. Kass, T. De Marco, P. Carson et al. "Cardiac-Resynchronization Therapy with or without an Implantable Defibrillator in Advanced Chronic Heart Failure." *New England Journal of Medicine* 350, no. 21 (2004): 2140–50.

Brodwin, Paul. *Biotechnology and Culture: Bodies, Anxieties, Ethics*. Theories of Contemporary Culture. Bloomington: Indiana University Press, 2000.

Broom, A., J. Adams, and P. Tovey. "Evidence-Based Healthcare in Practice: A Study of Clinician Resistance, Professional De-skilling, and Inter-specialty Differentiation in Oncology." *Social Science and Medicine* 68, no. 1 (2009): 192–200.

Brown, Nik. "Shifting Tenses—From 'Regimes of Truth' to 'Regimes of Hope.'" Paper presented at Shifting Politics—Politics of Technology—The Times They Are A-changin', Groningen, April 21–22, 2006.

Buchhalter, Lillian, Abigale Ottenberg, Tracy Webster, Keith Swetz, David Hayes, and Paul Mueller. "Features and Outcomes of Patients Who Underwent Cardiac Device Deactivation." *JAMA Internal Medicine* 174, no. 1 (2014): 80–85.

Butler, Katy. *Knocking on Heaven's Door: The Path to a Better Way of Death*. New York: Scribner, 2013.

Butler, Katy, and Sunita Puri. "Deathbed Shock: Causes and Cures." *JAMA Internal Medicine* 174, no. 1 (2014): 88–89.

Butler, R. N., and J. P. Nyberg. "Issue Brief: Clinical Trials and Older Persons: The Need for Greater Representation." Working paper. *International Longevity Center–USA* (2002).

Butler, Robert. "Do Health and Longevity Create Wealth?" Paper presented at the Lieberman Lecture, University of California, San Francisco, 2006.

Buxton, A. E. "Implantable Cardioverter-Defibrillators Should Be Used Routinely in the Elderly." *American Journal of Geriatric Cardiology* 15, no. 6 (2007): 361–64.

Callahan, Daniel. *Taming the Beloved Beast: How Medical Technology Costs Are Destroying Our Health Care System*. Princeton: Princeton University Press, 2009.

Callahan, Daniel. *What Price Better Health? Hazards of the Research Imperative*. California/Milbank Books on Health and the Public. Berkeley: University of California Press, 2003.

"Cancer Trends Progress Report." Bethesda, MD: National Cancer Institute, U.S. National Institutes of Health, DHHS, 2011.

Cardenas, A., and P. Gines. "Predicting Mortality in Cirrhosis—Serum Sodium Helps." *New England Journal of Medicine* 359, no. 10 (2008): 1060–62.

Carpenter, D., A. S. Kesselheim, and S. Joffe. "Reputation and Precedent in the Bevacizumab Decision." *New England Journal of Medicine* 365, no. 2 (2011): e3.

Carsten, Janet. *After Kinship*. New Departures in Anthropology. Cambridge: Cambridge University Press, 2004.

Cartwright, Lisa. *Screening the Body: Tracing Medicine's Visual Culture*. Minneapolis: University of Minnesota Press, 1995.

Cassell, Eric J. *The Nature of Suffering and the Goals of Medicine*. New York: Oxford University Press, 1991.

Caverly, T. J., S. M. Al-Khatib, J. S. Kutner, F. A. Masoudi, and D. D. Matlock. "Patient Preference in the Decision to Place Implantable Cardioverter-Defibrillators." *Archives of Internal Medicine* 172, no. 14 (2012): 1104–5.

Center on Budget and Policy Priorities. "Policy Basics: Where Do Our Federal Tax Dollars Go?" Washington, DC: Center on Budget and Policy Priorities, 2013.

Centers for Disease Control and Prevention. "Rate of all-listed procedures for discharges from short-stay hospitals, by procedure category and age: United States, 2010." Accessed August 12, 2014. http://www.cdc.gov/nchs/data/nhds/4procedures/2010pro4_numberprocedureage.pdf.

————. "Hepatitis B Information for Health Professionals." Accessed August 12, 2014. http://www.cdc.gov/hepatitis/HBV/HBVfaq.htm#overview.

———. "Surveillance for Acute Viral Hepatitis, United States, 2007." MMWR *Surveillance Summaries* 58, no. ss03 (2009): 1–27.

———. "Viral Hepatitis." Accessed June 19, 2009. http://www.cdc.gov/hepatitis/.

———. "Vital Signs: Health Insurance Coverage and Health Care Utilization—United States, 2006–2009 and January–March 2010." MMWR *Morbidity and Mortality Weekly Report* 59, no. 44 (2010): 1448–54.

Centers for Medicare and Medicaid Services. "Medicare Enrollment Reports." Accessed May 30, 2012. http://cms.gov/Research-Statistics-Data-and-Systems /Statistics-Trends-and-Reports/MedicareEnrpts/index.html.

———. "Medicare Evidence Development & Coverage Advisory Committee," August 1, 2014. Accessed August 12, 2014. http://www.cms.gov/Regulations-and-Guidance /Guidance/FACA/MEDCAC.html.

———. "NHE Fact Sheet." Accessed March 18, 2013. http://www.cms.gov/Research -Statistics-Data-and-Systems/Statistics-Trends-and-Reports/NationalHealthEx pendData/NHE-Fact-Sheet.html.

Chambers, J. D., and P. J. Neumann. "Listening to Provenge—What a Costly Cancer Treatment Says about Future Medicare Policy." *New England Journal of Medicine* 364, no. 18 (2011): 1687–89.

Chan, P. S., B. K. Nallamothu, J. A. Spertus, F. A. Masoudi, C. Bartone, D. J. Kereiakes, and T. Chow. "Impact of Age and Medical Comorbidity on the Effectiveness of Implantable Cardioverter-Defibrillators for Primary Prevention." *Circulation: Cardiovascular Quality and Outcomes* 2, no. 1 (2009): 16–24.

Chkhotua, A. B., T. Klein, E. Shabtai, A. Yussim, N. Bar-Nathan, E. Shaharabani, S. Lustig, and E. Mor. "Kidney Transplantation from Living-Unrelated Donors: Comparison of Outcome with Living-Related and Cadaveric Transplants under Current Immunosuppressive Protocols." *Urology* 62, no. 6 (2003): 1002–6.

Christakis, Nicholas A. *Death Foretold: Prophecy and Prognosis in Medical Care.* Chicago: University of Chicago Press, 1999.

———. "The Ellipsis of Prognosis in Modern Medical Thought." *Social Science and Medicine* 44, no. 3 (1997): 301–15.

Cleveland Clinic. "Bioethics Reflections." Cleveland Clinic Bioethics Department. Accessed December 5, 2011. http://my.clevelandclinic.org/Documents/Bioethics /reflections/fall10.pdf.

Cohen, L. M., and M. J. Germain. "Measuring Quality of Dying in End-Stage Renal Disease." *Seminars in Dialysis* 17, no. 5 (2004): 376–79.

Cohen, L. M., M. J. Germain, and D. M. Poppel. "Practical Considerations in Dialysis Withdrawal: 'To Have That Option Is a Blessing.'" JAMA *Internal Medicine* 289, no. 16 (2003): 2113–19.

Cohen, Lawrence. "Operability, Bioavailability, and Exception." In *Global Assemblages: Technology, Politics, and Ethics as Anthropological Problems,* edited by Aihwa Ong and Stephen J. Collier, 79–90. Malden, MA: Blackwell, 2005.

———. "Where It Hurts: Indian Material for an Ethics of Organ Transplantation." *Daedalus* 128, no. 4 (1999): 135–65.

Congressional Budget Office. "Medicare." Accessed March 18, 2013. http://www.cbo .gov/topics/retirement/medicare.

Corn, B. W. "Ending End-of-Life Phobia—A Prescription for Enlightened Health Care Reform." *New England Journal of Medicine* 361, no. 27 (2009): e63.

"The Costly War on Cancer." *Economist*, May 28, 2011, 2.

Coyne, Richard, Vilis Kilpe, and Jackie Sheridan. "Decision Memorandum: Liver Transplantation (Cag 00053n)." December 2, 1999. Accesssed March 19, 2013. http://www.cms.gov/medicare-coverage-database/details/nca-decision-memo .aspx?.

Crawford, R. "Health as a Meaningful Social Practice." *Health (London)* 10, no. 4 (2006): 401–20.

———. "Risk Ritual and the Management of Control and Anxiety in Medical Culture." *Health (London)* 8, no. 4 (2004): 505–28.

Cutler, Nicole. "Understanding Hepatitis C Interferon Therapy." Hepatitis Central. July 31, 2006. Accessed May 7, 2012. http://www.hepatitis-central.com/mt/archives /2006/07/understanding_h.html.

D'Agostino, R. B., Sr. "Changing End Points in Breast-Cancer Drug Approval—The Avastin Story." *New England Journal of Medicine* 365, no. 2 (2011): e2.

Danovitch, G. M. "Who Cares? A Lesson from Pakistan on the Health of Living Donors." *American Journal of Transplantation* 8, no. 7 (2008): 1361–62.

Davis, Connie L. "Evaluation of the Living Kidney Donor: Current Perspectives." *American Journal of Kidney Diseases* 43, no. 3 (2004): 508–30.

Davis, Connie L., and Francis L. Delmonico. "Living-Donor Kidney Transplantation: A Review of the Current Practices for the Live Donor." *Journal of the American Society of Nephrology* 16, no. 7 (2005): 2098–110.

Davison, S. N. "Quality End-of-Life Care in Dialysis Units." *Seminars in Dialysis* 15, no. 1 (2002): 41–44.

Davison, S. N., G. S. Jhangri, J. L. Holley, and A. H. Moss. "Nephrologists' Reported Preparedness for End-of-Life Decision-Making." *Clinical Journal of the American Society of Nephrology* 1, no. 6 (2006): 1256–62.

de Fijter, Johan W. "An Old Virtue to Improve Senior Programs." *Transplant International* 22, no. 3 (2009): 259–68.

de Lissovoy, G. "The Implantable Cardiac Defibrillator: Is the Glass Half Empty or Half Full?" *Medical Care* 45, no. 5 (2007): 371–73.

De Vries, R., and T. Lemmens. "The Social and Cultural Shaping of Medical Evidence: Case Studies from Pharmaceutical Research and Obstetric Science." *Social Science and Medicine* 62, no. 11 (2006): 2694–706.

Delmonico, Francis L., Robert Arnold, Nancy Scheper-Hughes, Laura A. Siminoff, Jeffrey Kahn, and Stuart J. Youngner. "Ethical Incentives—Not Payment—for Organ Donation." *New England Journal of Medicine* 346, no. 25 (2002): 2002–5.

Dickerson, S. S. "Redefining Life While Forestalling Death: Living with an Implantable Cardioverter Defibrillator after a Sudden Cardiac Death Experience." *Qualitative Health Research* 12, no. 3 (2002): 360.

Dienstag, J. L., and A. B. Cosimi. "Liver Transplantation—A Vision Realized." *The New England Journal of Medicine* 367, no. 16 (October 12, 2012): 1483–1485.

Dijck, José van. *The Transparent Body: A Cultural Analysis of Medical Imaging.* In Vivo. Seattle: University of Washington Press, 2005.

Dodson, John A., Terri R. Fried, Peter H. Van Ness, Nathan E. Goldstein, and Rachel Lampert. "Patient Preferences for Deactivation of Implantable Cardioverter-Defibrillators." *JAMA Internal Medicine* 173, no. 5 (2013): 377–79.

Dopson, S., L. Locock, J. Gabbay, E. Ferlie, and L. Fitzgerald. "Evidence-Based Medicine and the Implementation Gap." *Health* 7, no. 3 (2003): 311–30.

Dorsey, E. R., J. de Roulet, J. P. Thompson, J. I. Reminick, A. Thai, Z. White-Stellato, C. A. Beck, B. P. George, and H. Moses III. "Funding of U.S. Biomedical Research, 2003–2008." *JAMA Internal Medicine* 303, no. 2 (2010): 137–43.

Dumit, Joseph. "The Depsychiatrisation of Mental Illness." *Journal of Public Mental Health* 4, no. 3 (2005): 8–13.

———. *Drugs for Life: How Pharmaceutical Companies Define Our Health*. Experimental Futures. Durham, NC: Duke University Press, 2012.

———. "Normal Insecurities, Healthy Insecurities." In *The Insecure American: How We Got Here and What We Should Do about It*, edited by Hugh Gusterson and Catherine Lowe Besteman, 163–81. Berkeley: University of California Press, 2010.

Earle, C. C., B. A. Neville, M. B. Landrum, J. Z. Ayanian, S. D. Block, and J. C. Weeks. "Trends in the Aggressiveness of Cancer Care near the End of Life." *Journal of Clinical Oncology* 22, no. 2 (2004): 315–21.

Eckert, M., and T. Jones. "How Does an Implantable Cardioverter Defibrillator (ICD) Affect the Lives of Patients and Their Families?" *International Journal of Nursing Practice* 8, no. 3 (2002): 152–57.

Elliott, Carl. *White Coat, Black Hat: Adventures on the Dark Side of Medicine*. Boston: Beacon Press, 2010.

Epstein, Steven. *Impure Science: AIDS, Activism, and the Politics of Knowledge*. Medicine and Society. Berkeley: University of California Press, 1996.

———. *Inclusion: The Politics of Difference in Medical Research*. Chicago Studies in Practices of Meaning. Chicago: University of Chicago Press, 2007.

Evidence-Based Medicine Working Group. "Evidence-Based Medicine. A New Approach to Teaching the Practice of Medicine." *JAMA Internal Medicine* 268, no. 17 (1992): 2420–25.

Ferris, F. D., E. Bruera, N. Cherny, C. Cummings, D. Currow, D. Dudgeon, N. Janjan et al. "Palliative Cancer Care a Decade Later: Accomplishments, the Need, Next Steps—From the American Society of Clinical Oncology." *Journal of Clinical Oncology* 27, no. 18 (2009): 3052–58.

Field, Marilyn J., and Kathleen N. Lohr, eds. *Clinical Practice Guidelines: Directions for a New Program*. Institute of Medicine Committee to Advise the Public Health Service on Clinical Practice Guidelines, vol. 90–08. Washington, DC: National Academy Press, 1990.

Fisher, Jill A. *Medical Research for Hire: The Political Economy of Pharmaceutical Clinical Trials*. Critical Issues in Health and Medicine. New Brunswick, NJ: Rutgers University Press, 2009.

Fogoros, Richard M. "Controversy on Drug Eluting Stents Widens: New Information Suggests Long-Term Problems." Accessed June 8, 2011. http://heartdisease.about .com/od/angioplastystents/a/DESproblems.htm.

Foote, S. B. "Why Medicare Cannot Promulgate a National Coverage Rule: A Case of Regula Mortis." *Journal of Health Politics, Policy and Law* 27, no. 5 (2002): 707–30.

Fox, Renee C. "Afterthoughts: Continuing Reflections on Organ Transplantation." In *Organ Transplantation: Meanings and Realities*, edited by Stuart J. Youngner, Renee C. Fox, and Lawrence J. O'Connell, 252–72. Madison: University of Wisconsin Press, 1996.

———. "The Evolution of American Bioethics." In *Social Science Perspectives on Medical Ethics*, edited by George Weisz, 201–20. Dordrecht: Kluwer Academic, 1990.

Fox, Renée C., and Judith P. Swazey. *The Courage to Fail: A Social View of Organ Transplants and Dialysis*. 1974. New Brunswick, NJ: Transaction, 2002.

———. "Medical Morality Is Not Bioethics: Medical Ethics in China and the United States." In *Essays in Medical Sociology: Journeys into the Field*, edited by Renée C. Fox, 645–70. New Brunswick, NJ: Transaction, 1988.

———. *Spare Parts: Organ Replacement in American Society*. New York: Oxford University Press, 1992.

Frank, Arthur W. *The Renewal of Generosity: Illness, Medicine, and How to Live*. Chicago: University of Chicago Press, 2004.

Freise, Chris. "[Commentary on 'Outcome of Liver Transplantation in Septuagenarians: A Single-Center Experience']." *Archives of Surgery* 142, no. 8 (2007): 782.

Fuchs, V. R. "The Growing Demand for Medical Care." *New England Journal of Medicine* 279, no. 4 (1968): 190–95.

Gapstur, S. M., and M. J. Thun. "Progress in the War on Cancer." *JAMA Internal Medicine* 303, no. 11 (2010): 1084–85.

Germain, M. J., and L. M. Cohen. "Maintaining Quality of Life at the End of Life in the End-Stage Renal Disease Population." *Advances in Chronic Kidney Disease* 15, no. 2 (2008): 133–39.

Germain, M. J., S. N. Davison, and A. H. Moss. "When Enough Is Enough: The Nephrologist's Responsibility in Ordering Dialysis Treatments." *American Journal of Kidney Diseases* 58, no. 1 (2011): 135–43.

Giddens, Anthony. *The Consequences of Modernity*. Stanford, CA: Stanford University Press, 1990.

———. *Modernity and Self-Identity: Self and Society in the Late Modern Age*. Stanford, CA: Stanford University Press, 1991.

Gifford, Sandra M. "The Meaning of Lumps: A Case Study of the Ambiguities of Risk." In *Anthropology and Epidemiology: Interdisciplinary Approaches to the Study of Health and Disease*, edited by Craig R. Janes, Ron Stall, and Sandra M. Gifford, 213–44. Boston: Reidel, 1986.

Gillick, M. R. "Medicare Coverage for Technological Innovations—Time for New Criteria?" *New England Journal of Medicine* 350, no. 21 (2004): 2199–203.

———. "The Technological Imperative and the Battle for the Hearts of America." *Perspectives in Biology and Medicine* 50, no. 2 (2007): 276–94.

Goldberger, Z. D., and A. Fagerlin. "ICDs—Increasingly Complex Decisions." *Archives of Internal Medicine* 172, no. 14 (2012): 1106–7.

Goldenberg, I., A. J. Moss, W. J. Hall, S. McNitt, W. Zareba, M. L. Andrews, and D. S. Cannom. "Causes and Consequences of Heart Failure after Prophylactic Implantation of a Defibrillator in the Multicenter Automatic Defibrillator Implantation Trial II." *Circulation* 113, no. 24 (2006): 2810–17.

Goldman, D. P., B. Shang, J. Bhattacharya, A. M. Garber, M. Hurd, G. F. Joyce, D. N. Lakdawalla, C. Panis, and P. G. Shekelle. "Consequences of Health Trends and Medical Innovation for the Future Elderly." *Health Affairs* 24, Suppl. 2 (2005): W5R5–17.

Goldstein, N., M. Carlson, E. Livote, and J. S. Kutner. "Brief Communication: Management of Implantable Cardioverter-Defibrillators in Hospice: A Nationwide Survey." *Annals of Internal Medicine* 152, no. 5 (2010): 296–99.

Goldstein, N. E., R. Lampert, E. Bradley, J. Lynn, and H. M. Krumholz. "Management of Implantable Cardioverter Defibrillators in End-of-Life Care." *Annals of Internal Medicine* 141, no. 11 (2004): 835–38.

Goldstein, N. E., and J. Lynn. "Trajectory of End-Stage Heart Failure: The Influence of Technology and Implications for Policy Change." *Perspectives in Biology and Medicine* 49, no. 1 (2006): 10–18.

Goldstein, N. E., D. Mehta, S. Siddiqui, E. Teitelbaum, J. Zeidman, M. Singson, E. Pe, E. H. Bradley, and R. S. Morrison. "'That's Like an Act of Suicide': Patients' Attitudes toward Deactivation of Implantable Defibrillators." *Journal of General Internal Medicine* 23, Suppl. 1 (2008): 7–12.

Goldstein, N. E., D. Mehta, E. Teitelbaum, E. H. Bradley, and R. S. Morrison. "'It's Like Crossing a Bridge': Complexities Preventing Physicians from Discussing Deactivation of Implantable Defibrillators at the End of Life." *Journal of General Internal Medicine* 23, Suppl. 1 (2008): 2–6.

Gordon, Deborah. "Tenacious Assumptions in Western Medicine." In *Biomedicine Examined*, edited by Margaret M. Lock and Deborah Gordon, 19–56. Culture, Illness, and Healing. Boston: Kluwer Academic, 1988.

Gordon, E. J. "The Political Contexts of Evidence-Based Medicine: Policymaking for Daily Hemodialysis." *Social Science and Medicine* 62, no. 11 (2006): 2707–19.

Gordon, Elisa J., Joel Frader, Aviva M. Goldberg, Doug Penrod, Gwenn McNatt, and John E. Franklin. "In Response to Testa et al. 'Elective Surgical Patients as Living Organ Donors: A Clinical and Ethical Innovation.'" *American Journal of Transplantation* 10, no. 3 (2010): 704–5; author reply 06.

Gottlieb, D. J., W. Zhou, Y. Song, K. G. Andrews, J. S. Skinner, and J. M. Sutherland. "Prices Don't Drive Regional Medicare Spending Variations." *Health Affairs* 29, no. 3 (2010): 537–43.

Grant, M. "Ethical and Attitudinal Considerations for Critical Care Nurses Regarding Deactivation of Implantable Cardioverter-Defibrillators." *AACN Advanced Critical Care* 21, no. 2 (2010): 222–26.

Gruman, Gerald J. "Cultural Origins of Present-Day 'Age-ism': The Modernization of the Life Cycle." In *Aging and the Elderly: Humanistic Perspectives in Gerontology*, edited by Stuart F. Spicker, Kathleen M. Woodward, and David D. Van Tassel. Atlantic Highlands, NJ: Humanities Press, 1978.

Hammill, Stephen C., Mark S. Kremers, Lynne Warner Stevenson, Paul A. Heidenreich, Christine M. Lang, Jeptha P. Curtis, Yongfei Wang, et al. "Review of the

Registry's Fourth Year, Incorporating Lead Data and Pediatric ICD Procedures, and Use as a National Performance Measure." *Heart Rhythm* 7, no. 9 (2010): 1340–45.

Harrington, S. E., and T. J. Smith. "The Role of Chemotherapy at the End of Life: 'When Is Enough, Enough?'" *JAMA Internal Medicine* 299, no. 22 (2008): 2667–78.

Harvard Health Newsletters. "Who Needs an Implantable Cardioverter-Defibrillator?" June 1, 2011. Accessed February 17, 2012. http://harvardpartnersinternational .staywellsolutionsonline.com/HealthNewsLetters/69,H061id.

Harvey, David. *A Brief History of Neoliberalism*. Oxford: Oxford University Press, 2005.

Hawthorne, Fran. *Inside the FDA: The Business and Politics behind the Drugs We Take and the Food We Eat*. Hobokcn, NJ: Wiley, 2005.

Healy, David. "The New Medical Oikumene." In *Global Pharmaceuticals: Ethics, Markets, Practices*, edited by Adriana Petryna, Andrew Lakoff and Arthur Kleinman, 61–84. Durham, NC: Duke University Press, 2006.

Healy, Kieran Joseph. *Last Best Gifts: Altruism and the Market for Human Blood and Organs*. Chicago: University of Chicago Press, 2006.

Heart Failure Society of America. "HFSA 2006 Comprehensive Heart Failure Practice Guideline." *Journal of Cardiac Failure* 12, no. 1 (2006): e1–2.

Heidenreich, P. A., and V. Tsai. "Is Anyone Too Old for an Implantable Cardioverter-Defibrillator?" *Circulation: Cardiovascular Quality and Outcomes* 2, no. 1 (2009): 6–8.

Helft, P. R. "Necessary Collusion: Prognostic Communication with Advanced Cancer Patients." *Journal of Clinical Oncology* 23, no. 13 (2005): 3146–50.

Hernandez, A. F., A. M. Shea, C. A. Milano, J. G. Rogers, B. G. Hammill, C. M. O'Connor, K. A. Schulman, E. D. Peterson, and L. H. Curtis. "Long-Term Outcomes and Costs of Ventricular Assist Devices among Medicare Beneficiaries." *JAMA Internal Medicine* 300, no. 20 (2008): 2398–406.

Hirose, Ryutaro. "[Commentary on 'Outcome of Liver Transplantation in Septuagenarians: A Single-Center Experience']." *Archives of Surgery* 142, no. 8 (2007): 782.

Hlatky, M. A. "Evidence-Based Use of Cardiac Procedures and Devices." *New England Journal of Medicine* 350, no. 21 (2004): 2126–28.

Hoffmaster, Barry. "Can Ethnography Save the Life of Medical-Ethics?" *Social Science and Medicine* 35, no. 12 (1992): 1421–31.

Hoffmaster, C. Barry. *Bioethics in Social Context*. Philadelphia: Temple University Press, 2001.

Holmes, Seth M., Angela C. Jenks, and Scott Stonington. "Anthropologies of Clinical Training in the 21st Century." Special issue, *Culture, Medicine and Psychiatry* 35, no. 2 (2011).

Hubbard, J., and A. Jatoi. "Adjuvant Chemotherapy in Colon Cancer: Ageism or Appropriate Care?" *Journal of Clinical Oncology* 29, no. 24 (2011): 3209–10.

Hunt, S. A., W. T. Abraham, M. H. Chin, A. M. Feldman, G. S. Francis, T. G. Ganiats, M. Jessup et al. "ACC/AHA 2005 Guideline Update for the Diagnosis and Management of Chronic Heart Failure in the Adult: A Report of the American

College of Cardiology/American Heart Association Task Force on Practice Guidelines (Writing Committee to Update the 2001 Guidelines for the Evaluation and Management of Heart Failure)." *Circulation* 112, no. 12 (2005): e154–235.

Ioannidis, John P. A. "Why Most Published Research Findings Are False." *PLoS Medicine* 2, no. 8 (2005): 696–701.

Jackson, Michael. *Existential Anthropology: Events, Exigencies, and Effects.* New York: Berghahn Books, 2004.

Jacoby, Susan. *Never Say Die: The Myth and Marketing of the New Old Age.* New York: Pantheon Books, 2011.

Jain, S. L. "Living in Prognosis: Toward an Elegiac Politics." *Representations* 98, no. 1 (2007): 77–92.

James, John S. "DDC: AZT Combination Approval Recommended." *AIDS Treatment News*, no. 150 (May 1, 1992).

Jeffrey, Kirk. *Machines in Our Hearts: The Cardiac Pacemaker, the Implantable Defibrillator, and American Health Care.* Baltimore: Johns Hopkins University Press, 2001.

Johnson, J. R., Y. M. Ning, A. Farrell, R. Justice, P. Keegan, and R. Pazdur. "Accelerated Approval of Oncology Products: The Food and Drug Administration Experience." *Journal of the National Cancer Institute* 103, no. 8 (2011): 636–44.

Jonas, H. "Philosophical Reflections on Experimenting with Human Subjects." *Daedalus* 98, no. 2 (1969): 219–47.

Jonsen, Albert R. *The Birth of Bioethics.* New York: Oxford University Press, 1998.

Joseph, G., and D. Dohan. "Diversity of Participants in Clinical Trials in an Academic Medical Center: The Role of the 'Good Study Patient?'" *Cancer* 115, no. 3 (2009): 608–15.

Joyce, Kelly A. *Magnetic Appeal: MRI and the Myth of Transparency.* Ithaca, NY: Cornell University Press, 2008.

Kamphuis, H. C., N. W. Verhoeven, R. Leeuw, R. Derksen, R. N. Hauer, and J. A. Winnubst. "ICD: A Qualitative Study of Patient Experience the First Year after Implantation." *Journal of Clinical Nursing* 13, no. 8 (2004): 1008–16.

Katz, Stephen, and Barbara Marshall. "New Sex for Old: Lifestyle, Consumerism, and the Ethics of Aging Well." *Journal of Aging Studies* 17, no. 1 (2003): 3–16.

Kaufman, Sharon R. . . . *And a Time to Die: How American Hospitals Shape the End of Life.* New York: Scribner, 2005.

Kaufman, Sharon R. *The Healer's Tale: Transforming Medicine and Culture.* Life Course Studies. Madison: University of Wisconsin Press, 1993.

———. "In the Shadow of 'Death with Dignity': Medicine and Cultural Quandaries of the Vegetative State." *American Anthropologist* 102, no. 1 (2000): 69–83.

———. "Making Longevity in an Aging Society." *Perspectives in Biology and Medicine* 53 (2010): 407–24.

———. "The World War II Plutonium Experiments: Contested Stories and Their Lessons for Medical Research and Informed Consent." *Culture, Medicine and Psychiatry* 21, no. 2 (1997): 161–97.

Kaufman, Sharon R., and Lakshmi Fjord. "Making Longevity in an Aging Society: Linking Technology, Policy and Ethics." *Medische Antropologie* 23 (2011): 119–38.

————. "Medicare, Ethics and Reflexive Longevity: Governing Time and Treatment in an Aging Society." *Medical Anthropology Quarterly* 25 (2011): 209–31.

Kaufman, Sharon R., and Wendy Max. "Medicare's Embedded Ethics: The Challenge of Cost Control in an Aging Society." *Health Affairs Blog*, March 28, 2011. http://healthaffairs.org/blog/2011/03/28/medicares-embedded-ethics.

Kaufman, Sharon R., P. S. Mueller, A. L. Ottenberg, and B. A. Koenig. "Ironic Technology: Old Age and the Implantable Cardioverter Defibrillator in U.S. Health Care." *Social Science and Medicine* 72, no. 1 (2011): 6–14.

Kaufman, Sharon R., Janet K. Shim, and Ann J. Russ. "Old Age, Life Extension, and the Character of Medical Choice." *Journals of Gerontology* B: *Psychological Sciences* 61, no. 4 (2006): S175–84.

Keating, P., and A. Cambrosio. "Cancer Clinical Trials: The Emergence and Development of a New Style of Practice." *Bulletin of the History of Medicine* 81, no. 1 (2007): 197–223.

————. "From Screening to Clinical Research: The Cure of Leukemia and the Early Development of the Cooperative Oncology Groups, 1955–1966." *Bulletin of the History of Medicine* 76, no. 2 (2002): 299–334.

Keating, Peter, and Alberto Cambrosio. *Cancer on Trial: Oncology as a New Style of Practice*. Chicago: University of Chicago Press, 2012.

Keswani, R. N., A. Ahmed, and E. B. Keeffe. "Older Age and Liver Transplantation: A Review." *Liver Transplantation* 10, no. 8 (2004): 957–67.

"Kidney Failure." U.S. National Library of Medicine, U.S. Department of Health and Human Services, National Institutes of Health. Accessed October 10, 2012. http://www.nlm.nih.gov/medlineplus/kidneyfailure.html.

"Kidney Transplantation." U.S. National Library of Medicine, U.S. Department of Health and Human Services, National Institutes of Health. Accessed October 10, 2012. http://www.nlm.nih.gov/medlineplus/kidneytransplantation.html.

Kirkpatrick, J. N., and A. Y. Kim. "Ethical Issues in Heart Failure." *Perspectives in Biology and Medicine* 49, no. 1 (2006): 1–9.

Knauf, F., and P. S. Aronson. "ESRD as a Window into America's Cost Crisis in Health Care." *Journal of the American Society of Nephrology* 20, no. 10 (2009): 2093–97.

Koenig, B. A. "The Technological Imperative in Medical Practice." In *Biomedicine Examined*, edited by Margaret M. Lock and Deborah Gordon, 465–96. Boston: Kluwer Academic, 1988.

Konner, Melvin. *Becoming a Doctor: A Journey of Initiation in Medical School*. New York: Viking, 1987.

Kozak, L. J., M. J. Hall, and M. F. Owings. *National Hospital Discharge Survey: 2000 Annual Summary with Detailed Diagnosis and Procedure Data*. Vital and Health Statistics. Series 13, Data from the National Health Survey. Hyattsville, MD: National Center for Health Statistics, 2002.

Krahn, A. D., S. J. Connolly, R. S. Roberts, and M. Gent. "Diminishing Proportional Risk of Sudden Death with Advancing Age: Implications for Prevention of Sudden Death." *American Heart Journal* 147, no. 5 (2004): 837–40.

Kramer, D. B., A. E. Buxton, and P. J. Zimetbaum. "Time for a Change—A New Approach to ICD Replacement." *New England Journal of Medicine* 366, no. 4 (2012): 291–93.

Krimsky, Sheldon. *Science in the Private Interest: Has the Lure of Profits Corrupted Biomedical Research?* Lanham, MD: Rowman and Littlefield, 2003.

Kurella, M., K. E. Covinsky, A. J. Collins, and G. M. Chertow. "Octogenarians and Nonagenarians Starting Dialysis in the United States." *Annals of Internal Medicine* 146, no. 3 (2007): 177–83.

Kutner, N. G., and S. V. Jassal. "Quality of Life and Rehabilitation of Elderly Dialysis Patients." *Seminars in Dialysis* 15, no. 2 (2002): 107–12.

Lambert, Helen. "Accounting for EBM: Notions of Evidence in Medicine." *Social Science and Medicine* 62, no. 11 (2006): 2633–45.

Lambert, Helen, Elisa J. Gordon, and Elizabeth A. Bogdan-Lovis. "Introduction: Gift Horse or Trojan Horse? Social Science Perspectives on Evidence-Based Health Care." *Social Science and Medicine* 62, no. 11 (2006): 2613–20.

Landers, Susan J. "Trials of Treating the Elderly: Determining Drug Safety and Effectiveness." American Medical Association. September 17, 2007. Accessed February 15, 2011. http://www.ama-assn.org/amednews/2007/09/17/hlsa0917.htm.

Laqueur, Thomas W. "From Generation to Generation: Imagining Connectedness in the Age of Reproductive Technologies." In *Biotechnology and Culture: Bodies, Anxieties, Ethics*, edited by Paul Brodwin, 75–98. Bloomington: Indiana University Press, 2000.

Latour, B., and C. Venn. "Morality and Technology: The End of the Means." *Theory, Culture and Society* 19, nos. 5–6 (2002): 247–60.

Lefkowitz, R. J., and J. T. Willerson. "Prospects for Cardiovascular Research." *JAMA Internal Medicine* 285, no. 5 (2001): 581–87.

Lemmens, Trudo. "Piercing the Veil of Corporate Secrecy about Clinical Trials." *Hastings Center Report* 34, no. 5 (2004): 14–18.

Levy, Norman B. *Living or Dying: Adaptation to Hemodialysis.* Springfield, IL: Thomas, 1974.

Lin, G. A., R. A. Dudley, and R. F. Redberg. "Why Physicians Favor Use of Percutaneous Coronary Intervention to Medical Therapy: A Focus Group Study." *Journal of General Internal Medicine* 23, no. 9 (2008): 1458–63.

Lipshutz, G. S., J. Hiatt, R. M. Ghobrial, D. G. Farmer, M. M. Martinez, H. Yersiz, J. Gornbein, and R. W. Busuttil. "Outcome of Liver Transplantation in Septuagenarians: A Single-Center Experience." *Archives of Surgery* 142, no. 8 (2007): 775–81; discussion 81–84.

"Liver Transplantation NIH Consensus Statement Online 1983 Jun 20–23." 4, no. 7 (1983): 1–15. http://consensus.nih.gov/1983/1983livertransplantation036html.htm.

Lock, Margaret M. "The Quest for Human Organs and the Violence of Zeal." In *Violence and Subjectivity*, edited by Veena Das, Arthur Kleinman, Mamphela Ramphele, and Pamela Reynolds, 271–95. Berkeley: University of California Press, 2000.

2013. Accessed June 25, 2013. http://optn.transplant.hrsa.gov/news/newsDetail.asp?id=1600.

———. "Proposal to Substantially Revise the National Kidney Allocation System (Kidney Transplantation Committee)." Accessed October 16, 2012.http://optn.transplant.hrsa.gov/PublicComment/pubcommentPropSub_311.pdf.

Organ Procurement and Transplantation Network and Scientific Registry of Transplant Recipients. "OPTN/SRTR 2011 Annual Data Report." Rockville, MD: Department of Health and Human Services, Health Resources and Services Administration, Healthcare Systems Bureau, Division of Transplantation, 2012.

Parsons, T. "Illness and the Role of the Physician: A Sociological Perspective." *American Journal of Orthopsychiatry* 21, no. 3 (1951): 452–60.

Patel, Uptal D., and Kevin A. Schulman. "Invited Commentary—Can We Begin with the End in Mind? End-of-Life Care Preferences before Long-Term Dialysis: Comment on 'Treatment Intensity at the End-of-Life in Older Adults Receiving Long-Term Dialysis.'" *Archives of Internal Medicine* 172, no. 8 (2012): 663–64.

Petryna, Adriana. *When Experiments Travel: Clinical Trials and the Global Search for Human Subjects.* Princeton: Princeton University Press, 2009.

Petryna, Adriana, Andrew Lakoff, and Arthur Kleinman. *Global Pharmaceuticals: Ethics, Markets, Practices.* Durham, NC: Duke University Press, 2006.

Phurrough, Steve, JoAnna Farrell, and Joseph Chin. "Decision Memorandum: Implantable Cardioverter Defibrillators (Cag 00157n)." Centers for Medicare and Medicaid Services. June 6, 2003. Accessed May 5, 2012. http://www.cms.gov/medicare-coverage-database/details/nca-decision-memo.aspx?NCAId=39&fromdb=true.

Pine, Adrienne. "From Healing to Witchcraft: On Ritual Speech and Roboticization in the Hospital." *Culture, Medicine and Psychiatry* 35, no. 2 (2011): 262–84.

Pollock, Anne. "The Internal Cardiac Defibrillator." *Inner History of Devices* (2008): 98–111.

Poppel, D. M., L. M. Cohen, and M. J. Germain. "The Renal Palliative Care Initiative." *Journal of Palliative Medicine* 6, no. 2 (2003): 321–26.

Potetz, Lisa, Juliette Cubanski, and Tricia Neuman. "Medicare Spending and Financing: A Primer." Washington, DC: Henry J. Kaiser Foundation, 2011.

Prasad, Vinay, Adam Cifu, and John P. A. Ioannidis. "Reversals of Established Medical Practices: Evidence to Abandon Ship." *JAMA Internal Medicine* 307, no. 1 (2012): 37–38.

President's Council on Bioethics (U.S.). Report on Bioethics. "Beyond Therapy: Biotechnology and the Pursuit of Happiness." October 24, 2003. https://bioethicsarchive.georgetown.edu/pcbe/reports/beyondtherapy/index.html For access date, please use, October 15, 2005.

Prottas, Jeffrey. *The Most Useful Gift: Altruism and the Public Policy of Organ Transplants.* Jossey-Bass Health Series. San Francisco: Jossey-Bass, 1994.

Rajan, K. S. "Experimental Values: Indian Clinical Trials and Surplus Health." *New Left Review*, no. 45 (2007): 67–88.

———. *Twice Dead: Organ Transplants and the Reinvention of Death.* California Series in Public Anthropology. Berkeley: University of California Press, 2002.

Lock, Margaret M., and Deborah Gordon. *Biomedicine Examined.* Culture, Illness, and Healing. Boston: Kluwer Academic, 1988.

Lock, Margaret M., and Vinh-Kim Nguyen. *An Anthropology of Biomedicine.* Malden, MA: Wiley-Blackwell, 2010.

Lowy, Ilana. "'Nothing More to Be Done': Palliative Care versus Experimental Therapy in Advanced Cancer." *Science in Context* 8, no. 1 (1995): 209–30.

———. *Preventive Strikes: Women, Precancer, and Prophylactic Surgery.* Baltimore: Johns Hopkins University Press, 2010.

———. "Trustworthy Knowledge and Desperate Patients: Clinical Tests for New Drugs from Cancer to AIDS." In *Living and Working with the New Medical Technologies: Intersections of Inquiry*, edited by Margaret M. Lock, Allan Young, and Alberto Cambrosio, 49–81. Cambridge: Cambridge University Press, 2000.

Ly, K. N., J. Xing, R. M. Klevens, R. B. Jiles, J. W. Ward, and S. D. Holmberg. "The Increasing Burden of Mortality from Viral Hepatitis in the United States between 1999 and 2007." *Annals of Internal Medicine* 156, no. 4 (2012): 271–78.

Lynn, Joanne, H. R. Arkes, M. Stevens, F. Cohn, B. Koenig, E. Fox, N. V. Dawson et al. "Rethinking Fundamental Assumptions: Support's Implications for Future Reform. Study to Understand Prognoses and Preferences and Risks of Treatment." *Journal of the American Geriatrics Society* 48, no. 5 Suppl. (2000): S214–21.

Mandal, Aloke K., Jon J. Snyder, David T. Gilbertson, Allan J. Collins, and John R. Silkensen. "Does Cadaveric Donor Renal Transplantation Ever Provide Better Outcomes Than Live-Donor Renal Transplantation?" *Transplantation* 75, no. 4 (2003): 494–500.

Marks, Harry M. *The Progress of Experiment: Science and Therapeutic Reform in the United States, 1900–1990.* Cambridge History of Medicine. Cambridge: Cambridge University Press, 1997.

Marmor, T., and J. Oberlander. "From HMOs to ACOs: The Quest for the Holy Grail in U.S. Health Policy." *Journal of General Internal Medicine* 27, no. 9 (2012): 1215–18.

MatchingDonors.com. May 31, 2012. Accessed May 31, 2012. http://matchingdonors.com/life/index.cfm.

Matlock, D. D., P. N. Peterson, P. A. Heidenreich, F. L. Lucas, D. J. Malenka, Y. Wang, J. P. Curtis et al. "Regional Variation in the Use of Implantable Cardioverter-Defibrillators for Primary Prevention: Results from the National Cardiovascular Data Registry." *Circulation: Cardiovascular Quality and Outcomes* 4, no. 1 (2011): 114–21.

Matsuyama, R., S. Reddy, and T. J. Smith. "Why Do Patients Choose Chemotherapy Near the End of Life? A Review of the Perspective of Those Facing Death from Cancer." *Journal of Clinical Oncology* 24, no. 21 (2006): 3490–96.

Mauss, Marcel. *The Gift: Forms and Functions of Exchange in Archaic Societies.* Glencoe, IL: Free Press, 1954.

Mayo Clinic Staff. "Drug-Eluting Stents: Do They Increase Heart Attack Risk?" Accessed June 8, 2011. http://www.mayoclinic.com/health/drug-eluting-stents/HB00090.

———. "HIV/AIDS Tests and Diagnosis." Accessed November 12, 2012. http://www .mayoclinic.com/health/hiv-aids/DS00005/DSECTION=tests-and-diagnosis.

———. "Tests and Procedures: Creatinine Test." Accessed November 6, 2012. http://www.mayoclinic.org/tests-procedures/creatinine/basics/definition/PRC -20014534.

McCray, A. T., and N. C. Ide. "Design and Implementation of a National Clinical Trials Registry." *Journal of the American Medical Informatics Association* 7, no. 3 (2000): 313–23.

Medicare.gov. Accessed May 31, 2012. http://www.medicare.gov/.

Medicare Rights. Accessed May 31, 2012. http://www.medicarerights.org.

MedicineNet. "Left Ventricular Assist Device (LVAD) for Heart Failure." Accessed February 13, 2012. http://www.medicinenet.com/left_ventricular_assist_device _lvad/article.htm.

———. "Liver Cancer." Accessed June 19, 2009. http://www.medicinenet.com /liver_cancer/page2.htm.

Mendelson, D., and T. V. Carino. "Evidence-Based Medicine in the United States—De Rigueur or Dream Deferred?" *Health Affairs* 24, no. 1 (2005): 133–36.

Metzger, R. A., F. L. Delmonico, S. Feng, F. K. Port, J. J. Wynn, and R. M. Merion. "Expanded Criteria Donors for Kidney Transplantation." *American Journal of Transplantation* 3, Suppl. 4 (2003): 114–25.

Moniruzzaman, M. "'Living Cadavers' in Bangladesh: Bioviolence in the Human Organ Bazaar." *Medical Anthropology Quarterly* 26, no. 1 (2012): 69–91.

Montero, A. J., and C. Vogel. "Fighting Fire with Fire: Rekindling the Bevacizumab Debate." *New England Journal of Medicine* 366, no. 4 (2012): 374–75.

Moriates, C., K. Soni, A. Lai, and S. Ranji. "The Value in the Evidence: Teaching Residents to 'Choose Wisely.'" *JAMA Internal Medicine* 173, no. 4 (2013): 308–10.

Morrissey, Paul E., and Angelito F. Yango. "Renal Transplantation: Older Recipients and Donors." *Clinics in Geriatric Medicine* 22, no. 3 (2006): 687–707.

Mortier, Freddy, and Xavier Rogiers. "Living Donation, Are There Limits?" *American Journal of Transplantation* 10, no. 5 (2010): 1330; author reply 31.

Moscucci, M. "Behavioral Factors, Bias, and Practice Guidelines in the Decision to Use Percutaneous Coronary Interventions for Stable Coronary Artery Disease." *Archives of Internal Medicine* 167, no. 15 (2007): 1573–75.

Moses, H., 3rd, E. R. Dorsey, D. H. Matheson, and S. O. Thier. "Financial Anatomy of Biomedical Research." *JAMA Internal Medicine* 294, no. 11 (2005): 1333–42.

Moses, H., 3rd, and J. B. Martin. "Biomedical Research and Health Advances." *New England Journal of Medicine* 364, no. 6 (2011): 567–71.

Moss, A. J., W. Zareba, W. J. Hall, H. Klein, D. J. Wilber, D. S. Cannom, J. P. Daubert et al. "Prophylactic Implantation of a Defibrillator in Patients with Myocardial Infarction and Reduced Ejection Fraction." *New England Journal of Medicine* 346, no. 12 (2002): 877–83.

Mueller, P. S., S. M. Jenkins, K. A. Bramstedt, and D. L. Hayes. "Deactivating Implanted Cardiac Devices in Terminally Ill Patients: Practices and Attitudes." *Pacing and Clinical Electrophysiology* 31, no. 5 (2008): 560–68.

Mukherjee, Siddhartha. *The Emperor of All Maladies: A Biography of Cancer.* New York: Scribner, 2010.

Nathan, H. M., S. L. Conrad, P. J. Held, K. P. McCullough, R. E. Pietroski, L. A. Siminoff, and A. O. Ojo. "Organ Donation in the United States." *American Journal of Transplantation* 3, Suppl. 4 (2003): 29–40.

National Comprehensive Cancer Network. Accessed March 21, 2012. http://www .nccn.org.

National Kidney Foundation. "A to Z Health Guide." Accessed May 31, 2012. http://www.kidney.org/atoz/.

Nease, Robert F., Sharon Glave Frazee, Larry Zarin, and Steven B. Miller. "Choice Architecture Is a Better Strategy Than Engaging Patients to Spur Behavior Change." *Health Affairs* 32, no. 2 (2013): 242–49.

Nensi, A., and N. Chandok. "Liver Transplantation in Older Adults." *Journal of the American Geriatrics Society* 60, no. 2 (2012): 400.

Neumann, P. J., and J. D. Chambers. "Medicare's Enduring Struggle to Define 'Reasonable and Necessary' Care." *New England Journal of Medicine* 367, no. 19 (2012): 1775–77.

Neumann, P. J., A. B. Rosen, and M. C. Weinstein. "Medicare and Cost-Effectiveness Analysis." *New England Journal of Medicine* 353, no. 14 (2005): 1516–22.

Nolan, M. T., B. Walton-Moss, L. Taylor, and K. Dane. "Living Kidney Donor Decision Making: State of the Science and Directions for Future Research." *Progress in Transplantation* 14, no. 3 (2004): 201–9.

Nordin, A. J., D. J. Chinn, I. Moloney, R. Naik, A. de Barros Lopes, and J. M. Monaghan. "Do Elderly Cancer Patients Care about Cure? Attitudes to Radical Gynecologic Oncology Surgery in the Elderly." *Gynecologic Oncology* 81, no. 3 (2001): 447–55.

O'Hare, A. M., A. I. Choi, W. J. Boscardin, W. L. Clinton, I. Zawadzki, P. L. Hebert, M. Kurella Tamura, L. Taylor, and E. B. Larson. "Trends in Timing of Initiation of Chronic Dialysis in the United States." *Archives of Internal Medicine* 171, no. 18 (2011): 1663–69.

O'Hare, A. M., R. A. Rodriguez, S. M. Hailpern, E. B. Larson, and M. Kurella Tamura. "Regional Variation in Health Care Intensity and Treatment Practices for End-Stage Renal Disease in Older Adults." *JAMA Internal Medicine* 304, no. 2 (2010): 180–86.

Ojo, A. O. "Expanded Criteria Donors: Process and Outcomes." *Seminars in Dialysis* 18, no. 6 (2005): 463–68.

Oreopoulos, D. G., and N. Dimkovic. "Geriatric Nephrology Is Coming of Age." *Journal of the American Society of Nephrology* 14, no. 4 (2003): 1099–101.

Organ Procurement and Transplantation Network. "Concepts for Kidney Allocation." February 16, 2011. http://optn.transplant.hrsa.gov/SharedContentDocuments /KidneyConceptDocument.PDF.

———. "Data." Accessed January 30, 2014. http://optn.transplant.hrsa.gov/.

Organ Procurement and Transplantation Network. "OPTN/UNOS Board Approves Significant Revisions to Deceased Donor Kidney Allocation Policy." June 25,

Rector, T. S., B. C. Taylor, N. Greer, I. Rutks, and T. J. Wilt. "Use of Left Ventricular Assist Devices as Destination Therapy in End-Stage Congestive Heart Failure: A Systematic Review." Washington, DC, 2012.

Redberg, Rita F. "Editor's Note in 'The Impact of New Cardiovascular Device Technology on Health Care Costs.'" *Archives of Internal Medicine* 171, no. 14 (2011): 1289–91.

———. "Getting to Best Care at Lower Cost." *JAMA Internal Medicine* 173, no. 2 (2013): 91–92.

Relman, Arnold S. "The New Medical-Industrial Complex." *New England Journal of Medicine* 303, no. 17 (1980): 963–70.

Rieff, David. *Swimming in a Sea of Death: A Son's Memoir.* New York: Simon and Schuster, 2008.

Rosansky, S. J., P. Eggers, K. Jackson, R. Glassock, and W. F. Clark. "Early Start of Hemodialysis May Be Harmful." *Archives of Internal Medicine* 171, no. 5 (2011): 396–403.

Rose, Nikolas. *The Politics of Life Itself: Biomedicine, Power, and Subjectivity in the Twenty-first Century.* Princeton, NJ: Princeton University Press, 2007.

Rosenberg, Charles E. *Our Present Complaint: American Medicine, Then and Now.* Baltimore: Johns Hopkins University Press, 2007.

Ross, Lainie Friedman, William Parker, Robert M. Veatch, Sommer E Gentry, and J. Richard Thistlethwaite. "Equal Opportunity Supplemented by Fair Innings: Equity and Efficiency in Allocating Deceased Donor Kidneys." *American Journal of Transplantation* 12, no. 8 (2012): 2115–24.

Rothman, David J. *Beginnings Count: The Technological Imperative in American Health Care.* New York: Oxford University Press, 1997.

———. *Strangers at the Bedside: A History of How Law and Bioethics Transformed Medical Decision Making.* New York: Basic Books, 1991.

Rubin, Lillian B. "Let's Talk about Dying." Salon.com, December 26, 2012. Accessed December 27, 2012. http://www.salon.com/2012/12/27/lets_talk_about_dying/.

Russ, Ann J., Janet K. Shim, and Sharon R. Kaufman. "'Is There Life on Dialysis?' Time and Aging in a Clinically Sustained Existence." *Medical Anthropology* 24, no. 4 (2005): 297–324.

Sackett, David L., R. Brian Haynes, G. H. Guyatt, and Peter Tugwell. *Clinical Epidemiology: A Basic Science for Clinical Medicine.* Boston: Little, Brown, 1985.

Sackett, David L., William M. C. Rosenberg, J. A. Muir Gray, R. Brian Haynes, and W. Scott Richardson. "Evidence Based Medicine: What It Is and What It Isn't—It's about Integrating Individual Clinical Expertise and the Best External Evidence." *British Medical Journal* 312, no. 7023 (1996): 71–72.

Samstein, B., and J. Emond. "Liver Transplants from Living Related Donors." *Annual Review of Medicine* 52 (2001): 147–60.

Sandel, Michael J. *Justice: What's the Right Thing to Do?* New York: Farrar, Straus and Giroux, 2009.

———. *What Money Can't Buy: The Moral Limits of Markets.* New York: Farrar, Straus and Giroux, 2012.

Satel, Sally. "Supply, Demand and Kidney Transplants: A Bad Incentive Structure Creates a Dire Shortage." In *Policy Review*. Hoover Institution, Stanford University, 2007.

Saxena, Ramesh, Xueqing Yu, Mauricio Giraldo, Juan Arenas, Miguel Vazquez, Christopher Y. Lu, Nosratola D. Vaziri, Fred G. Silva, and Xin J. Zhou. "Renal Transplantation in the Elderly." *International Urology and Nephrology* 41, no. 1 (2009): 195–210.

Schell, J. O., M. J. Germain, F. O. Finkelstein, J. A. Tulsky, and L. M. Cohen. "An Integrative Approach to Advanced Kidney Disease in the Elderly." *Advances in Chronic Kidney Disease* 17, no. 4 (2010): 368–77.

Scheper-Hughes, Nancy. "The Global Traffic in Human Organs." *Current Anthropology* 41, no. 2 (2000): 191–224.

———. "Keeping an Eye on the Global Traffic in Human Organs." *Lancet* 361, no. 9369 (2003): 1645–48.

———. "The Last Commodity: Post-human Ethics and the Global Traffic." In *Global Assemblages: Technology, Politics, and Ethics as Anthropological Problems*, edited by Aihwa Ong and Stephen J. Collier, 145–67. Malden, MA: Blackwell, 2004.

———. "Parts Unknown: Undercover Ethnography of the Organs-Trafficking Underworld." *Ethnography* 5, no. 1 (2004): 29–73.

Schmucker, D. L., and E. S. Vesell. "Are the Elderly Underrepresented in Clinical Drug Trials?" *Journal of Clinical Pharmacology* 39, no. 11 (1999): 1103–8.

Schratzberger, G., and G. Mayer. "Age and Renal Transplantation: An Interim Analysis." *Nephrology, Dialysis, Transplantation* 18, no. 3 (2003): 471–76.

Schroeder, S. A. "Personal Reflections on the High Cost of American Medical Care: Many Causes but Few Politically Sustainable Solutions." *Archives of Internal Medicine* 171, no. 8 (2011): 722–27.

Segev, Dorry L., Sommer E. Gentry, Daniel S. Warren, Brigitte Reeb, and Robert A. Montgomery. "Kidney Paired Donation and Optimizing the Use of Live Donor Organs." *JAMA Internal Medicine* 293, no. 15 (2005): 1883–90.

Sharp, Lesley Alexandra. *Strange Harvest: Organ Transplants, Denatured Bodies, and the Transformed Self.* Berkeley: University of California Press, 2006.

Shim, Janet K., Ann J. Russ, and Sharon R. Kaufman. "Clinical Life: Expectation and the Double Edge of Medical Promise." *Health (London)* 11, no. 2 (2007): 245–64.

———. "Risk, Life Extension and the Pursuit of Medical Possibility." *Sociology of Health and Illness* 28, no. 4 (2006): 479–502.

Shimazono, Y. "The State of the International Organ Trade: A Provisional Picture Based on Integration of Available Information." *Bulletin of the World Health Organization* 85, no. 12 (2007): 955–62.

Shore, Cris, and Susan Wright. *Anthropology of Policy: Critical Perspectives on Governance and Power.* London: Routledge, 1997.

Shorter, Edward. *Bedside Manners: The Troubled History of Doctors and Patients.* New York: Simon and Schuster, 1985.

Siminoff, L. A., and K. Chillag. "The Fallacy of the 'Gift of Life.'" *Hastings Center Report* 29, no. 6 (1999): 34–41.

Sims, R. J., M. J. Cassidy, and T. Masud. "The Increasing Number of Older Patients with Renal Disease." *British Medical Journal* 327, no. 7413 (2003): 463–64.

Skinner, J., and E. S. Fisher. "Reflections on Geographic Variations in U.S. Health Care." Dartmouth Institute for Health Policy and Clinical Practice. May 12, 2010. Accessed May 30, 2012. http://www.dartmouthatlas.org/downloads/press /Skinner_Fisher_DA_05_10.pdf.

Slaughter, M. S., R. Bostic, K. Tong, M. Russo, and J. G. Rogers. "Temporal Changes in Hospital Costs for Left Ventricular Assist Device Implantation." *Journal of Cardiac Surgery* 26, no. 5 (2011): 535–41.

Sohail, M. R., C. A. Henrikson, M. J. Braid-Forbes, K. F. Forbes, and D. J. Lerner. "Mortality and Cost Associated with Cardiovascular Implantable Electronic Device Infections." *Archives of Internal Medicine* 171, no. 20 (2011): 1821–28.

Starr, Paul. *The Social Transformation of American Medicine.* New York: Basic Books, 1982.

Starzl, Thomas E., Anthony J. Demetris, and David H. Van Thiel. "Liver Transplantation." *New England Journal of Medicine* 321, no. 15 (1989): 1014–22.

Stegall, M. D. "The Right Kidney for the Right Recipient: The Status of Deceased Donor Kidney Allocation Reform." *Seminars in Dialysis* 23, no. 3 (2010): 248–52.

Steinbrook, Robert. "Public Solicitation of Organ Donors." *New England Journal of Medicine* 353, no. 5 (2005): 441–44.

Strathern, Marilyn. *Reproducing the Future: Essays on Anthropology, Kinship, and the New Reproductive Technologies.* Manchester, UK: Manchester University Press, 1992.

Sulmasy, D. P. "Within You/Without You: Biotechnology, Ontology, and Ethics." *Journal of General Internal Medicine* 23 (2007): 69–72.

Summers, D. M., R. J. Johnson, J. Allen, S. V. Fuggle, D. Collett, C. J. Watson, and J. A. Bradley. "Analysis of Factors That Affect Outcome after Transplantation of Kidneys Donated after Cardiac Death in the UK: A Cohort Study." *Lancet* 376, no. 9749 (2010): 1303–11.

SUPPORT Principal Investigators. "A Controlled Trial to Improve Care for Seriously Ill Hospitalized Patients: The Study to Understand Prognoses and Preferences for Outcomes and Risks of Treatments (Support)." *JAMA Internal Medicine* 274, no. 20 (1995): 1591–98.

Swindle, J. P., M. W. Rich, P. McCann, T. E. Burroughs, and P. J. Hauptman. "Implantable Cardiac Device Procedures in Older Patients: Use and in-Hospital Outcomes." *Archives of Internal Medicine* 170, no. 7 (2010): 631–37.

Tan, Jane C., and Glenn M. Chertow. "Cautious Optimism Concerning Long-Term Safety of Kidney Donation." *New England Journal of Medicine* 360, no. 5 (2009): 522–23.

Taylor, J. S., S. M. DeMers, E. K. Vig, and S. Borson. "The Disappearing Subject: Exclusion of People with Cognitive Impairment and Dementia from Geriatrics Research." *Journal of the American Geriatrics Society* 60, no. 3 (2012): 413–19.

Testa, Giuliano, Peter Angelos, Megan Crowley-Matoka, and Mark Siegler. "Elective Surgical Patients as Living Organ Donors: A Clinical and Ethical Innovation." *American Journal of Transplantation* 9, no. 10 (2009): 2400–5.

Thoratec Corporation. "Heartmate II Clinical Outcomes." Accessed May 31, 2012. http://www.thoratec.com/vad-trials-outcomes/clinical-outcomes/hm2-bridge -to-transplant.aspx.

Timmermans, Stefan. *Sudden Death and the Myth of CPR.* Philadelphia: Temple University Press, 1999.

Timmermans, Stefan, and Marc Berg. *The Gold Standard: The Challenge of Evidence-Based Medicine and Standardization in Health Care.* Philadelphia: Temple University Press, 2003.

Timmermans, Stefan, and M. Buchbinder. "Patients-in-Waiting: Living between Sickness and Health in the Genomics Era." *Journal of Health and Social Behavior* 51, no. 4 (2010): 408–23.

Timmermans, Stefan, and A. Mauck. "The Promises and Pitfalls of Evidence-Based Medicine." *Health Affairs* 24, no. 1 (2005): 18–28.

Tunis, S. R. "Why Medicare Has Not Established Criteria for Coverage Decisions." *New England Journal of Medicine* 350, no. 21 (2004): 2196–98.

United Network of Organ Sharing. "Awareness and Promotion." Accessed October 8, 2012. http://www.unos.org/donation/index.php?topic=awareness.

U.S. Department of Health and Human Services, Food and Drug Administration, Center for Biologics Evaluation and Research, and Center for Drug Evaluation and Research. "Guidance for Industry: Information Program on Clinical Trials for Serious or Life-Threatening Diseases and Conditions." Washington, DC, 2002.

U.S. Department of Health and Human Services, Food and Drug Administration, Center for Drug Evaluation and Research, and Center for Biologics Evaluation and Research. "Guidance for Industry: Clinical Trial Endpoints for the Approval of Cancer Drugs and Biologics." Washington, DC, 2007.

U.S. National Institutes of Health. Accessed May 30, 2012, and May 15, 2014. ClinicalTrials.gov.

———. "OPTN." Accessed October 17, 2012. http://www.unos.org/donation/index .php?topic=optn.

U.S. Renal Data System. "Incident and Prevalent Counts by Quarter." National Institutes of Health, National Institute of Diabetes and Digestive and Kidney Diseases. Accessed August 12, 2014. http://www.usrds.org/qtr/default.aspx.

———. "USRDS 2011 Annual Data Report: Atlas of Chronic Kidney Disease and End-Stage Renal Disease in the United States." Bethesda, MD: National Institutes of Health, National Institute of Diabetes and Digestive and Kidney Diseases, 2011.

———. "USRDS 2012 Annual Data Report: Atlas of Chronic Kidney Disease and End-Stage Renal Disease in the United States." Bethesda, MD: National Institutes of Health, National Institute of Diabetes and Digestive and Kidney Diseases 2012.

University of Alabama at Birmingham School of Medicine. Intermacs. Accessed November 28, 2012. http://www.uab.edu/medicine/intermacs/.

University of Minnesota Medical Center. "Transplant, Solid Organ." Fairview Health Services. Accessed March 29, 2011. http://www.uofmtransplant.org/Adult/Kidney Transplant/livingdonorblog/index.asp?p=1&t=3406.

Weber, M. A., N. K. Wenger, and S. Scheidt. "Who Should Be Treated with Implantable Cardioverter-Defibrillators?" *American Journal of Geriatric Cardiology* 15, no. 6 (2006): 336–37.

Weeks, J. C., P. J. Catalano, A. Cronin, M. D. Finkelman, J. W. Mack, N. L. Keating, and D. Schrag. "Patients' Expectations about Effects of Chemotherapy for Advanced Cancer." *New England Journal of Medicine* 367, no. 17 (2012): 1616–25.

Weeks, J. C., E. F. Cook, S. J. O'Day, L. M. Peterson, N. Wenger, D. Reding, F. E. Harrell et al. "Relationship between Cancer Patients' Predictions of Prognosis and Their Treatment Preferences." *JAMA Internal Medicine* 279, no. 21 (1998): 1709–14.

Wilk, Richard. "It's about Time: A Commentary on Guyer." *American Ethnologist* 34, no. 3 (2007): 440–43.

Withell, B. "Patient Consent and Implantable Cardioverter Defibrillators: Some Palliative Care Implications." *International Journal of Palliative Nursing* 12, no. 10 (2006): 470–75.

Wolfe, Robert A., Valarie B. Ashby, Edgar L. Milford, Akinlolu O. Ojo, Robert E. Ettenger, Lawrence Y.C. Agodoa, Philip J. Held, and Friedrich K. Port. "Comparison of Mortality in All Patients on Dialysis, Patients on Dialysis Awaiting Transplantation, and Recipients of a First Cadaveric Transplant." *New England Journal of Medicine* 341, no. 23 (1999): 1725–30.

Woodward, Kathleen M. "Statistical Panic." *Differences: A Journal of Feminist Cultural Studies* 11, no. 2 (1999): 177–203.

———. *Statistical Panic: Cultural Politics and Poetics of the Emotions.* Durham, NC: Duke University Press, 2009.

Yarnoz, M. J., and A. B. Curtis. "Why Cardioverter-Defibrillator Implantation Might Not Be the Best Idea for Your Elderly Patient." *American Journal of Geriatric Cardiology* 15, no. 6 (2007): 367–71.

Zalman, D. M., J. B. Sussman, X. Chen, C. T. Cigolle, C. S. Blaum, and R. A. Hayward. "Examining the Evidence: A Systematic Review of the Inclusion and Analysis of Older Adults in Randomized controlled Trials." *Journal of General Internal Medicine* 26, no. 7 (2011): 783–90.

INDEX

chemoembolization procedures, 160–61, 162, 275n84

Chin, Ming, 161–63

cirrhosis, 159–60

clinical trials: best treatments and, 55–57; drug companies and, 79–94; emergence of, 16, 28; evidentiary value of, 24, 28, 57–73, 259n19; generalizability issues of, 70–73, 94–98; good enough evidence and, 87–94; growth of, 53–54; indication creep and, 55–57; industrial scope of, 3–4, 7, 54–55, 79–82, 241–42; Medicare and, 24, 27, 72, 105–7, 111–14, 123; patient activism and, 82–84, 87–94, 108; physician-patient relationship and, 73–78; quantification and, 12, 34; risk awareness and, 32–36; technological imperative and, 114–22; tested populations and, 71–73, 94–98, 114, 137. See also research industry

clinicaltrials.gov, 83, 85, 113

Clinton, Bill, 95

CMS (Centers for Medicare and Medicaid Services), 105–7

common goods, 8–9, 54, 217–18, 223–36, 238–39, 246–47

"Concepts for Kidney Allocation" (OPTN/UNOS), 220–21

creatinine, 34, 150, 181, 257n22, 278n37

cyclosporine, 67

Dang, Van, 40–45, 48, 111, 160, 211

Dartmouth Atlas of Health Care, 77

death: cancer therapies and, 87–94; demands of longevity and, 39–43; hope and, 149–55; hospice care and, 12, 22–23, 28, 130, 144, 147, 149; life's value and, 4–5; Medicare policy and, 107–10, 114–15; medicine's cultural role and, 131–32; patients' familial obligations and, 171, 184–87; prematurity of, 131–32, 142–43; prognoses and, 17, 195–216; the quandary and, 2–3, 37–39; risk awareness and, 26,

32–36; technology's prolonging of, 1, 11, 14, 22–23, 26, 28–36, 49–50, 100, 110, 120–24, 245

decision-making: Medicare's influence on, 6, 16, 45–47, 65–66, 99–100, 107–10, 114–15, 140–44, 155–57, 161–63, 170–71; ordinary medicine and, 21–26, 62–68; patients' roles in, 73–78, 149–55, 161–63, 184–85, 199–202, 207, 243–45, 284n20; physicians and, 21–23, 45–47, 62–78, 94–98, 136–37, 143–57, 243–45; research industry and, 62–70, 73–78

Department of Health and Human Services, 222

DESS (drug eluting stents), 112, 121. See also stents

destination therapies, 114–22, 133–64. See also dialysis (of kidneys)

diabetes, 167, 204

diagnostic tests. See screening

dialysis (of kidneys), 13; age considerations and, 146–49, 155–57; as bridge technology, 166–67; description of, 145–46; as destination therapy, 143–57; experiences of, 149–55; interactions with other therapies of, 31; maintenance dialysis and, 49–50, 273n57; Medicare coverage for, 144–45, 147–48, 221; organ donations and, 175–76, 178, 180–87; standardization of, 16–17

doctors. See physicians

Donate Life America, 227

drugs and drug companies: AIDS epidemic and, 82–84; cancer treatments and, 1, 83–87; clinical trials and, 3, 53–57, 69–70, 72–73, 94–98, 259n19; costs of, 1, 101, 243, 263n37, 263n42; expanded uses of, 55–57; indication creep and, 81–82, 262n19; market logic of, 83–94; physicians' relationships with, 1, 54; research agendas and, 16, 28, 57–68, 72–73, 79–82

Dunbar, Lewis, 205–7

health care drivers (*continued*)
and, 12–13, 22–26; reform efforts
and, 242–47; research industry and,
7, 24, 53–54, 62–70; technology as,
24, 127–28

health care policies: the common good
and, 18–19, 217–18, 223–39; definitions of, 266n8; ethical field and,
36–40, 43–47; fairness issues and,
217–18, 226–33; Medicare reimbursement and, 14, 99–100, 105–7; patient
expectations and, 12–13, 240–42;
reform efforts and, 44, 236–37,
242–47

heart failure. *See* DESS (drug eluting
stents); ICD (implantable cardiac
defibrillator); LVAD (left ventricular
assist device); stents

Heart Failure Society, 119

HeartMate, 119

Heath, Hattie, 200–202, 204

hepatitis B, 158–64, 209

hepatitis C, 45–47, 159–60, 163–64,
209, 266n5

Herceptin (drug), 87

HMOS, 242

Holy Fire (Sterling), 235

hope, 149–55, 214

hospice care, 12, 22–23, 28, 77, 130, 144,
147, 149, 240

ICD (implantable cardiac defibrillator): age considerations and, 29–32,
56–57, 71, 84, 142–43; chronic conditions and, 134–43; clinical trials and,
106; costs of, 5, 119; criteria for use
of, 57–61; definitions of, 22, 256n2,
256n12; efficacy of, 141–42; Medicare approval of, 4, 56, 116–18, 218;
ordinary medicine and, 12–13; physicians' discourses about, 11–12, 57–61;
prognosis and, 199; standards of
care and, 16–17, 26–36, 128, 137–40,
270n21

ICUS (intensive care units), 13

indication creep, 72–73, 81–82, 84,
87–94, 114, 262n19

individual rights, 108–9, 149–55,
161–63, 184–85, 199–202, 207,
243–47, 284n20

industry. *See* clinical trials; drugs and
drug companies; research industry

Institute of Medicine, 72

insurance (medical): clinical decisions
and, 16, 24; health care policy and,
36–39; standard of care and, 7, 9–10,
100–104, 110–14, 122–24, 185. *See also*
Medicare

interferon, 45, 103, 257n35

Intermacs (Interagency Registry for
Mechanically Assisted Circulatory
Support), 268n45

Ishiguro, Kazuo, 235

Jackson, Michael, 127

Jones, Claude, 135–37, 142, 198–99

*Journal of the American Medical Associa-
tion*, 167

Keating, Peter, 86

kidneys: dialysis and, 13, 31, 49–50,
145–57, 166–67, 175–87, 221, 273n57;
family donors and, 166–69, 171–75,
187–94, 275n7; ICDs and, 31; as
scarce resource, 167–68, 170–71,
175–77, 194, 218–36, 276n9, 281n28,
282n29; standards of care and,
16–17, 204, 233–36. *See also* organ
donation; transplants

Kidney Transplantation Committee
(UNOS), 220

Koenig, Barbara, 115

Konner, Melvin, 67, 69

Kravinsky, Zell, 229, 231

Latour, Bruno, 130

lithium, 67–68

livers: family donors and, 165–75; medical eligibility for, 159–63; Medicare
reimbursement for, 45–48, 102–4,

157–63; physician-patient discourses and, 40–43; prognoses and, 208–11; as scarce resources, 134, 158–59, 162, 170–71, 175–77, 194, 226–33; standardization of, 16–17; technological advancements and, 67–68, 133–34, 274n77

living donors, 17, 166–73, 176–92, 226–33, 275n7

longevity: clinical trials and, 87–94; demands of, 39–43; as determinant of life's value, 4–5, 28–36, 241; Medicare policy and, 100–104, 107–10, 123–24; organ donation and, 168–75; prognoses and, 195–216; quantification drive and, 34–35, 94–98, 163–64, 204–5; rationality of, 15; technological developments and, 9, 133–64, 182

Los Angeles Times, 223–24

Lupron (drug), 132

LVAD (left ventricular assist device): approval of, 4, 118; costs of, 5, 119, 269n46; standard of care and, 26, 118–23

magnetic resonance imaging, 68

maintenance dialysis. *See* dialysis (of kidneys)

MatchingDonors.com, 229–30, 232

Mauss, Marcel, 170

Medicaid, 276n13

medical-industrial complex, 54, 57–68, 79–82. *See also* clinical trials; drugs and drug companies; patients; physicians; technology

Medicare: aging population and, 27–28, 49–50, 114–15, 220–23, 281n17; clinical trials and, 24, 27, 56, 72, 85, 95, 100–104; CMS and, 105–7; cost-blindness of, 15, 28, 119–20, 266n3; creation of, 65, 86, 100–104, 106–7; decision-making influence of, 6, 16, 45–47, 65–66, 99–100, 107–10, 114–15, 140–42, 144, 155–57, 161–63,

170–71; eligibility requirements of, 9–11, 45, 57–61, 87, 99–110, 118–22, 159–63, 276n13; FDA approval and, 87, 93; as health care driver, 7, 9–10, 36–37, 44, 236–37; liver transplants and, 157–63, 170, 173–75, 185; private insurance and, 87, 99–102, 105–7; reform efforts and, 12, 44, 218; standards of care and, 100–104, 110–14, 122–24, 185; technological imperative and, 114–22, 137–40

medicine: the common good and, 8–9, 54, 217–18, 223–36, 238–39, 246–47; contemporary state of, 21–22; costs of, 1, 5, 8–9, 12, 26, 44, 70, 105, 155–57, 218, 238–40, 242–44, 260n50, 263n42, 266n3; evidence in, 3–4, 16, 57–68, 79–82, 111–14; health care policy and, 12–13, 36–39; the law and, 130, 156; market-based approaches to, 8–9, 16, 25–26, 54–55, 66, 79–94, 99–100, 113, 203–8, 218–19, 226–33, 235–37, 242–44, 246–47, 260n50, 276n9; prognosis and, 17, 195–216; risk awareness and, 17, 26–36, 57–61, 103, 135–42, 181–82, 195–216, 243–45; technology and, 1, 3–4, 63–68, 114–22, 127–28. *See also* evidence-based medicine (EBM); health care policies; ordinary medicine; patients; physicians; technology

Meier, Diane, 213–14

Mukherjee, Siddhartha, 240

National Cancer Institute, 81, 85

National Comprehensive Cancer Network, 85, 93–94, 101, 262n29

National Institute on Aging, 33, 95

National Kidney Foundation, 273n57

nephrology. *See* kidneys

Never Let Me Go (Ishiguro), 235

New England Journal of Medicine, 54

New York Times, 113

NIH (National Institutes of Health), 28, 56, 61–63, 80–85, 95–96, 118–19, 158

Nixon, Richard, 86
Nocera, Joe, 265n73
numbers. *See* quantification

Obama, Barack, 242
off-label uses, 262n19. *See also* indication creep
ordinary medicine: clinical trials and, 61–68; decision-making and, 21–23, 25–26, 62–68; definitions of, 2–3, 6–9, 21–23, 26; drivers of, 6–7, 22–26; ethical field and, 7–11, 25–26, 28; evidence of therapeutic value and, 3–4, 54–61, 73–78, 100–104, 113–14, 195–216; fairness paradigms and, 217–37; patients' ages and, 13–18; the quandary and, 8–10, 239–42; standards of care and, 7, 26–28
organ donation, 165–69, 171–73, 177–83, 187–94, 226–36
Organ Procurement and Transplantation Network, 159, 220

pacemakers, 31–32, 116, 119–20, 134, 140–41. *See also* ICD (implantable cardiac defibrillator)
palliative care, 92, 213. *See also* hospice care
Parsons, Talcott, 277n15
patients: age considerations and, 11–13, 29, 192–94; consumer activism of, 28, 82–84, 87–94, 144–45, 164, 203–8; decision-making of, 73–78, 149–55, 161–63, 184–85, 199–202, 207, 243–45, 284n20; expectations of, 22, 24, 37–39, 71–73, 109–10, 122–24, 131–32, 140–42, 240–42; families of, 8–9, 17, 165–73, 176–92; Medicare eligibility and, 9–11, 57–61, 87, 99–104, 107–10, 118–22, 159–63; physician expertise and, 17, 28–29, 36–37, 198–216; quality of life and, 116–18, 149–55; recovery definitions and, 131–32; risk awareness and, 32–36, 195–98, 279n8; time left and, 17, 37–39, 208–11

Patient Self-Determination Act, 108, 244
pharmaceuticals and pharmaceutical companies. *See* drugs and drug companies
physicians: decision-making and, 21–23, 45–47, 62–78, 94–98, 136–37, 143–57, 243–45; drug companies' relation to, 1, 54, 140–42; education of, 67–70, 242–43; evidence-based medicine and, 55–61, 94–98; families' relation to, 38, 42, 136–37, 188–89, 211–16; health care policy and, 12–13, 15, 240; Medicare eligibility and, 13, 45–47, 65–66, 99–100, 105–15, 137–40; patients' expectations and, 37–43, 73–78, 94–98, 148, 207; prognoses and, 17, 28–29, 32–36, 195–98, 203–8, 213–16; the quandary and, 11–12, 28–29
postprogress, 13–18, 47–50, 94–98, 129, 143, 149–55
poverty, 243–44
preventive medicine, 17–18, 26–27, 94
private industry. *See* clinical trials; drugs and drug companies; research industry
prognoses: family negotiations and, 211–16; the quandary and, 200–202; risk awareness and, 203–8; temporal negotiations and, 17, 195–98, 208–11
progress (medical). *See* medicine; postprogress; technology
progression-free survival trials, 91
Provenge (drug), 87
PSA test, 260n46

quandary, the (too much versus not enough): ambivalent feelings and, 10, 21, 24; chronic conditions and, 133–64; clinical trials and, 94–98; definitions of, 2–3, 5–6, 255n3; equity issues and, 17, 217–19, 242–47; evidence-based medicine and, 77–78; families and, 13–18, 129–31; life quality and, 39–43; Medicare policy and, 122–24; ordinary medicine and, 8–9; organ donations and, 183–94; physician-patient relationship and, 37–39, 73–78; technological advances and, 16–17, 129–31

quantification, 12, 34, 37–39, 87–94, 163–64, 195–98, 213–14, 221, 241

Quinlan, Karen Ann, 129–31, 146, 156, 255n2

racism, 243–44

rationing (of health care), 44, 59, 63, 170–71, 219, 221, 238–40

RCTS (randomized controlled trials), 64, 258n14. See also clinical trials

recoveries (from medical conditions), 131–32, 135–37. See also death; patients; technology

Redberg, Rita, 112–14

Relman, Arnold, 54, 79

research industry: approval process and, 82–84; best treatments and, 55–57; clinical trials and, 70–73, 241–42; government funding and, 61–68; health care drivers and, 7, 24, 53–54, 62–70; Medicare and, 27; physicians' decision-making and, 62–70, 73–78; risk awareness and, 32–36; technological imperative and, 114–22, 158–59. See also clinical trials; drugs and drug companies; technology

Rieff, David, 212–13, 215–16

rights. See individual rights

risk awareness: health care reform and, 243–44; ICDs and, 28–36, 57–61, 135–37, 140–42; Medicare and, 103; organ donation and, 181–82; prognoses and, 17, 195–216, 244–45; quantification and, 17, 34, 195–216; technology and, 26–28, 203–7, 216

Rosenberg, Charles E., 217, 242

Rothman, David, 36

Rubin, Lillian, 241

Russ, Ann, 255n1

Sandel, Michael J., 217

screening, 34, 195–98, 203–11, 243. See also risk awareness

Segev, Dorry L., 165, 167

Shields, J. Dunbar, 65–66, 68

Shim, Janet, 255n1, 258n6

social goods. See common goods

solicitation (of organ donors), 226–33

Sontag, Susan, 212–13, 215

standard of care: health care drivers and, 26–36; Medicare reimbursement and, 7, 9, 100–104, 110–14, 122–24, 184–85; technology and, 114–22, 127–31, 133–64, 184–85

statistical methodologies, 63–67. See also clinical trials

Statistical Panic (Woodward), 35

stents, 77, 111–13, 121, 267n22

Sterling, Bruce, 235

stranger donations, 166–69, 176–77, 185, 226, 282n34

Strathern, Marilyn, 235, 269n3

successful treatment definitions, 17, 47, 133–35, 164, 241–43

SUPPORT study, 244

surgical solicitation, 232–35

Swazey, Judith, 146–47, 171, 281n28

Swimming in a Sea of Death (Rieff), 212–13, 215–16

technology: American attitudes toward, 5, 8, 61–68, 100–101, 110, 114–22; costs of, 8–9, 119; death's prolonging by, 1, 3–4, 9, 13–14, 27–36, 49–50, 129–31, 133–64, 240–41; ethical field and, 36–37, 133–64; as health care driver, 24, 127–28; market forces and, 134, 140–42, 144–45; Medicare reimbursements and, 7, 57–61, 100–104, 122–24, 137–40; ordinary medicine and, 127–28, 240, 245; patient expectations and, 122–24; patients' ages and, 10, 15–16; physician-patient relationship and, 62–68, 136–37; risk awareness and, 203–7,

technology (*continued*)
216; standards of care and, 114–22, 127–31, 133–64, 184–85
therapies: age-blindness and, 9–10, 114–15, 220–23; clinical trials industry and, 55–68, 83–87, 263n37; destination therapies and, 114–22, 133–64; ethical field and, 7–8, 133–64; patient activism and, 82–84; prognoses and, 17, 195–98, 203–7; the quandary and, 8–9, 14, 122–24, 155–57; risk awareness and, 56–57; standard of care and, 7, 12–13, 15–16, 100–104, 110–14, 122–24, 185; success definitions and, 17, 47, 133–35, 164, 241–43. *See also* clinical trials; *specific devices*
Thoratec (company), 119
time (left): cancer drugs and, 84–87; control of, 17; death's prematurity and, 131–32, 142–43, 266n4; dialysis procedures and, 149–55; organ donations and, 173–75; physician-patient relationship and, 37–39, 74–76; prognoses and, 195–98; quantification drive and, 34–35
Timmermans, Stefan, 271n34
Tolleson, Sam, 29–32, 37–38, 111, 135, 142
transplants: destination therapies and, 118–22; fairness issues and, 217–26; family obligations and, 17, 166–71, 176–92; gift exchanges and, 171–73, 177–82, 226–33; of kidneys, 5, 144–45, 167–68, 170–71, 175–77, 194, 218–36, 281n28, 282n29; of livers, 27–28, 40–43, 45–48, 102–4, 133–34, 157–63, 165–77, 208–11, 226–33; market-based understandings of,

228–33, 281n28, 282n29; medical eligibility for, 159–63, 277n28; Medicare reimbursement and, 87, 99–104; patient age and, 10; technological improvements and, 129, 158–59, 166–69, 172, 234
Trin, Thao, 208–11

United States: aging population of, 4–5, 9–10, 27; death's timing and, 131–32; health care policy in, 12–13, 44–47, 217–23; individualism and, 149–55, 161–63, 184–85, 199–202, 207, 243–45, 284n20; medical "breakthroughs" and, 114–22, 133–64; research funding and, 57–68; risk awareness and, 26, 32–36, 103. *See also* clinical trials; drugs and drug companies; health care drivers; health care policies; Medicare; technology
University of Minnesota Medical Center, 231
UNOS (United Network for Organ Sharing), 103–4, 162, 167, 173, 178, 180, 220–28, 230, 266n5

values (ethical). *See* ethical field
Venn, Couze, 130
ventilator (iron lung), 36–37, 128–31

Walters, Martha, 22–25, 29, 38, 49
Waxman, Henry, 90
website solicitation (of organs), 229–31
Woodward, Kathleen, 35

Zaltrap (drug), 263n42